DEEP BRAIN STIMULATION

DEEP BRAIN STIMULATION

A Case-Based Approach

EDITED BY

SHILPA CHITNIS, MD, PHD

PRAVIN KHEMANI, MD

AND MICHAEL S. OKUN, MD

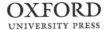

OXFORD
UNIVERSITY PRESS

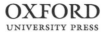

OXFORD
UNIVERSITY PRESS

Oxford University Press is a department of the University of Oxford. It furthers
the University's objective of excellence in research, scholarship, and education
by publishing worldwide. Oxford is a registered trade mark of Oxford University
Press in the UK and certain other countries.

Published in the United States of America by Oxford University Press
198 Madison Avenue, New York, NY 10016, United States of America.

© Oxford University Press 2020

Library of Congress Cataloging-in-Publication Data
Names: Chitnis, Shilpa, Khemani, Pravin and Okun, Michael S., editors.
Title: Deep brain stimulation : a case-based approach / Shilpa Chitnis, Pravin Khemani and Michael S. Okun.
Description: New York, NY : Oxford University Press, [2020] |
Includes bibliographical references and index.
Identifiers: LCCN 2019059948 (print) | LCCN 2019059949 (ebook) |
ISBN 9780190647209 (hardback) | ISBN 9780190647223 (epub) |
ISBN 9780190647230 (other)
Subjects: LCSH: Brain stimulation—Therapeutic use—Case studies. |
Extrapyramidal disorders—Treatment—Case studies. |
Tremor—Treatment—Case studies. | Nervous system—Surgery—Case studies.
Classification: LCC RC350.B72 D437 2020 (print) | LCC RC350.B72 (ebook) |
DDC 616.8—dc23
LC record available at https://lccn.loc.gov/2019059948
LC ebook record available at https://lccn.loc.gov/2019059949

A successful academic career can't happen without dedicated mentorship. We are grateful to our amazing mentors in the field of movement disorders. Our patients teach us important lessons in humility, clinical care, compassion, and tolerance. Our clinical staff and teams toil endlessly to provide us the much-needed background support in the clinical and research arenas. Lastly, our movement disorders fellows work hard, and their training sets up the foundation for our continual learning and mentorship. This book is dedicated to all of these amazing people who make a daily difference in our lives.

—Shilpa, Pravin, Michael

Shilpa

This book is dedicated to my wonderful family, who exhibit patience, tolerance, love, and encouragement year after year. I am especially grateful for the unconditional love and sacrifices of my parents. Dr. Jayaraman Rao and Dr. Krishna Agrawal, my mentors now lost to the ravages of time, who were role models for exemplary mentorship. I am grateful for their guidance and friendship. Lastly, I am thankful for the love and support of my wonderful friends.

Pravin

I dedicate this book to everyone who has supported and encouraged me in my professional journey—my family, friends, teachers, and colleagues, and my patients who have entrusted their care to me.

Michael

This book is dedicated to my wonderful wife Leslie and my beautiful and talented children, Jack and Grace.

CONTENTS

CONTRIBUTORS

Mitra Afshari, MD, MPH
Assistant Professor of Neurological Sciences
Department of Neurological Sciences
Rush University
Chicago, IL

Jawad A. Bajwa, MD
Assistant Professor, Neurology
National Neuroscience Institute
King Fahad Medical City
Riyadh, Riyadh Province

Oscar Bernal-Pacheco, MD
Neurologist-Movement Disorders
Department of Neurology
Instituto Roosevelt
Chia, Cundin

Sagari Bette, MD
Movement Disorders Neurologist
Parkinson's Disease and Movement Disorders
Center of Boca Raton
Boca Raton, FL

Brent Bluett, DO
Clinical Assistant Professor
Department of Neurology and Neurological
Sciences
Stanford Movement Disorders Center
Palo Alto, CA

Helen Bronte-Stewart, MD, MSE, FAAN, FANA
Director, Stanford Movement Disorders Center
Department of Neurology and Neurological
Sciences
Stanford University School of Medicine
Stanford, CA

Ethan G. Brown, MD
Assistant Professor of Neurology
UCSF Movement Disorders and
Neuromodulation Center
Weill Institute of Neurosciences
Department of Neurology
University of California San Francisco
San Francisco, CA

Ankur Butala, MD
Assistant Professor of Neurology, Psychiatry and
Behavioral Sciences
Parkinson Disease and Movement
Disorders Center
Johns Hopkins University School of Medicine
Baltimore, MD

Elena Call, MD
Movement Disorders Specialist
Department of Neurology
Kaiser Permanente
Redwood City, CA

Lana Chahine, MD
Assistant Professor
Department of Neurology
University of Pittsburgh
Pittsburgh, PA

David Charles, MD
Professor and Vice-Chair
Department of Neurology
Vanderbilt University
Nashville, TN

Shilpa Chitnis, MD, PhD
Professor of Neurology and Neurotherapeutics
University of Texas Southwestern
Medical Center
Dallas, TX

Kelly A. Mills, MD, MHS
Assistant Professor of Neurology
Department of Neurology
Movement Disorders
Johns Hopkins University School of Medicine
Baltimore, MD

Svjetlana Miocinovic, MD, PhD
Assistant Professor
Department of Neurology
Emory University
Atlanta, GA

Kyle T. Mitchell, MD
Assistant Professor
Department of Neurology
Movement Disorders
Duke University School of Medicine
Durham, NC

Takashi Morishita, MD, PhD
Associate Professor
Department of Neurosurgery
Fukuoka University
Fukuoka, Japan

Mariana Moscovich, MD, PhD
Department of Neurology
Klinik für Neurologie
UKSH, Campus Kiel
Curitiba, Paraná

Padraig O'Suilleabhain, MD
Professor
Department of Neurology
University of Texas Southwestern
Dallas, TX

Michael S. Okun, MD
Adelaide Lackner Chair of Neurology, Executive
Director Fixel Institute for Neurological
Diseases, Neurology and Neurosurgery
University of Florida Health
Gainesville, FL

Jill L. Ostrem, MD
Carlin and Ellen Wiegner Endowed Professor of
Neurology
UCSF Movement Disorders and
Neuromodulation Center
Weill Institute of Neurosciences
Department of Neurology
University of California San Francisco
San Francisco, CA

Genko Oyama, MD, PhD, FAAN
Department of Neurology
Juntendo University Faculty of Medicine
Tokyo, Japan

Rajesh Pahwa, MD
Laverne and Joyce Rider Professor
Department of Neurology
University of Kansas Medical Center
Kansas City, KS

Gian Pal, MD, MS
Assistant Professor
Section of Movement Disorders, Department of
Neurological Sciences
Rush University Medical Center
Edison, NJ

Valeriy Parfenov, MD
Neurologist
Department of Neurology
Brigham and Women's Hospital
Weymouth, MA

Adriana Martinez Perez, MD
Neurologist/Epileptologist, Epileptologist
FOSCAL
Floridablanca, Santander

Javier R. Pérez-Sánchez, MD, PhD
Consultant Neurologist
Movement Disorders Unit
Hospital General Universitario Gregorio
Marañón
Madrid, Madrid

Adolfo Ramirez-Zamora, MD
Associate Professor of Neurology
University of Florida
Fixel Center for Neurological Diseases
Gainesville, FL

Meagen R. Salinas, MD
Assistant Professor
Department of Neurology and
Neurotherapeutics
University of Texas Southwestern Medical
Center Dallas
Dallas, TX

Fuyuko Sasaki, MD
Department of Neurology
Juntendo University Faculty of Medicine
Tokyo, Japan

Susanne Schneider, MD, PhD
Consultant Neurologist
Department of Neurology
Ludwig Maximilians University
Munich, Germany

Andi Nugraha Sendjaja, MD
Neurosurgeon, Neurosurgery
Rumah Sakit BP Batam
Batam, Indonesia

Kathleen Shannon, MD
Chair
Department of Neurology
University of Wisconsin School of Medicine and
Public Health
Madison, WI

Vibhash D. Sharma, MD
Assistant Professor
Department of Neurology
University of Kansas Medical Center
Kansas City, KS

Yasushi Shimo, MD
Department of Neurology
Juntendo University Faculty of Medicine
Tokyo, Japan

Danielle S. Shpiner, MD
Assistant Professor of Clinical Neurology
Department of Neurology, Division of
Parkinson's Disease and Movement Disorders
University of Miami Miller School of Medicine
Miami, FL

Aparna Wagle Shukla, MD
Associate Professor of Neurology
Norman Fixel Institute for Neurological Diseases
University of Florida
Gainesville, FL

Junaid Siddiqui, MD, MRCP
Assistant Professor, Neurology, Movement
Disorders
Department of Neurology
University of Missouri
Columbia, MO

Mustafa S. Siddiqui, MD
Professor of Neurology
Department of Neurology
Wake Forest School of Medicine
Clemmons, NC

Konstantin Slavin, MD
Professor
Department of Neurosurgery
University of Illinois
Chicago, IL

Meredith Spindler, MD
Assistant Professor of Clinical Neurology
Perelman School of Medicine of the University
of Pennsylvania
Philadelphia, PA

Philip A. Starr, MD, PhD
Professor in Residence of Neurological Surgery
Dolores Cakebread Endowed Chair in
Neurological Surgery
Co-Director Functional Neurosurgery Program
UCSF Movement Disorders and
Neuromodulation Center
Weill Institute of Neurosciences
Department of Neurological Surgery
University of California San Francisco
San Francisco, CA

Arjun Tarakad, MD
Assistant Professor of Neurology
Director of Deep Brain Stimulation Program
Parkinson's Disease Center and Movement
Disorders Clinic
Baylor College of Medicine
Houston, TX

Stephen B. Tatter, MD, PhD
Professor of Neurosurgery
Department of Neurosurgery
Wake Forest School of Medicine
Winston-Salem, NC

Teri R. Thomsen, MD, JD
Associate Professor, Clinical
Department of Neurology
Carver College of Medicine
University of Iowa Hospitals and Clinics
Iowa City, IA

Michael Ullman, BS
Cornea and External Disease Fellow
Department of Ophthalmology and Visual
Sciences
Washington University in St. Louis
St. Louis, Missouri

Atsushi Umemura, MD, PhD
Department of Neurosurgery
Juntendo University Faculty of Medicine
Tokyo, Japan

Nora Vanegas-Arroyave, MD
Assistant Professor of Neurology
Department of Neurology
Columbia University
New York, NY

Vinata Vedam-Mai, PhD
Assistant Professor
Department of Neurology
University of FL
Gainesville, FL

Dhanya Vijayakumar, MD
Assistant Professor
The University of South Carolina School of
Medicine Greenville
Prisma Health Upstate;
Neuroscience Associates
Department of Internal Medicine
Greenville, SC

Monica Volz, FNP-BC, MSN, RN
Department of Neurology
UCSF Movement Disorders and
Neuromodulation Center (MDNC)
Weill Institute of Neurosciences
University of California San Francisco
San Francisco, CA

Rebecca Whiddon, MD
Neurologist
Department of Neurology
The NeuroMedical Center Clinic
Baton Rouge, LA

Anthony T. Yachnis, MD
Professor and Program Director
Department of Pathology, Immunology, and
Laboratory Medicine
University of Florida College of Medicine
Gainesville, FL

Laurice Yang, MD, MHA
Clinical Assistant Professor
Department of Neurology
Stanford University School of Medicine
Palo Alto, CA

Umar Yazdani, MD
Department of Neurology and
Neurotherapeutics, Movement Disorder Section
University of Texas Southwestern
Dallas, TX

Pamela R. Zeilman, MSN, APRN-BC
Nurse Practitioner, DBS Clinical and Study
Coordinator
Department of Neurology, Movement Disorders
& Neurorestoration Program
UF Norman Fixel Institute for Neurological
Diseases
Gainesville, FL

Qiang Zhang, MD
Movement Disorder Fellow
Department of Neurology
University of Iowa Hospitals and Clinics
Iowa City, IA

SECTION 1

Introduction

Common Programming Strategies for Deep Brain Stimulation

FUNDAMENTALS OF THE ELECTRICAL IMPULSE

Electrical current is delivered through a deep brain stimulation (DBS) electrode or lead, usually from the **cathode** (the negatively charged contact) to the **anode** (positively charged contact).[1] Each electrical pulse is defined by its duration (**pulse width**), average amount of current or voltage (**amplitude**), and number of cycles delivered in a period of time (**frequency**) (Figure I.1).[2] The **duty cycle** refers to the time frame during which the patient is receiving electrical stimulation from the DBS, and the cycle can be adjusted, sometimes in complex scenarios (e.g., *X* seconds, minutes, or hours *on; X* seconds, minutes, or hours *off; off* during sleep; *on* during work or high-stress hours).[3]

GENERATION AND UNIQUE PROPERTIES OF THE ELECTRICAL IMPULSE IN DEEP BRAIN STIMULATION

The DBS pulse has a cathodal and anodal phase. The **cathodal phase** occurs when negative electrical charges exit from an electrical contact point. The **anodal phase** occurs when the negative electrical charges flow into an electrical contact point.

Phase terminology is distinct from and should not be interchanged with current or the designation of cathode and anode.[1] **Cathodal current** describes the flow of negative electrical charge from the cathode to the anode. The **anodal current** is the counterflow from the anode to the cathode and has a lower electrical current but longer duration compared with the primary cathodal current. Although the majority of axonal stimulation arises from cathodal stimulation,

programmers should be familiar with anodal stimulation (Figure I.2).[4]

VOLUME OF TISSUE ACTIVATION

The **volume of tissue activation** (VTA) is the area of "excited" axons that is created by electrical stimulation.[1] The ability to sculpt the volume of tissue activation is useful to optimize benefit and reduce side effects. A number of strategies are available to sculpt the electrical field and to influence the VTA. Contact point selection and non-monopolar stimulation options allow shaping of the field and are discussed later. When traditional ring-shaped contacts are stimulated, the electrical field can be sculpted in the same axis as the lead. However, perpendicular directional steering requires segmented leads. Segmented leads allow for current steering, potentially away from neighboring structures.

ELECTRODE ARCHITECTURE: CONTACT POINT DESIGN

The traditional DBS lead that has been used for several decades consists of four **circumferential** contact points (Figure I.3). Newer **segmented leads** allow current to be directed away from nearby tissue whose stimulation may lead to side effects. Commercially available leads have three segments.

PROGRAMMING MODALITIES

Monopolar stimulation (Figure I.4A) has one contact point as the cathode (negative) and the implanted pulse generator (IPG) as the anode (positive). Often, this is the technique used to review

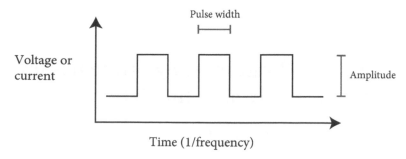

FIGURE I.1. A waveform of current delivered by deep brain stimulation showing intrinsic properties of amplitude, pulse width, and frequency.

the contact points to determine the optimal contact point that has the greatest benefit (often, at the lowest current) and the least amount of stimulation induced side effects. The shape of the electrical field is spherical when applying monopolar stimulation. **Anodic stimulation** has recently been demonstrated as another possibility. In this paradigm, the cathode is the case and the anode is the stimulation contact. The reverse in polarity is hypothesized to render the neighboring axon hyperpolarized.

Multiple monopolar stimulation (Figure I.4B) assigns more than one contact point on the lead as cathodes while the IPG remains the anode.

Bipolar stimulation occurs when the cathode and anode are both present on the lead and the shape of the electrical field is elliptical. **Wide bipolar stimulation** (Figure I.4C) uses the most dorsal and ventral contact points. Typically, the better contact point found on the monopolar review is set as the cathode. However, this can be inverted to reverse the current in an attempt

to activate a different set of axons. Wide bipolar stimulation has a field shape more similar to monopolar stimulation. **Intermediate bipolar stimulation** (Figure I.4D) occurs when the cathode and anode are separated by one contact point on the lead. **Narrow bipolar stimulation** (Figure I.4E) has the cathode and anode on adjacent contact points and forms the typical elliptical electrical field shape. The charge density is the highest with wide bipolar configurations followed by intermediate bipolar stimulation and is the least with narrow bipolar settings.

Tripolar stimulation (Figure I.4F) has two anodes and one cathode on the lead with a typical configuration placing two anodes on either side of the cathode.

Interleaving is a strategy that is used to take advantage of two different programs that deliver stimulation pulse trains offset by time (Figure I.5).[5] Each program can deliver unique stimulation (because of the different configurations). By having

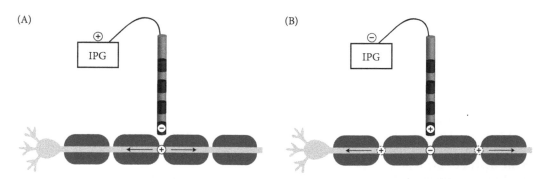

FIGURE I.2. Cathodal stimulation (A) with the implantable pulse generator (IPG) as the anode and a contact point on the deep brain stimulation (DBS) lead as the cathode. The electric field induced by the cathode depolarizes the nearby axon and leads to an action potential that propagates in the directions indicated by the *arrows*. Anodal stimulation (B) with the DBS lead contact point as the anode and the IPG as the cathode. The electric field induced by the anode hyperpolarizes the nearby axon, generating positive charge density at neighboring nodes of Ranvier, which, if of sufficient magnitude, will lead to action potentials that will then propagate in the directions shown.

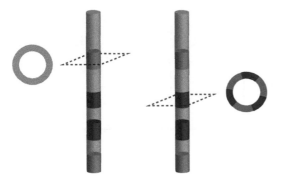

FIGURE I.3. Example of a lead with circumferential contact points (*light gray*) is shown on the *left* and segmented contacts (*dark gray*) on the *right*. Note the typical positioning of the segmented leads between two circumferential leads.

two programs, one can gain benefits that may be unique to a particular configuration but not sufficient to address improvement in other symptom areas. For example, if the ventral-most contact point provides excellent tremor relief but no improvement in rigidity, then having a second program with a unique configuration involving a more dorsal

contact can potentially provide improvement in rigidity. Another use of interleaving can be to avoid stimulation-induced side effects. When the implantation of the lead is suboptimal, programmers may be faced with narrow therapeutic windows that may only provide partial relief when a single program is used. By having two programs, interleaving allows more axons to be stimulated owing to two pulse trains that are offset by time. One drawback to interleaving is faster battery depletion.

INDEPENDENT SOURCES AND OTHER PROGRAMMING TECHNIQUES

Single-source programming occurs when the stimulation rate and pulse width remain the same between contact points, and this has been the classic model for DBS (Figure I.6A).[1] **Multiple independent current control (MICC)** has facilitated a specific amplitude and pulse width for each of the contact points on the same lead (Figure I.6B). The benefit of multiple independent sources is to allow for more precise steering of current, and this technique can potentially improve benefits

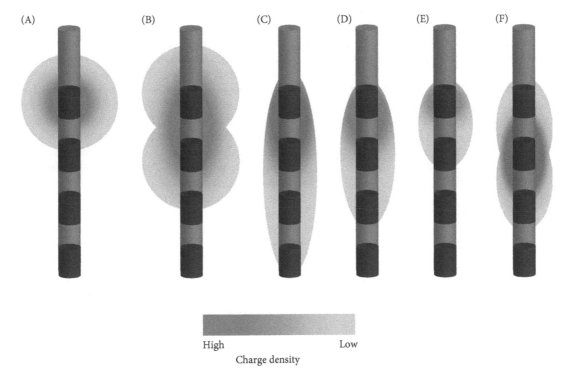

High   Low

Charge density

FIGURE I.4. Multiple programming modalities are shown, including monopolar stimulation (A), multiple monopolar stimulation (B), wide bipolar stimulation (C), intermediate bipolar stimulation (D), narrow bipolar stimulation (E), and tripolar stimulation (F).

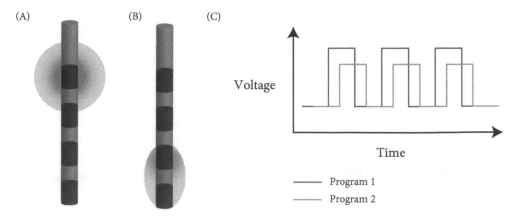

FIGURE I.5. Program 1 (A) and program 2 (B) are depicted with their offset waveforms demonstrating interleaving (C).

while minimizing side effects. There is also the potential to stimulate two different brain regions simultaneously.

Duty cycle stimulation allows for an open-loop model that can deliver stimulation at predetermined times.[3] This can be advantageous to allow for an overall lower amount of stimulation than traditional continuous stimulation. It has been used in many settings, including recently as a successful strategy in Tourette syndrome and also in patients who may benefit from turning devices off at night (e.g., tremor). Recent research has suggested that more complex duty cycles may be possible for treatment of some symptoms.

FUTURE OUTLOOK

Sensing capabilities as part of closed-loop stimulation (adaptive DBS) and also remote tele-programming represent active areas of research.

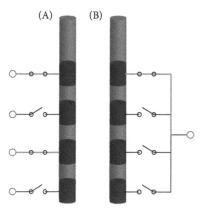

FIGURE I.6. Diagrammatic representation of multiple independent sources (A) and single source of programming (B), with viable current paths emphasized in *light gray*.

Closed-loop stimulation requires continuous sensing of various physiologic parameters, which can be analyzed and acted on based on a predetermined algorithm that uses real-time physiology for feedback control.[6] This constant-sensing system can facilitate stimulation only when pathologic physiologic signals are detected, thus potentially providing patients with stimulation when they have more symptoms. This approach may be particularly valuable as "preset" duty cycle stimulation or other open-loop parameters remain static relative to an individual patient's needs. Closed-loop approaches have many challenges, including induction of side effects, ramping time, and complexity of symptoms with differing physiologic signatures. Another technique under investigation is **coordinated reset**. This technique uses multiple contacts across structures stimulated in a fixed or varied sequence. Data have been emerging on the usefulness of this technique. **Current shaping** (e.g., biphasic pulses) has been another promising approach. Finally, changes in **stimulation pattern** could also offer superior outcomes. Technologic advances and a deeper understanding of the physiology will likely guide the next generation of DBS programming techniques.

REFERENCES

1. E. B. Montgomery, Deep brain stimulation programming: mechanisms, principles, and practice, Second ed., Oxford University Press, Oxford; New York, 2017.
2. W. J. Marks, Deep brain stimulation management, Second ed., Cambridge University Press, Cambridge; New York, 2015.

3. P. J. Rossi, E. Opri, J. B. Shute, R. Molina, D. Bowers, H. Ward, K. D. Foote, A. Gunduz, M. S. Okun, Scheduled, intermittent stimulation of the thalamus reduces tics in Tourette syndrome, Parkinsonism Relat Disord 29 (2016) 35–41.

4. A. D. Kirsch, S. Hassin-Baer, C. Matthies, J. Volkmann, F. Steigerwald, Anodic versus cathodic neurostimulation of the subthalamic nucleus: A randomized-controlled study of acute clinical effects, Parkinsonism Relat Disord 55 (2018) 61–67.

5. S. Miocinovic, P. Khemani, R. Whiddon, P. Zeilman, D. Martinez-Ramirez, M. S. Okun, S. Chitnis, Outcomes, management, and potential mechanisms of interleaving deep brain stimulation settings, Parkinsonism Relat Disord 20(12) (2014) 1434–1437.

6. P. Ghasemi, T. Sahraee, A. Mohammadi, Closed- and open-loop deep brain stimulation: Methods, challenges, current and future aspects, J Biomed Phys Eng 8(2) (2018) 209–216.

SECTION 2

Tremor Disorders

Case 1

Patient Selection Criteria for Deep Brain Stimulation for Essential Tremor

LAURA S. SURILLO DAHDAH, UMAR YAZDANI, RICHARD B. DEWEY, JR.,
PADRAIG O'SUILLEABHAIN, AND SHILPA CHITNIS

CANDIDATE SELECTION AND SCREENING

Deep brain stimulation (DBS) of the ventral intermediate (Vim) nucleus of the thalamus has been shown to be an effective and safe treatment in patients with medication-refractory essential tremor (ET).[1-5] The decision to proceed with DBS for tremor is complex and multifaceted. The first questions are whether medications are useful for ET and have been tried without success at the highest tolerated dose and if the tremor is disabling. If these basic issues are addressed, DBS may be indicated. When deciding whether to proceed with DBS in those who have failed appropriate medication trials, the two critical points of importance are correctly identifying the movement disorder (i.e., tremor, dystonic tremor, myoclonus, or ataxia) and being certain that patients do not have a functional (psychogenic) tremor or Parkinson disease (PD). Some patients with ET may have rest tremor,[6,7] and some degree of asymmetry is not rare.[8] Frequency also decreases with disease duration.[9] In these circumstances, ET may be misdiagnosed as PD. A dopamine transporter scan (DaTscan) can reliably distinguish between these two entities but will not separate ET from dystonic tremor.[10] A DaTscan is therefore rarely useful for surgical selection, especially when a neurologist trained in movement undertakes the screening.

Careful screening and selection criteria commonly used when screening ET patients for DBS include establishing the diagnosis of ET and demonstrating that the patient has moderate to severe action and/or postural tremor that is disabling in one or more activities of daily living or a reduction in quality of life. Impaired functions may include writing, typing, feeding, personal hygiene, or social embarrassment due to severe tremor. The disability due to ET may depend heavily on the patient's occupation and social circumstances but also social embarrassment.

Potential candidates should have failed appropriate medication trials before considering stereotactic neurosurgery. First-line treatments that should be tried in all patients without a contraindication are propranolol (or other nonselective beta blockers) and primidone. Second-line drugs that should also be considered include topiramate and gabapentin, being cognizant of the potential side effects of these medications.[11,12] It should be kept in mind that oral drugs for tremor, even when effective for an individual, generally only improve tremor amplitude in an average of 50%.[7] Practitioners should also consult the recent American Academy of Neurology guidelines for the medical treatment of tremor. By contrast, studies have shown that Vim DBS, when successful, can improve contralateral tremor scores by 75%, and this is often an enduring benefit lasting 5 years or longer.[8] Favilla and colleagues, however, recently showed that ET will progress despite DBS treatment, which is different than in PD tremor.[13] Medical comorbidities, imaging, neurologic, neurosurgical, neuropsychological, and psychiatric evaluations should be reviewed as part of the planning process for DBS. Presurgical videotaping of the tremor examination can be helpful to assess baseline severity and for later postoperative comparison.

DIAGNOSIS OF ESSENTIAL TREMOR

Revised diagnostic criteria for ET include an isolated action tremor syndrome of bilateral upper extremities with at least 3 years' duration, with or without tremor in other locations such as the head, voice, or lower extremities, in the absence of other neurologic signs, such as dystonia, ataxia, or parkinsonism.[12,14]

SYMPTOMS THAT RESPOND TO DEEP BRAIN STIMULATION

Patients may undergo unilateral or bilateral DBS for ET. Unilateral stimulation reliably results in marked improvement of contralateral action, postural, and resting tremor, and in some cases, DBS may have a mild ipsilateral benefit.[4,15,16] Unilateral Vim stimulation does not reliably improve voice tremor but may improve head tremor.[17-19,20] Voice tremor therefore should not be a primary indication for DBS. Unilateral and bilateral DBS treatments have resulted in inconsistent improvements in head tremor, but the trajectory angle has been used as a potential factor affecting outcome.[1,17,19,21]

RISKS AND EXPECTATIONS OF DEEP BRAIN STIMULATION SURGERY

DBS surgery, when successful, can achieve improvements in tremor amplitude by up to 85%.[12] However, as discussed previously, voice and head tremor do not respond as reliably to DBS as does extremity tremor. It is important to keep in mind that proximal tremor does not respond well to DBS, so the regionality of the tremor should be assessed preoperatively and should be included in the patient and family discussions. Patients should also be aware that ET is a progressive disease and that regular follow-up visits for DBS programming to address any re-emerging or worsening tremor may be necessary because disease progression is common (despite DBS). Video recordings of baseline tremor are useful records if preoperative tremor severity needs to be reviewed by the patient or examiner.

Surgical risks of DBS in ET are similar to those in PD. Additionally, in Vim DBS for ET, patients should be counseled that speech and gait abnormalities are the most common side effects of thalamic stimulation, more so with bilateral implantations.[22] Many patients elect to receive bilateral DBS because of disabling bilateral hand and arm tremors. Staging DBS surgeries and performing the first procedure on either the dominant hand or the more affected side can allow for sufficient time to consider a second implantation, which may or may not be necessary.[23] Recently, several groups have documented significant cognitive abnormalities in patients with Vim DBS. Therefore, patients should be counseled accordingly, and neuropsychological performance should be considered.[24,25]

MEDICAL COMORBIDITIES AND DEEP BRAIN STIMULATION

Patients with multiple comorbidities increasing their risk for surgery should be cleared by their general physician and subspecialists. There are no universally agreed-on inclusion or exclusion criteria for the selection of DBS candidates, although the guidelines discussed here are commonly accepted among experts. Identified medical comorbidities must be evaluated carefully when making the choice between frame-based or frameless approaches and between awake and asleep DBS techniques, and when deciding whether to employ microelectrode recording (MER). Cardiac, pulmonary, and other conditions such as obesity may increase surgical risk. Patients with hypertension are at increased risk for hemorrhage with MER.[19] The existence of comorbid diabetes or immunosuppression can increase the operative risk for infection and other complications following the surgical procedure. In general, healthy and cooperative patients are needed for a successful awake surgery. There is no specific age above which DBS for ET is contraindicated, but all other things being equal, younger patients tend to tolerate DBS surgery better than older patients. Older patients typically exhibit a higher risk for surgical complications compared with younger patients.[26-31]

NEUROPSYCHIATRIC ILLNESS AND DEEP BRAIN STIMULATION

Psychiatric comorbidities may limit the success of DBS, and thus screening should be performed.[32] Typically, this battery of testing is performed as part of neuropsychological testing that is performed preoperatively, but in complex cases, formal psychiatric consultation should occur during the planning stage. Some centers routinely include both neuropsychology and psychiatry, but all expert centers will involve psychiatry if there is preexisting psychiatric disease or history of suicide. Only patients with stable and fully optimized psychiatric disease should undergo DBS surgery, and there should be a plan for postoperative monitoring.

DEMENTIA AND DEEP BRAIN STIMULATION

As part of the evaluation of candidacy for DBS, neuropsychological testing should be performed and thoughtfully reviewed by the multidisciplinary team. Neuropsychological performance is one factor in the decision as to whether to proceed with DBS and also as to what the postoperative management should be. Patients with poor performance in neuropsychological testing, especially in frontal lobe and memory domains, may not be suitable candidates because of the high risk for worsening cognitive function with DBS surgery.[33] Medications such as benzodiazepines, sleep aids, antiepileptics, and pain relievers can confound performance on neuropsychological measures; therefore, test administrators should be cognizant of the patient's

medication regimen. One common mistake is to test patients with ET on maximal doses of primidone and benzodiazepines and label them as cognitively impaired.[23]

ABNORMAL PREOPERATIVE MAGNETIC RESONANCE IMAGING

Performing brain magnetic resonance imaging (MRI) in the evaluation of a patient's candidacy for DBS is important not only for confirmation of a treatable diagnosis but also for the assessment of surgical risks. Patients with major vascular disease may be at increased risk for brain hemorrhage or stroke. Global cerebral atrophy increases the risk for suboptimal lead location due to brain shift during implantation as well as the risk for postoperative subdural hematoma. Preoperative MRI can be useful for planning the target for lead implantation. Preoperatively, the use of contrast to define venous anatomy can prevent postoperative venous infarction.[34] Structural lesions such as vascular malformations along the track of lead implantation may be a contraindication.[35]

PEARLS

- Patients may undergo unilateral or bilateral DBS for ET.
- Unilateral stimulation reliably results in marked improvement of contralateral action, postural, and resting tremor and in some cases may have a mild ipsilateral effect.
- Unilateral Vim stimulation does not reliably improve voice tremor. Voice tremor therefore should not be a primary indication for DBS.
- Head tremor has revealed inconsistent improvements from unilateral and bilateral stimulation but does occasionally respond to DBS, and this may be related to trajectory angle.
- Head and voice tremor are unpredictable in their responsiveness to DBS and thus may fail to meet patient expectations.
- Many patients elect to receive bilateral stimulation. These patients should be warned that speech impairment and gait ataxia are known side effects observed more commonly after the second implantation.
- With staged procedures, a second implantation can be delayed or deferred, depending on the outcome of the first surgery.
- Cognition and mood do not commonly deteriorate following thalamic stimulation, although preoperative cognitive impairment and uncontrolled mood or thought disorders can worsen after DBS.
- The single most important factor that is critical to the success of DBS for ET is the use of multidisciplinary screening. Multidisciplinary screening can yield an important risk-to-benefit profile that can be used in the preoperative discussions.
- Finally, DBS for ET has more success in distal tremor than proximal tremor, and in most cases, the tremor will progress over time despite the DBS therapy.

REFERENCES

1. Pahwa, R., Lyons, K. E., Wilkinson, S. B., Tröster, A. I., Overman, J., Kieltyka, J., & Koller, W. C. (2001). Comparison of thalamotomy to deep brain stimulation of the thalamus in essential tremor. *Movement Disorders: Official Journal of the Movement Disorder Society, 16*(1), 140–143.
2. Vaillancourt, D. E., Sturman, M. M., Metman, L. V., Bakay, R. A. E., & Corcos, D. M. (2003). Deep brain stimulation of the VIM thalamic nucleus modifies several features of essential tremor. *Neurology, 61*(7), 919–925.
3. Koller, W., Pahwa, R., Busenbark, K., Hubble, J., Wilkinson, S., Lang, A., & Malapira, T. (1997). High-frequency unilateral thalamic stimulation in the treatment of essential and parkinsonian tremor. *Annals of Neurology: Official Journal of the American Neurological Association and the Child Neurology Society, 42*(3), 292–299.
4. Lyons, K. E., & Pahwa, R. (2005). Long-term benefits in quality of life provided by bilateral subthalamic stimulation in patients with Parkinson disease. *Journal of Neurosurgery, 103*(2), 252–255.
5. Schuurman, P. R., Bosch, D. A., Bossuyt, P. M., Bonsel, G. J., Van Someren, E. J., De Bie, R. M., & Speelman, J. D. (2000). A comparison of continuous thalamic stimulation and thalamotomy for suppression of severe tremor. *New England Journal of Medicine, 342*(7), 461–468.
6. Cohen, O., Pullman, S., Jurewicz, E., Watner, D., & Louis, E. D. (2003). Rest tremor in patients with essential tremor: prevalence, clinical correlates, and electrophysiologic characteristics. *Archives of Neurology, 60*(3), 405–410.
7. Martinelli, P., Gabellini, A. S., Gulli, M. R., & Lugaresi, E. (1987). Different clinical features of essential tremor: a 200-patient study. *Acta Neurologica Scandinavica, 75*(2), 106–111.
8. Pahwa, R., Lyons, K. E., Wilkinson, S. B., Simpson Jr., R. K., Ondo, W. G., Tarsy, D., Norregaard, T., Hubble, J. P., Smith, D. A., Hauser, R. A., & Jankovic, J. (2006). Long term evaluation of deep brain stimulation of the thalamus. *Journal of Neurosurgery, 104*(4), 506–512.
9. Elble, R. J. (2000). Essential tremor frequency decreases with time. *Neurology, 55*(10), 1547–1551.
10. Tatsch, K., & Poepperl, G. (2013). Nigrostriatal dopamine terminal imaging with dopamine transporter SPECT: an update. *Journal of Nuclear Medicine, 54*(8), 1331–1338.
11. Munhoz, R. P., Picillo, M., Fox, S. H., Bruno, V., Panisset, M., Honey, C. R., & Fasano, A. (2016). Eligibility criteria for deep brain stimulation in Parkinson's disease, tremor, and dystonia. *Canadian Journal of Neurological Sciences, 43*(4), 462–471.

12. Marks Jr., W. J. (Ed.). (2015). *Deep brain stimulation management*. Cambridge, UK: Cambridge University Press.
13. Favilla, C. G., Ullman, D., Wagle Shukla, A., Foote, K. D., Jacobson IV, C. E., & Okun, M. S. (2012). Worsening essential tremor following deep brain stimulation: disease progression versus tolerance. *Brain, 135*(5), 1455–1462.
14. Bhatia, K. P., Bain, P., Bajaj, N., Elble, R. J., Hallett, M., Louis, E. D., . . . Tremor Task Force of the International Parkinson and Movement Disorder Society. (2018). Consensus statement on the classification of tremors. From the Task Force on Tremor of the International Parkinson and Movement Disorder Society. *Movement Disorders, 33*(1), 75–87.
15. Ondo, W., Jankovic, J., Schwartz, K., Almaguer, M., & Simpson, R. K. (1998). Unilateral thalamic deep brain stimulation for refractory essential tremor and Parkinson's disease tremor. *Neurology, 51*(4), 1063–1069.
16. Obwegeser, A. A., Uitti, R. J., Witte, R. J., Lucas, J. A., Turk, M. F., & Wharen Jr., R. E. (2001). Quantitative and qualitative outcome measures after thalamic deep brain stimulation to treat disabling tremors. *Neurosurgery, 48*(2), 274–284.
17. Sydow, O., Thobois, S., Alesch, F., & Speelman, J. D. (2003). Multicentre European study of thalamic stimulation in essential tremor: a six year follow up. *Journal of Neurology, Neurosurgery & Psychiatry, 74*(10), 1387–1391.
18. Carpenter, M. A., Pahwa, R., Miyawaki, K. L., Wilkinson, S. B., Searl, J. P., & Koller, W. C. (1998). Reduction in voice tremor under thalamic stimulation. *Neurology, 50*(3), 796–798.
19. Obwegeser, A. A., Uitti, R. J., Turk, M. F., Strongosky, A. J., & Wharen, R. E. (2000). Thalamic stimulation for the treatment of midline tremors in essential tremor patients. *Neurology, 54*(12), 2342–2344.
20. Moscovich, M., Morishita, T., Foote, K. D., Favilla, C. G., Chen, Z. P., & Okun, M. S. (2013). Effect of lead trajectory on the response of essential head tremor to deep brain stimulation. *Parkinsonism and Related Disorders, 19*(9), 789–794.
21. Pahwa, R., Lyons, K. L., Wilkinson, S. B., Carpenter, M. A., Tröster, A. I., Searl, J. P., & Koller, W. C. (1999). Bilateral thalamic stimulation for the treatment of essential tremor. *Neurology, 53*(7), 1447–1447.
22. Gorgulho, A., De Salles, A. A. F., Frighetto, L., & Behnke, E. (2005). Incidence of hemorrhage associated with electrophysiological studies performed using macroelectrodes and microelectrodes in functional neurosurgery. *Journal of Neurosurgery, 102*(5), 888–896.

23. Rodriguez, R. L., Fernandez, H. H., Haq, I., & Okun, M. S. (2007). Pearls in patient selection for deep brain stimulation. *Neurologist, 13*(5), 253–260.

24. Lombardi, W. J., Woolston, D. J., Roberts, J. W., & Gross, R. E. (2001). Cognitive deficits in patients with essential tremor. *Neurology, 57*(5), 785–790.

25. Leehey, M. A. (2009). Fragile X-associated tremor/ataxia syndrome: clinical phenotype, diagnosis, and treatment. *Journal of Investigative Medicine, 57*(8), 830–836.

26. Welter, M. L., Houeto, J. L., Tezenas du Montcel, S., Mesnage, V., Bonnet, A. M., Pillon, B., & Agid, Y. (2002). Clinical predictive factors of subthalamic stimulation in Parkinson's disease. *Brain, 125*(3), 575–583.

27. Rodriguez, R. L., Miller, K., Bowers, D., Crucian, G., Wint, D., Fernandez, H., . . . Okun, M. S. (2005). Mood and cognitive changes with deep brain stimulation: what we know and where we should go. *Minerva Medica, 96*(3), 125–144.

28. Russmann, H., Ghika, J., Villemure, J. G., Robert, B., Bogousslavsky, J., Burkhard, P. R., & Vingerhoets, F. J. G. (2004). Subthalamic nucleus deep brain stimulation in Parkinson disease patients over age 70 years. *Neurology, 63*(10), 1952–1954.

29. Kleiner-Fisman, G., Fisman, D. N., Sime, E., Saint-Cyr, J. A., Lozano, A. M., & Lang, A. E. (2003). Long-term follow up of bilateral deep brain stimulation of the subthalamic nucleus in patients with advanced Parkinson disease. *Journal of Neurosurgery, 99*(3), 489–495.

30. Jaggi, J. L., Umemura, A., Hurtig, H. I., Siderowf, A. D., Colcher, A., Stern, M. B., & Baltuch, G. H. (2004). Bilateral stimulation of the subthalamic nucleus in Parkinson's disease: surgical efficacy and prediction of outcome. *Stereotactic and Functional Neurosurgery, 82*(2–3), 104–114.

31. Guehl, D., Cuny, E., Benazzouz, A., Rougier, A., Tison, F., Machado, S., & Burbaud, P. (2006). Side-effects of subthalamic stimulation in Parkinson's disease: clinical evolution and predictive factors. *European Journal of Neurology, 13*(9), 963–971.

32. Cyron, D. (2016). Mental side effects of deep brain stimulation (DBS) for movement disorders: the futility of denial. *Frontiers in Integrative Neuroscience, 10*, 17.

33. Saint-Cyr, J. A., Trépanier, L. L., Kumar, R., Lozano, A. M., & Lang, A. E. (2000). Neuropsychological consequences of chronic bilateral stimulation of the subthalamic nucleus in Parkinson's disease. *Brain, 123*(10), 2091–2108.

34. Morishita, T., Okun, M. S., Burdick, A., Jacobson IV, C. E., & Foote, K. D. (2013). Cerebral venous infarction: a potentially avoidable complication of deep brain stimulation surgery. *Neuromodulation, 16*(5), 407–413.

35. Lang, A. E., Houeto, J. L., Krack, P., Kubu, C., Lyons, K. E., Moro, E., & Uitti, R. (2006). Deep brain stimulation: preoperative issues. *Movement Disorders: Official Journal of the Movement Disorder Society, 21*(S14), S171–S196.

Case 2

Deep Brain Stimulation for Essential Tremor

Basic Programming Pearls

BRENT BLUETT

INTRODUCTION

Essential tremor (ET) is one of the most common movement disorders, with an estimated prevalence between 0.4% and 5% in the general population.[1] Differentiating ET from other disorders, such as an enhanced physiologic tremor or Parkinson disease, is necessary for subsequent management. ET is typically characterized by a chronic postural and kinetic bilateral upper limb tremor and can be associated with tremor in the head, voice, or lower limbs.[2] ET is rhythmic and oscillatory, with a typical frequency of 4 to 7 Hz. Importantly, clinical features of parkinsonism, ataxia, or dystonia should be absent. ET can be evaluated clinically using the validated Fahn–Tolosa–Marin Tremor Rating Scale[3] and/or components of the Unified Parkinson's Disease Rating Scale (UPDRS) Part III.[4] Standard evaluation includes having patients hold both arms outstretched in front of them (hands pronated) to evaluate for a postural tremor, using finger-to-nose or finger-to-finger maneuvers to evaluate for a kinetic or intention tremor, and additional measures such as drawing an Archimedes spiral, pouring a cup of water into another cup, or attempting to perform other daily activities for which a tremor would worsen voluntary movement.

First-line treatment for ET involves using medications such as propranolol or primidone, but approximately 25% to 55% of patients will have medication-refractory ET.[5] For eligible patients, surgical interventions, including deep brain stimulation (DBS) and thalamotomy (radiofrequency and magnetic resonance imaging–guided focused ultrasound) are available.[6] The overall efficacy is similar for thalamotomy and DBS of the thalamus for ET, but thalamotomy is associated with a higher complication rate.[7] DBS also offers the advantage of being reversible and externally programmable, and it can adapt to tremor progression and can also be performed bilaterally. The choice of surgical intervention depends on each patient's unique characteristics and should be determined by a multidisciplinary team in conjunction with the patient's wishes.

DBS of the ventral intermediate (Vim) nucleus for ET was approved by the US Food and Drug Administration in 1997.[8] It has proved to be a safe and effective long-term therapy for refractory ET,[9] although the efficacy of Vim DBS tends to wane significantly after several years, possibly owing to disease progression.[10,11] Bilateral implantation of the Vim tends to result in more side effects than unilateral stimulation, with paresthesias, dysarthria, and gait disturbances being the most common adverse events.[12]

Current DBS systems for ET operate in an open-loop system, where stimulation parameters are set once programmed and are not adaptable to the patient's clinical symptoms in real time.[13] Adaptive closed-loop systems are being developed but are not discussed in this chapter because they are not currently available for ET. There are several open-loop DBS systems currently available for treatment of tremor. These systems differ in their power source (voltage or current), ability to shape the stimulation field (based on electrode design and polarity configuration), range of stimulation parameters, and ability to perform interleaving.[14] This chapter focuses on programming for high-frequency open-loop DBS systems currently available for medication-refractory ET.

CURRENT APPROACHES TO DEEP BRAIN STIMULATION PROGRAMMING FOR ESSENTIAL TREMOR

The overall goals of DBS programming for ET are (1) to maximize control of tremor, (2) to minimize adverse side effects, and (3) to prolong the neurostimulator battery life.[15]

For ET, DBS programming is determined by the positioning of the leads in the Vim—if optimal, less side effects occur and lower stimulation parameters are in general needed to obtain the desired outcome. The outcome is a result of the tissue stimulated by the electrodes (which stimulates a circuit), which is based on the accuracy of surgical implantation and the programming parameters—voltage, frequency, and pulse width. Most DBS side effects are due to current spreading into brain regions adjacent to the target area.

Newer neurostimulation systems allow the programmer to steer the current in horizontal directions using segmented leads and on multiple independent current control (MICC), with the hope of increasing the therapeutic window of effective stimulation without adverse effects.[16,17] The increase in possible programming parameters also can increase the time to effectively program, especially at the first programming session, and patient fatigue can be an issue.

INITIATION OF PROGRAMMING

At some centers, DBS may be activated and programmed before discharge from the hospital. More commonly, programming of the implantable pulse generator (IPG) is performed in the outpatient setting a few weeks after surgical implantation of the DBS leads in order to let edema resolve.

Initial programming in the outpatient setting is typically performed 2 to 4 weeks after implantation of the leads to allow for resolution of brain tissue edema (which can alter impedances) and the "microlesion effect"—an initial improvement of symptoms by surgical placement of the lead in the proper neuroanatomic structure.[18] Patient education should be provided at this visit, including how to use the patient programmer, what to do in case of an emergency, and how to avoid accidentally turning off the stimulator.

During initial programming, a monopolar review is typically performed first. The goal is to find the therapeutic window—the lowest voltage that best ameliorates tremor, and alternatively, the higher voltage that induces side effects.[19] The monopolar review is performed by first selecting the IPG case as the anode (positive sign), and then individually testing each contact of the DBS electrode as the cathode (negative sign). In DBS systems with segmented electrodes, all (three) ring electrodes are activated.[20] Generally, pulse width is set to 60 to 90 μsec and frequency to 130 Hz, and the voltage for each electrode is gradually increased by 0.1 to 0.5 V (0.1–0.5 mA in segmented electrodes) to a maximum of 5 V (or 5 mA), unless side effects occur first.[21] For segmented electrodes, after the most efficacious ring electrode is identified, single contacts of the ring can be evaluated individually by gradually increasing current in lower increments, typically 0.1 to 0.2 mA.[22] Ultimately, the contact and voltage that best improve tremor without side effects are selected.

If the monopolar review alone does not identify the optimal stimulation parameters, the pulse width and then frequency (typically at the optimal contact identified in monopolar review) can be gradually increased until the optimal outcome is identified.[19] This is done in a similar manner to that discussed earlier, except that the voltage (and either the pulse width or frequency) is kept constant. If a low voltage results in adverse effects, bipolar stimulation—stimulation of more than one contact at a time—can be attempted. Bipolar stimulation narrows the spread of current and can help avoid stimulation of adjacent tissue for which spread may cause adverse effects.[22]

INITIAL PROGRAMMING SETTINGS

A multicenter European study in 1999 found that monopolar stimulation, with an average voltage of 2 V, was used in 38 of 46 cases of DBS for ET.[23] A study of 14 patients with DBS of the Vim for ET found that the effect on tremor at frequencies of 90 to 100 Hz was not significantly different from that at 160 to 170 Hz, but the therapeutic window decreased significantly and power consumption increased as the frequency was increased beyond 100 Hz.[24] Optimal tremor control was usually achieved by increasing the amplitude to 2 to 3 V and could be further improved by approximately one-third with longer pulse widths (90–120 μsec).[25] Monopolar stimulation was typically used for ET, with bipolar stimulation typically reserved for when adverse effects occurred with lower voltage on monopolar settings.[19]

Existing open-loop DBS systems facilitate the creation of groups with different settings. Select patients should be given the opportunity to choose between groups that may provide the desired outcome based on their setting—for example, if optimal control of the tremor without any adverse effects cannot be identified during initial programming, one group can be created that completely controls the tremor with mild dysarthria, while another group can be created that has good tremor control but no dysarthria. The patient can switch between the two groups based on individual preference. Additionally, most patients are given parameters by which they can adjust an individual parameter on their own—most frequently the voltage. If tremor control fluctuates using group A at a voltage of 3 V, the patient can adjust the voltage, typically no more than 0.5 V in either direction, to obtain the optimal outcome.

MEDICATION MANAGEMENT AFTER INITIAL PROGRAMMING

The goal of DBS for ET is to reduce symptoms and potentially eliminate the need for medications, which often cause side effects of sedation and fatigue. When there is a robust and sustained response to initial programming, medications can be reduced if the patient wishes. The patient's blood pressure and heart rate should be considered when reducing propranolol. Coordination with the patient's cardiologist or other prescribing physician is advised to avoid adverse cardiovascular events. Primidone, topiramate, and/or gabapentin should be tapered off slowly and gradually in order to avoid withdrawal or the theoretical potential of inducing a seizure (although this is more relevant for patients taking these medications for epilepsy).

SUBSEQUENT PROGRAMMING

During the first 6 months, it may take several programming sessions before the optimal outcome is achieved. Most patients return for follow-up programming within 3 months of the initial session in order to modify existing parameters.

In a study on the long-term efficacy of DBS of the Vim in 34 patients with ET, most required a gradual increase in stimulation parameters within 5 years after surgery.[26] The diminishing effect of DBS on tremor control was thought to be

due in part to developing a tolerance or habituation to chronic brain stimulation, although disease progression may be the most common reason for worsening symptoms.[9,11] Studies have found that alternating stimulation patterns may reduce habituation to chronic Vim stimulation in ET or may address the disease progression.[27,28] Alternatively, turning off the stimulator at night may reduce the worsening[9] but may prove uncomfortable for the patient.

The most frequent temporary adverse effect during programming is paresthesia, which occurs if excessive tissue stimulation reaches dorsal thalamic sensory nuclei (ventralis caudalis, or Vc).[16] Overstimulation reaching fibers lateral and ventral to the Vim can result in imbalance and gait ataxia, which in some cases may be avoided by choosing more dorsal or medial contacts with a lower amplitude or by reducing pulse width.

Dysarthria, a common side effect after bilateral Vim implantation, can occur with excessive stimulation of ventral contacts reaching cerebellothalamic fibers or lateral stimulation of the internal capsule.[29] If dysarthria occurs after initial programming, subsequent programming should first re-evaluate the stimulation parameters by lowering the voltage or by considering a more dorsal or medial contact, or alternatively by lowering the pulse width. If this side effect continues despite the previous issues, bipolar settings or, eventually, interleaving stimulation can be considered. Dysarthria and imbalance may not always be adequately addressed by DBS programming and in some cases results from a microlesion effect.

Interleaving consists of rapid, alternating activation of two electrode contacts with the same frequency (up to 125 Hz) but with separate amplitudes and pulse widths.[16] Current-shaping interleaving—performed by programming different current amplitudes on different contacts—may now be used as well. Reducing the amplitude of one contact below the threshold of inducing dysarthria, combined with activating a more dorsally located contact with higher stimulation amplitude, has been shown in a small number of cases to suppress tremor while reducing dysarthria.[30] Because interleaving consists of using two independent programming settings, it can drain the battery more quickly, and this factor should be considered before implementation.[31]

Because of the previous common side effects, while programming DBS for ET, it is important during programming adjustments to continually examine the patient's tremor, gait, and speech and to inquire about the presence of temporary adverse effects such as paresthesia.[19] A final examination is generally performed at the end of programming to ensure an optimal outcome.

IMPEDANCE CHECK

Impedance is a measure of resistance to current flow in an alternating-current system.[32] Intraoperatively, impedance is typically altered by brain edema. Studies of impedance in DBS of the Vim for ET have found that it tends to increase by 33% and eventually to stabilize in most cases 3 months after implantation.[33]

It is important to measure and to compare the lead integrity impedance (LII) and the therapeutic impedance. LII assesses impedance at each contact with the DBS manufacturers predefined stimulation parameters. The typical range for LII is 500 to 1,500 ohm, and a significant increase is often due to an open electrical circuit, while a significant decrease typically indicates a short circuit. Therapeutic impedance is determined at each contact based on the programmed stimulation parameters and therefore is a more accurate real-world measurement of energy use and, subsequently, battery life. It is important to note that therapeutic impedances are usually consistent with LII if typical stimulation parameters are used, but stimulation with a lower voltage may result in a somewhat falsely elevated therapeutic impedance. If there is a large discrepancy between LII and therapeutic impedance, testing at a higher voltage may resolve this issue.[34]

To have a baseline reference, it is important at the initial programming visit for the impedance be evaluated individually at each contact.[18] Measuring impedance in a unipolar configuration with standard parameters helps to confine the impedance measurement to an individual electrode[15] and facilitates comparison of future measurements with the baseline.

Constant Voltage Versus Constant Current Stimulation. The total current delivered depends on both voltage and impedance, and because the amount of voltage delivered does not vary with constant voltage stimulation (CVS), potential variations in current over time are assumed to be a consequence of alterations in impedance. Constant current stimulation (CCS) may provide more stable stimulation in cases in which impedance varies, such as when programming within 3 months of implantation, during which impedance usually gradually increases.[35]

PROGRAMMING THRESHOLDS

Typical DBS parameter setting ranges for ET include a pulse width of 60 to 210 μsec, a frequency of 130 to 185 Hz, and voltage range of 1 to 3.5 V or mA.[24] Tremor is most responsive to increases in amplitude, and may be further improved by 25% by using pulse widths of 90 to 120 μsec.[16] However, maintaining a lower pulse width tends to lessen the occurrence of ataxia and dysarthria as a side effect.[36] Studies of the effect of varying frequencies have found that postural and kinetic tremors usually do not improve

---

PEARLS

- Vim DBS is a safe and effective treatment for medication-refractory ET.
- Multidisciplinary evaluation should be performed to determine the optimal candidates for DBS.
- Initiation of programming is typically performed 2 to 4 weeks after surgical implantation of leads.
- A monopolar review is usually performed at the initial programming session in order to identify the therapeutic window of each contact.
- Segmented electrodes facilitate current steering, which may reduce the incidence of side effects and increase the therapeutic window.
- Interleaving can be performed in difficult cases, but consideration should be given to battery life.
- Many cases of habituation are due to disease progression, and patients should be counseled preoperatively about likely postprocedure worsening over time.

significantly when increased beyond 130 Hz, but increases beyond this frequency can lower battery life significantly.[37] Clinical bedside programmers should appreciate that individual differences may occur in programming and that the previously mentioned mean parameters may not apply to every patient.

REFERENCES

1. Flora ED, Perera CL, Cameron AL, Maddern GJ. Deep brain stimulation for essential tremor: a systematic review. *Mov Disord.* 2010;25(11):1550–1559.
2. Bhatia KP, Bain P, Bajaj N, et al. Consensus statement on the classification of tremors. From the Task Force on Tremor of the International Parkinson and Movement Disorder Society. *Mov Disord.* 2018;33(1):75–87.
3. Ondo W, Hashem V, LeWitt PA, et al. Comparison of the Fahn-Tolosa-Marin Clinical Rating Scale and the Essential Tremor Rating Assessment Scale. *Mov Disord Clin Pract.* 2018;5(1):60–65.
4. Forjaz MJ, Ayala A, Testa CM, et al. Proposing a Parkinson's disease-specific tremor scale from the MDS-UPDRS. *Mov Disord.* 2015;30(8):1139–1143.
5. Louis ED. Clinical practice: essential tremor. *N Engl J Med.* 2001;345(12):887–891.
6. Ferreira JJ, Mestre TA, Lyons KE, et al. MDS evidence-based review of treatments for essential tremor. *Mov Disord.* 2019;34(7):950–958.
7. Pahwa R, Lyons KE, Wilkinson SB, et al. Comparison of thalamotomy to deep brain stimulation of the thalamus in essential tremor. *Mov Disord.* 2001;16(1):140–143.
8. Lozano AM, Lipsman N, Bergman H, et al. Deep brain stimulation: current challenges and future directions. *Nat Rev Neurol.* 2019;15(3):148–160.
9. Baizabal-Carvallo JF, Kagnoff MN, Jimenez-Shahed J, Fekete R, Jankovic J. The safety and efficacy of thalamic deep brain stimulation in essential tremor: 10 years and beyond. *J Neurol Neurosurg Psychiatry.* 2014;85(5):567–572.
10. Paschen S, Forstenpointner J, Becktepe J, et al. Long-term efficacy of deep brain stimulation for essential tremor: an observer-blinded study. *Neurology.* 2019;92(12):e1378–e1386.
11. Favilla CG, Ullman D, Wagle Shukla A, Foote KD, Jacobson CE, Okun MS. Worsening essential tremor following deep brain stimulation: disease progression versus tolerance. *Brain.* 2012;135(Pt 5):1455–1462.
12. Buhmann C, Huckhagel T, Engel K, et al. Adverse events in deep brain stimulation: a retrospective long-term analysis of neurological, psychiatric and other occurrences. *PLoS One.* 2017;12(7):e0178984.
13. Hell F, Palleis C, Mehrkens JH, Koeglsperger T, Botzel K. Deep brain stimulation programming 2.0: future perspectives for target identification and adaptive closed loop stimulation. *Front Neurol.* 2019;10:314.
14. Amon A, Alesch F. Systems for deep brain stimulation: review of technical features. *J Neural Transm (Vienna).* 2017;124(9):1083–1091.
15. Volkmann J, Herzog J, Kopper F, Deuschl G. Introduction to the programming of deep brain stimulators. *Mov Disord.* 2002;17(Suppl 3):S181–187.
16. Koeglsperger T, Palleis C, Hell F, Mehrkens JH, Botzel K. Deep brain stimulation programming for movement disorders: current concepts and evidence-based strategies. *Front Neurol.* 2019;10:410.
17. Steigerwald F, Muller L, Johannes S, Matthies C, Volkmann J. Directional deep brain stimulation of the subthalamic nucleus: a pilot study using a novel neurostimulation device. *Mov Disord.* 2016;31(8):1240–1243.
18. Wagle Shukla A, Zeilman P, Fernandez H, Bajwa JA, Mehanna R. DBS programming: an evolving approach for patients with Parkinson's disease. *Parkinson Dis.* 2017;2017:8492619.
19. Dowsey-Limousin P. Postoperative management of Vim DBS for tremor. *Mov Disord.* 2002;17(Suppl 3):S208–211.
20. Dembek TA, Reker P, Visser-Vandewalle V, et al. Directional DBS increases side-effect thresholds: a prospective, double-blind trial. *Mov Disord.* 2017;32(10):1380–1388.
21. Volkmann J, Moro E, Pahwa R. Basic algorithms for the programming of deep brain stimulation in Parkinson's disease. *Mov Disord.* 2006;21(Suppl 14):S284–289.
22. Hartmann CJ, Fliegen S, Groiss SJ, Wojtecki L, Schnitzler A. An update on best practice of deep brain stimulation in Parkinson's disease. *Ther Adv Neurol Disord.* 2019;12:1756286419838096.
23. Limousin P, Speelman JD, Gielen F, Janssens M. Multicentre European study of thalamic stimulation in parkinsonian and essential tremor. *J Neurol Neurosurg Psychiatry.* 1999;66(3):289–296.
24. Kuncel AM, Cooper SE, Wolgamuth BR, et al. Clinical response to varying the stimulus parameters in deep brain stimulation for essential tremor. *Mov Disord.* 2006;21(11):1920–1928.
25. Picillo M, Lozano AM, Kou N, Munhoz RP, Fasano A. Programming deep brain stimulation for tremor and dystonia: the Toronto Western Hospital algorithms. *Brain Stimul.* 2016;9(3):438–452.
26. Zhang K, Bhatia S, Oh MY, Cohen D, Angle C, Whiting D. Long-term results of thalamic deep brain stimulation for essential tremor. *J Neurosurg.* 2010;112(6):1271–1276.

27. Barbe MT, Liebhart L, Runge M, et al. Deep brain stimulation in the nucleus ventralis intermedius in patients with essential tremor: habituation of tremor suppression. *J Neurol.* 2011;258(3):434–439.
28. Seier M, Hiller A, Quinn J, Murchison C, Brodsky M, Anderson S. Alternating thalamic deep brain stimulation for essential tremor: a trial to reduce habituation. *Mov Disord Clin Pract.* 2018;5(6):620–626.
29. Mucke D, Becker J, Barbe MT, et al. The effect of deep brain stimulation on the speech motor system. *J Speech Lang Hear Res.* 2014;57(4):1206–1218.
30. Barbe MT, Dembek TA, Becker J, et al. Individualized current-shaping reduces DBS-induced dysarthria in patients with essential tremor. *Neurology.* 2014;82(7):614–619.
31. Almeida L, Rawal PV, Ditty B, et al. Deep brain stimulation battery longevity: comparison of monopolar versus bipolar stimulation modes. *Mov Disord Clin Pract.* 2016;3(4):359–366.
32. Farris S, Vitek J, Giroux ML. Deep brain stimulation hardware complications: the role of electrode impedance and current measurements. *Mov Disord.* 2008;23(5):755–760.
33. Benabid AL, Pollak P, Gao D, et al. Chronic electrical stimulation of the ventralis intermedius nucleus of the thalamus as a treatment of movement disorders. *J Neurosurg.* 1996;84(2):203–214.
34. Deeb W, Patel A, Okun MS, Gunduz A. Management of elevated therapeutic impedances on deep brain stimulation leads. *Tremor Other Hyperkinet Mov (NY).* 2017;7:493.
35. Beaulieu-Boire I, Fasano A. Current or voltage? Another Shakespearean dilemma. *Eur J Neurol.* 2015;22(6):887–888.
36. Groppa S, Herzog J, Falk D, Riedel C, Deuschl G, Volkmann J. Physiological and anatomical decomposition of subthalamic neurostimulation effects in essential tremor. *Brain.* 2014;137(Pt 1):109–121.
37. Ushe M, Mink JW, Tabbal SD, et al. Postural tremor suppression is dependent on thalamic stimulation frequency. *Mov Disord.* 2006;21(8):1290–1292.

Case 3

Using Deep Brain Stimulation to Improve Orthostatic Tremor

ANHAR HASSAN

INDICATION FOR DEEP BRAIN STIMULATION
Medication-refractory orthostatic tremor (OT)

CLINICAL HISTORY AND RELEVANT EXAM

A 79-year-old woman presented with a diagnosis of OT that was made at age 64 years, after presenting with several years' history of progressively worse leg shaking on standing. The tremor occurred within 30 seconds of standing and spread to the trunk and arms within 1 minute. A surface electromyography (EMG) study confirmed OT with a 15- to 16-Hz tremor in the lower limbs, paraspinals, and upper limbs on standing (Figure 3.1). Medication trials of clonazepam, valproic acid, and gabapentin were ineffective or limited by sedation. The symptoms progressed, with limited standing ability and difficulty holding objects when standing, because of arm tremor. At the time of deep brain stimulation (DBS) evaluation, she reported leg tremor within seconds on standing. She was unable to stand for a conversation, take a shower, go through a buffet line, or stand to teach watercolor painting. She reported taking a stepping stool almost everywhere she traveled to compensate for standing. Preoperative evaluation was remarkable for lower limb tremor that was visible and palpable within a few seconds of standing. It was discussed with the patient that additional medication trials were unlikely to provide benefit, having already failed several medications, including clonazepam and given the disabling nature of the tremor. DBS was discussed as a potential therapeutic option based on several favorable case reports in the literature using bilateral ventromedial (Vim) thalamic DBS to treat medication-refractory OT. Therefore, she underwent multidisciplinary DBS evaluation with a DBS neurologist, neurosurgeon, neuropsychologist, speech pathologist, and nurse educator, and videos were taken of the patient seated and standing. Her case was presented at our DBS committee meeting. Neuropsychometric testing was within normal limits for age, with no cognitive contraindication identified for DBS. Brain magnetic resonance imaging showed a chronic lacunar infarct in the anterior right basal ganglia and moderate to severe chronic small vessel ischemic changes, which were thought to be incidental findings. Paired single-photon emission computed tomography was additionally performed to look for a novel DBS target for OT; this showed relative bilateral thalamic and medial right cerebellar hyperperfusion on standing with tremor compared with sitting. She was ultimately approved by the DBS review committee for bilateral Vim thalamic DBS implantation in an effort to treat medication-refractory OT.

COMPLICATIONS

There were no perioperative or postoperative complications. An experienced functional neurosurgery team performed bilateral DBS surgery plus battery placement in a single procedure. Electrophysiologic monitoring was performed to assist with surgical lead placement. Intraoperative fluoroscopic imaging confirmed the DBS leads to be at target (Figure 3.2). The left thalamic lead was placed first. Test stimulation of the left electrode (contact 0 negative, 3 positive, pulse width 60 msec, rate 135 Hz) produced transient mild paresthesia in the right lips and tongue at 2 V. There were no other side effects. The right thalamic lead was placed next. Test stimulation (contact 0 negative, 3 positive, pulse width 60 msec, rate 135 Hz) produced no side effects at 2 V. The leads were externalized. The patient stood

(A)

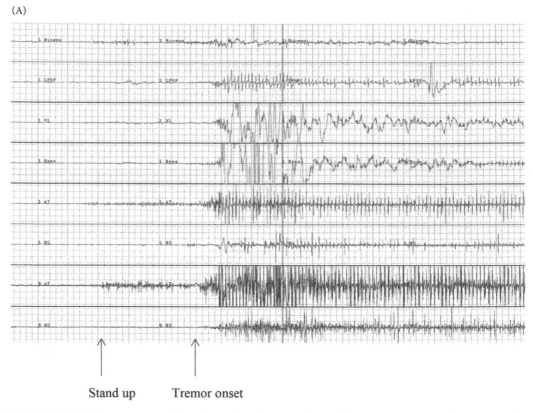

Stand up   Tremor onset

FIGURE 3.1. (A) Preoperative surface electrophysiology recordings of 15- to 16-Hz tremor burst potentials in bilateral lower limb and paraspinals muscles, with latency of approximately 1,500 msec, after standing up. Each small box division is equivalent to 100 msec. (B) Time frequency analysis showing 15- to 16-Hz tremor band (*red horizontal line*) in lower limbs, paraspinals, and upper limbs with standing. Vertical axis (Hz). Horizontal axis lists different test conditions. AT = anterior tibialis; Hams = hamstrings; L posture = leg posture; LPSP = lumbar paraspinals; MG = medial gastrocnemius; VL = vastus lateralis.

up in the operating room, and a bilateral microlesional effect was observed, with no initial tremors and mild bilateral leg tremor after a few minutes. With test stimulation on both sides (contact 0 negative, 3 positive, pulse width 60 msec, rate 135 Hz), the patient noted diffuse paresthesia but no other side effects.

TROUBLESHOOTING AND MANAGEMENT

The first DBS programming session was performed 2 weeks after lead placement. The patient reported that the microlesional effect was lost within 24 hours. On arrival, she stood for less than 10 seconds before OT emerged. The DBS was turned on and a monopolar review was performed (see Table 3.1 for thresholds and Table 3.2 for programming settings). After programming, the patient could stand for 45 seconds before tremor onset. There was very mild dysarthria at voltages of 1.5 V bilaterally, which resolved after decreasing voltage in the left stimulator to 1 V, suggesting the therapeutic threshold was narrow. The patient returned for the second programming session 1 year later. She had been unable to return earlier and had not had any programming changes. At the annual visit, she reported satisfaction with increased standing time and had returned to teaching watercolor painting. She was able to stand for 5 minutes or more before feeling unsteady and needing to sit down. She turned the device off overnight and back on in the morning, with mild transient paresthesias and mild dysarthria. Programming with a few different bipolar and monopolar configurations did not improve standing time. Therefore, only a slight voltage increase was made. During telephone follow-up

(B)

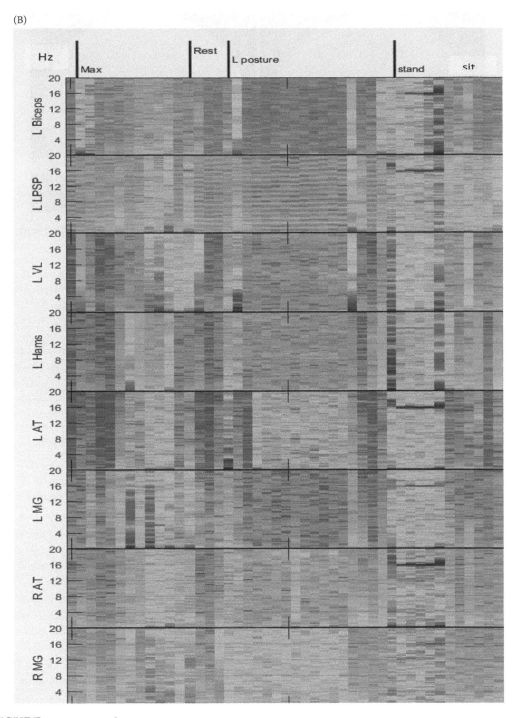

FIGURE 3.1. Continued

18 months after surgery, the patient reported "much improvement." Her next follow-up was 2 years after surgery. She was still able to stand for 5 minutes and could now stand for a conversation, stand in the shower, and go through a buffet line. No programming adjustments were made. At the final follow-up visit 3 years after surgery, at age 82 years, she reported that DBS was "life-changing." She was able to stand for 10 to 15 minutes for a conversation, with very

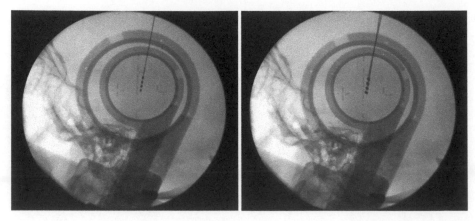

FIGURE 3.2. Intraoperative fluoroscopic imaging confirmation of thalamic lead placement (*left*: left lead; *right*: right lead).

minor shifts in stance position, and could stand to wash dishes, stand in the shower, and stand in a buffet line. She continued to turn the DBS device off overnight (with re-emergence of OT that limited standing or walking at this time) and back on in the morning. She reported mild postural arm tremor, which resolved after a minor increase in voltage bilaterally.

OUTCOME

A repeat surface EMG was performed at the 1-year annual visit. This showed a stable 16-Hz

TABLE 3.1. DEEP BRAIN STIMULATION THRESHOLDS

Side	Electrode	PW (μsec)	Frequency (Hz)	Amplitude (V)	Therapeutic Effects	Adverse Effects
Left	+C –0	60	130	0.5 V max		0.7 V tingling in hand
Left	+C –1	60	130	1.2 V max		1.2 V tongue numbness
Left	+C –2	60	130	2.0 V max	1.0 V tolerated standing for 45 sec	1.1 V facial tightness, 1.7 slurred speech, right head tight
Left	+C –3	60	130	3.0 V max		2.5 V slurred speech, 2.1 V neck tightness
Right	+C –8	60	130	1.5 V max		0.7 V transient tingling in fingers, 1.5 V whole arm tingling and tongue numbness but fading in face
Right	+C –9	60	130	1.3 V max		1.0 V hand tingling, 1.3 V facial numbness, slurred speech, 1.2 V facial numbness gone
Right	+C –10	60	130	2.0 V max	1.50 V tolerated standing for 45 secs	1.4 hand discomfort, 2.0 V pain, numbness, tingling in whole arm and face
Right	+C –11	60	130	2.8 V max		2.3 V tingling in thigh, 2.9 V transient thigh tightness, 3.0 V whole left side pulling and "nervous feeling"

TABLE 3.2. DEEP BRAIN STIMULATION PROGRAMMING PARAMETERS

Programming Session	Left Contacts	Right Contacts
1 (2 wk postoperative)	C+, 2–, 60 PW, 130 Hz, 1.00 V	C+, 10–, 60 PW, 130 Hz, 1.50 V
2 (1-yr visit)	C+, 2–, 60 PW, 130 Hz, 1.50 V	C+, 10–, 60 PW, 130 Hz, 2.00 V
3 (2-yr visit)	C+, 2–, 60 PW, 130 Hz, 1.50 V	C+, 10–, 60 PW, 130 Hz, 2.00 V
4 (3-yr visit)	C+, 2–, 60 PW, 130 Hz, 1.60 V	C+, 10–, 60 PW, 130 Hz, 2.10 V

PW = pulse width; V = voltage.

OT with the stimulator turned off, and with the stimulator turned on there was a more gradual onset of tremor with lower amplitude, providing some evidence of objective improvement of OT with DBS. After programming adjustments at the last visit 3 years after surgery, the patient could stand for up to 15 minutes with minimal visible tremor of the lower limbs. There was no postural or kinetic arm tremor, and speech and gait were reported as normal.

DISCUSSION

This case illustrates the benefit of Vim thalamic DBS for medication-refractory and disabling OT. OT is an uncommon tremor disorder, typically observed in elderly females. The most efficacious medication reported is clonazepam, but benefit can be limited by side effects or tremor progression.[1] There are a number of case reports documenting improvement of OT following bilateral Vim thalamic DBS.[2] A recent multicenter study collated 17 patients with medication-refractory OT treated with thalamic DBS (all bilateral except one).[3] The latency of symptoms on standing was significantly improved in both the short term (<48 months) and long term (>48 months). There was a 21.6% improvement in activities of daily living scores, although this lessened to 12.5% in a subgroup of patients with available long-term follow-up. Three patients obtained no or minimal benefit from the procedure, of which one had unilateral DBS, suggesting that bilateral stimulation may be required for symptomatic relief. Overall, DBS was safe and well-tolerated. The pathophysiologic underpinning for OT is believed to be centrally generated, although the exact location of the oscillator is unknown. It is thought to lie within the cerebellothalamocortical network, based on tremor improvement with Vim thalamic DBS (similar to other tremors), functional neuroimaging, and electrophysiology.[2,4,5] However, a spinal cord generator has also been hypothesized. Spinal cord stimulation for medication-refractory OT has been reported in a small number of cases, with sustained long-term benefit.[6] In future, head-to-head studies of deep brain versus spinal cord stimulation would be helpful to compare risk and benefit outcomes, as would functional imaging studies of larger numbers of subjects to define whether there is a better target and optimal programming parameters. In the meantime, the greatest experience reported is for thalamic DBS, which appears to be safe and well-tolerated in selected patients.

PEARLS

- Consider bilateral thalamic Vim DBS for medication-refractory OT.
- Although this case had long-term benefit, other cases reported in the literature have not had similar benefits. Mild to modest benefit has generated discussion as to where the central tremor oscillator is located and whether other brain or spinal cord targets may also provide relief.

REFERENCES

1. Hassan A, Ahlskog JE, Matsumoto JY, Milber JM, Bower JH, Wilkinson JR. Orthostatic tremor: clinical, electrophysiologic, and treatment findings in 184 patients. Neurology 2016;86:458–464.
2. Hassan A, van Gerpen JA. Orthostatic tremor and orthostatic myoclonus: weight-bearing hyperkinetic disorders. A systematic review, new insights, and unresolved questions. Tremor Other Hyperkinet Mov (NY) 2016;6:417.
3. Merola A, Fasano A, Hassan A, et al. Thalamic deep brain stimulation for orthostatic tremor: a multicenter international registry. Mov Disord 2017;32:1240–1244.
4. Gallea C, Popa T, Garcia-Lorenzo D, et al. Orthostatic tremor: a cerebellar pathology? Brain 2016;139:2182–2197.
5. Espay AJ, Duker AP, Chen R, et al. Deep brain stimulation of the ventral intermediate nucleus of the thalamus in medically refractory orthostatic tremor: preliminary observations. Mov Disord 2008;23:2357–2362.
6. Blahak C, Sauer T, Baezner H, et al. Long-term follow-up of chronic spinal cord stimulation for medically intractable orthostatic tremor. J Neurol 2016;263:2224–2228.

Case 4

Bilateral Ventral Intermediate Thalamic Deep Brain Stimulation for Medication-Refractory Orthostatic Tremor

MITRA AFSHARI, PHILIP A. STARR, AND JILL L. OSTREM

INDICATIONS FOR DEEP BRAIN STIMULATION

Orthostatic tremor, essential tremor

CLINICAL HISTORY AND EXAM

A 61-year-old right-handed woman presented to our institution with a 20-year history of mild bilateral kinetic hand tremor and a 10-year history of progressive gait imbalance on standing. The unsteadiness was relieved with walking. She was diagnosed with essential tremor (ET) and orthostatic tremor (OT). Her hand tremor initially responded to treatment with propranolol, but later worsened despite dose optimization.

On examination, she had mild bilateral, high-frequency, low-amplitude distal hand tremor. She could only stand in place for 50 seconds before developing a feeling of imbalance and a strong desire to sit down. A high-frequency tremor was also palpable in the anterior thighs. There was no evidence of head or voice tremor, cerebellar ataxia, parkinsonism, peripheral neuropathy, or muscle weakness. Brain magnetic resonance imaging (MRI) was unremarkable. Surface electromyogram (EMG) revealed a 14-Hz tremor in the legs and lumbar paraspinal muscles that was present only on standing. There was also a 7-Hz bilateral postural tremor in the arms.

COMPLICATIONS

While her ET was not terribly disabling, the patient's OT resulted in falls and interfered with many activities of daily living, including grooming, grocery shopping, preparing meals, and working as a caregiver. Medication trials to treat the OT with clonazepam, gabapentin, pramipexole, and levetiracetam either were ineffective or resulted in side effects.

TROUBLESHOOTING AND MANAGEMENT

After a detailed discussion with the patient about treatment options, multidisciplinary care coordination, and a review of the literature on surgical treatment of OT, the patient was evaluated for deep brain stimulation (DBS). She consented to simultaneous implantation of bilateral ventral intermediate (Vim) thalamic DBS leads (Medtronic 3387) with the goal of primarily treating the OT but also with expected benefit for the ET. The morning of the operation, the patient underwent repeat surface EMG recordings, which confirmed leg tremors of 15-Hz. In the axial plane, targets for the leads were 10.5 to 11 mm lateral to the ipsilateral border of the third ventricle and 6 to 6.5 mm anterior to the posterior commissure at the level of the anterior commissure–posterior plane. The targets were also 0.5 to 1 mm lateral to the typical target for ET to promote proximity to the lower extremity territory. The patient was awakened from sedation before inserting one of the DBS electrodes to its final target and asked to reproduce her leg tremor by pressing her foot against a foot board in a variety of different positions. EMG was able to record some bursts of 15- to 20-Hz activity, and the DBS lead was passed to the target. Of note, tremor improved with different foot positions after lead insertion, suggesting a potential microlesioning effect. Brain MRI was obtained on postoperative day 1, showing accurate lead placement without hemorrhage or edema, and the patient was discharged on postoperative day 2.

OUTCOME

During DBS programming, a benefit in standing time was seen immediately, and the patient experienced increasing benefit in standing over time. Following stable stimulation settings for 1 week, standing time improved from 2.5 to 5 minutes as measured after the first 30-day period without changes in DBS parameters. At 16 months, her postoperative standing time improved from her baseline of 50 seconds to 15 minutes. Her postoperative EMG showed the same leg and paraspinal muscle preoperative tremor frequency of 14-Hz; however, there was a delay in tremor onset, lower EMG amplitude, and periods of EMG quiescence. Her final stimulation parameters were: left hemisphere, 1+ 2−, 3 V, 60 µsec, 140 Hz; right hemisphere: 9+ 10−, 2.6 V, 60 µsec, 140 Hz. The patient's arm tremor also improved, and she was able to return to independently performing her activities of daily living.

DISCUSSION

OT is a rare and disabling disorder characterized by 13- to 18-Hz leg tremor during isometric muscle contraction, causing instability on standing that improves with sitting and ambulation. The first-line pharmacotherapy of OT includes GABAergic medications like benzodiazepines, including clonazepam, and more recently, gabapentin, often at high doses that may cause side effects and with waning benefit.[1,2] OT and ET have been thought to lie on the same spectrum of disease, and it has been suggested that the presence of arm tremor is a positive prognosticator for successful DBS surgery for OT.[2] It has been reported that the frequency of the arm tremor in these patients is likely a subharmonic of the leg tremor frequency.[2]

This case adds to the evidence that bilateral Vim DBS can be used to successfully treat OT. There are now several published cases in which bilateral Vim DBS, historically the preferred DBS target for ET, improved the latency of tremor onset and activities of daily living in OT.[3-5] It has also been hypothesized that in the setting of OT, Vim DBS therapy can potentially be optimized with more precise targeting according to the somatotopic arrangement of the lower extremity thalamic fibers.[6,7]

There are no validated scales for assessing OT-related severity or disability, and currently the best outcome measure is standing time. Therefore, this case also illustrates that objective measures like preoperative and postoperative EMG are potentially an effective way to measure success of surgery in the current absence of other objective scales. Of note, the EMG results conflict with the hypothesis that a single central tremor generator underpins OT because Vim DBS often delays the onset and reduces tremor amplitude but does not abolish tremor completely nor change its frequency.[8,9] Vim DBS may therefore modulate the cerebellothalamocortical loop, but more studies are needed to uncover the pathogenic mechanism of OT in order to reveal more directed therapy.

PEARLS

- OT may lie on the same spectrum of disease as ET, and like ET, refractory cases may benefit from bilateral Vim thalamic DBS.
- Preoperative and postoperative surface EMG of the lower extremities after DBS therapy for OT can provide additional objective measures of benefit, including those of tremor latency, EMG amplitude, and periods of EMG quiescence. Currently, the only objective outcome measure for OT treatment has been *standing time*.

REFERENCES

1. Hassan A, Ahlskog JE, Matsumoto JY, et al. Orthostatic tremor: clinical, electrophysiologic, and treatment findings in 184 patients. *Neurology* 2016;86:458–464.
2. Yaltho TC, Ondo WG. Orthostatic tremor: a review of 45 cases. *Parkinsonism Relat Disord* 2014;20:723–725.
3. Merola A, Fasano A, Hassan A, et al. Thalamic deep brain stimulation for orthostatic tremor: multicenter international registry. *Mov Disord* 2017;32(8):1240–1244.
4. Espay AJ, Duker AP, Chen R, et al. Deep brain stimulation of the ventral intermediate nucleus of the thalamus in medically refractory orthostatic tremor: preliminary observations. *Mov Disord* 2008;23:2357–2362.
5. Guridi J, Rodriguez-Oroz MC, Arbizu J, et al. Successful thalamic deep brain stimulation for orthostatic tremor. *Mov Disord* 2008;23:1808–1811.
6. Lyons MK, Behbahani M, Boucher OK, et al. Orthostatic tremor responds to bilateral thalamic deep brain stimulation. *Tremor Other Hyperkinet Mov* 2012;2012:2.
7. Contarino MF, Bour LJ, Schuurman PR, et al. Thalamic deep brain stimulation for orthostatic tremor: clinical and neurophysiological correlates. *Parkinsonism Relat Disord* 2015;21:1005–1007.
8. Muthuraman M, Hellriegel H, Paschen S, et al. The central oscillatory network of orthostatic tremor. *Mov Disord* 2013;28:1424–1430.
9. Magariños-Ascone C, Ruiz FM, Millán AS, et al. Electrophysiological evaluation of thalamic DBS for orthostatic tremor. *Mov Disord* 2010;25:2476–2477.

Case 5

Rebound Tremor Following a Suboptimally Placed Ventral Intermediate Nucleus Deep Brain Stimulation

PARUL JINDAL AND JOOHI JIMENEZ-SHAHED

INDICATION FOR DEEP BRAIN STIMULATION

Essential tremor refractory to medical management

CLINICAL HISTORY AND RELEVANT EXAM

A 73-year-old woman with medication-refractory essential tremor (ET) underwent bilateral ventral intermediate (Vim) deep brain stimulation (DBS) implantation by an experienced functional neurosurgery team. Intraoperative testing confirmed successful bilateral control of tremor without side effects. The patient did not have dysarthria or gait ataxia related to ET at the time of DBS placement. She did not experience any immediate postoperative complications.

COMPLICATIONS

The right hand tremor responded well to DBS stimulation of the left Vim in a monopolar configuration even at low voltages. Initially, the left hand tremor suppression was also adequate when programmed in monopolar configuration (Table 5.1). However, during subsequent programming sessions, the patient started noticing loss of tremor control in the left hand along with dysarthria and gait ataxia on higher stimulation settings.

During subsequent sessions, the patient was noted to develop high electrode impedance at contact 8 (see Table 5.1), which was present at only low voltage settings. This was a new finding that was not present at previous programming sessions. It was felt that inadequate tremor suppression in the left hand could be related to high impedances because optimal programming generally involved this contact.

TROUBLESHOOTING AND MANAGEMENT

The right Vim electrode was programmed in monopolar, bipolar, and interleaved configurations (see Table 5.1) with the objective of improving tremor control, and the patient was also asked to turn the stimulator off at night. These measures would result in only transient benefit, followed by return of symptoms to their previous severity within days or weeks. During DBS programming, it was noted that when the right Vim was turned off, the patient had marked "rebound" tremor with a rest component in the left hand, which subsided but was followed by prominent left hand postural and kinetic tremor of almost the same severity as her preoperative tremor. The patient would notice this marked rebound tremor every night when she turned off the DBS.

Suspecting a suboptimally placed electrode, a computed tomography scan of the head was ordered to check for electrode placement, which was merged back to the preoperative magnetic resonance image using the StealthStation Surgical Navigation System (Medtronic, Inc.). This showed the right Vim electrode position approximately 2 mm anteromedial from the optimal location. The left Vim was accurately placed. The patient subsequently underwent revision of the right Vim without any complications.

OUTCOME

After surgery, the right Vim electrode remained off for a period of 4 weeks, during which time tremor persisted. After programming, the patient had marked improvement in the left hand tremor at low amplitudes in a monopolar configuration (Table 5.1). She did not have any programming-related gait ataxia or dysarthria. She no longer

TABLE 5.1. RIGHT VENTRAL INTERMEDIATE PROGRAMMING PARAMETERS BEFORE AND AFTER ELECTRODE REVISION

	Polarity	Amplitude (V)	Pulse Width (μsec)	Frequency (Hz)
	BEFORE REVISION			
First programming session	C+ 10–	1.0	60	130
Maximum monopolar settings	C+ 10–	2.2	60	150
Maximum bipolar configuration	9+ 10–	2.5	60	150
Maximum interleaved configuration*	Vim1 C+ 10–	3.0	60	125
	Vim2 C+ 9	2.6	60	125
	AFTER REVISION			
First programming session	C+ 10	2.0	60	130
9 mo	C+ 10	2.8	60	170

*At the time of this electrode configuration, the patient developed a position-dependent open circuit (impedances >40,000 ohm) involving contact 8.
Vim = ventral intermediate.

experienced rebound tremor after turning off the DBS at night. Her DBS parameters were adjusted to maintain tremor benefit without speech or gait side effects.

DISCUSSION

This case illustrates the phenomenon of rebound tremor from a suboptimally placed DBS electrode. Habituation refers to the loss of sustained tremor control over days to weeks after DBS programming and has been demonstrated in up to 73% of individuals with Vim DBS to treat ET.[1] Although there may have been a component of this feature in our patient, the more salient feature was the rebound tremor due to a suboptimally placed lead. Rebound tremor is a temporary increase of tremor intensity over the preoperative state occurring a few seconds after switching off DBS. In our patient, rebound tremor was noted 8 to 9 months after surgery. Rebound tremor can occur both in the short term after DBS surgery and during long-term follow-up, although the time frames are not specifically defined. Some studies suggest that this may happen over a period of 10 weeks as the pathological tremor network seems to adapt to stimulation settings.[2] In a study by Pilitsis and colleagues, clinical outcomes were studied from 31 Vim leads in 27 patients with ET.[3] Loss of efficacy of stimulation, defined as loss of meaningful tremor relief and leads requiring voltages greater than 3.6 V for effective tremor control, was

seen in four patients at a mean follow-up of 39 months. Twenty-two patients continued to have meaningful tremor control with stimulation. The two groups did not have any difference in demographics or disease severity. In patients with loss of efficacy of stimulation during the perioperative stage, suboptimal anteroposterior positioning as evidenced on intraoperative fluoroscopy occurred more frequently ($p = 0.018$), and in these patients, fluoroscopy revealed suboptimal positioning more frequently ($p = 0.0005$). In this study, patients with more laterally placed electrodes tended to have less satisfactory efficacy.[3]

Although short-term worsening has been attributed to a decrease in the microlesioning effect and/or inadequate electrode placement,[2] late-onset worsening and rebound have been attributed to progression of the underlying disease, comorbidities such as demyelinating sensorimotor peripheral neuropathy, or adaptation of the biologic response of the stimulated neuronal network.[4]

In our patient, tremor worsening occurred in the setting of a suboptimally placed lead and was eliminated after lead revision surgery, which resulted in recapture of tremor control. Studies have proposed that suboptimal electrode placement, which increases the distance from dentatorubrothalamic tract (DRTT), may result in worsening of the stimulation effect, suggesting that diffusion tensor imaging (DTI)-based fiber tracking may be a valuable tool to supplement atlas-based targeting.[5] A recent study investigated direct targeting of the DRT fiber tract using DTI,[6] with the authors suggesting that this technology may particularly be helpful in patients with distorted thalamic anatomy and a dilated third ventricle. This approach has advantages over atlas-based targeting.

"DBS holidays," when patients turn off the stimulator for a few days or a week, have been reported to improve the tremor-suppressing effect and reduce DBS-induced side effects compared with chronic stimulation in patients with symptom worsening.[7,8] This strategy did not work

with our patient, who experienced persistent tremor during the few weeks when the right Vim electrode remained off after revision. However, revision of the suboptimally placed electrode eliminated tremor worsening, tremor rebound, and programming-related side effects. Potential habituation and rebound should be carefully assessed before action is taken because disease progression and suboptimal lead placement may be major factors in many patients with worsening tremor following DBS.[9] Further definition of habituation and tolerance in the literature needs to be undertaken.

PEARLS

- If a patient reports loss of tremor suppression benefit within days to weeks of DBS adjustments, consider that worsening may be due to a suboptimal lead placement.
- Tremor rebound (worsening tremor after stimulation is turned off) may occur and could also be due to suboptimally placed DBS leads. Appropriate brain imaging, as well as thresholds for programming, will usually reveal the issue.
- Turning DBS off at night may be helpful in some patients but may also be intolerable because of the rebound effect.
- Disease progression may account for many cases of apparent "tolerance" or "habituation," and the diagnostic possibilities should be carefully assessed before action is taken.

REFERENCES

1. Shih LC, LaFaver K, Lim C, Papavassiliou E, Tarsy D. (2013). Loss of benefit in VIM thalamic deep brain stimulation (DBS) for essential tremor: how prevalent is it? Parkinsonism & Related Disorders, 19(7), 676–679.
2. Barbe MT, Liebhart L, Runge M, Pauls KAM, Wojtecki L, Schnitzler A, Timmermann L. (2011). Deep brain stimulation in the nucleus ventralis intermedius in patients with essential tremor: habituation of tremor suppression. Journal of Neurology, 258(3), 434–439. https://doi.org/10.1007/s00415-010-5773-3
3. Pilitsis JG, Metman LV, Toleikis, JR, Hughes LE, Sani SB, Bakay RAE. (2008). Factors involved in long-term efficacy of deep brain stimulation of the thalamus for essential tremor. Journal of Neurosurgery, 109(4), 640–646. https://doi.org/10.3171/JNS/2008/109/10/0640
4. Patel N, Ondo W, Jimenez-Shahed, J. (2014). Habituation and rebound to thalamic deep brain stimulation in long-term management of tremor associated with demyelinating neuropathy. International Journal of Neuroscience, 124(12), 919–925. https://doi.org/10.3109/00207454.2014.895345
5. Anthofer JM, Steib K, Lange M, Rothenfusser E, Fellner C, Brawanski A, Schlaier J. (2017). Distance between active electrode contacts and dentatorubrothalamic tract in patients with habituation of stimulation effect of deep brain stimulation in essential tremor. Journal of Neurological Surgery. Part A, Central European Neurosurgery, 78(4), 350–357. https://doi.org/10.1055/s-0036-1597894
6. Fenoy AJ, Schiess MC. (2017). Deep brain stimulation of the dentato-rubro-thalamic tract: outcomes of direct targeting for tremor. Neuromodulation: Journal of the International Neuromodulation Society, 20(5), 429–436. https://doi.org/10.1111/ner.12585
7. Garcia Ruiz P, Muniz de Igneson J, Lopez Ferro O, Martin C, Magarinos Ascone C. (2001). Deep brain stimulation holidays in essential tremor. Journal of Neurology, 248(8), 725–726.
8. Kronenbuerger M, Fromm C, Block F, Coenen VA, Rohde I, Rohde V, Noth J. (2006). On-demand

deep brain stimulation for essential tremor: a report on four cases. Movement Disorders, 21(3), 401–405. doi:10.1002/mds.20714

9. Favilla CG, Ullman D, Wagle Shukla A, Foote KD, Jacobson CE, Okun MS. (2012). Worsening essential tremor following deep brain stimulation: disease progression versus tolerance. Brain, 135(Pt 5), 1455–1462. doi:10.1093/brain/aws026

Case 6

Symptomatic Cystic Lesion Following Deep Brain Stimulation Surgery

VIBHASH D. SHARMA AND SHILPA CHITNIS

INDICATION FOR DEEP BRAIN STIMULATION
Essential tremor

CLINICAL HISTORY AND RELEVANT EXAM
A 71-year-old left-handed man with a history of essential tremor for 16 years was evaluated for deep brain stimulation (DBS) surgery. He had progressive bilateral hand tremors, first noticed in the left hand. Over time, his tremor worsened and significantly interfered with activities of daily living. His tremor response was inadequate to multiple medications, including propranolol 160 mg three times per day, primidone 250 mg three times per day, and gabapentin 300 mg three times per day. Brain magnetic resonance imaging (MRI), neuropsychological, and psychiatric evaluations were all normal. After an interdisciplinary DBS evaluation, he was considered an excellent candidate for DBS surgery. He underwent bilateral thalamic ventral intermediate (Vim) nucleus implantation with intraoperative microelectrode recording (MER) to enhance targeting. Three simultaneous MER tracks were used on both sides of the brain. There were no intraoperative complications. A postoperative head computed tomography (CT) scan confirmed appropriate placement of leads without any acute complications. He had mild, transient dysarthria and gait imbalance 12 hours after surgery; however, these symptoms resolved within 24 hours. At the time of discharge, his neurologic exam was normal. When seen for initial DBS programming 3 weeks after implantation, he reported no new symptoms. There was complete suppression of tremor with DBS stimulation without any side effects with parameters.

COMPLICATIONS
Six weeks after DBS surgery, the patient presented to the emergency department with new onset of dysarthria, left arm weakness, and gait difficulty. He was afebrile, and his mental status was normal, but his neurologic examination showed left-sided hemiparesis, left arm ataxia, and mild gait ataxia. There was no tremor in the left hand and only a mild tremor in the right hand. A CT scan of head revealed a new hypodense area in the right thalamocapsular region, with mass effect on the right ventricle. His right stimulator was turned off without re-emergence of left-hand tremor.

TROUBLESHOOTING AND MANAGEMENT
The patient was admitted to the hospital for an evaluation. His right DBS stimulator was turned off. His initial laboratory studies, including complete blood count, C-reactive protein, and basic metabolic profile, were unremarkable. MRI of the brain revealed a cystic lesion (1.8 × 1.6 cm) located at the distal tip of the right DBS lead, which was hypointense on T1-weighted and hyperintense on T2-weighted images. There was increased fluid-attenuated inversion recovery (FLAIR) signal surrounding the cystic lesion (Figure 6.1A) and no restricted diffusion or contrast enhancement (Figure 6.1B–D).Based on the imaging findings, stroke and hemorrhage were ruled out, and a diagnosis of cystic lesion was made. Because the suspicion for infection was very low, the patient was not treated with antibiotics. Although steroids could have been given, owing to the limited literature on treatment of cystic lesions with steroids, we opted to manage the patient conservatively. He underwent physical therapy, and his neurologic symptoms improved gradually over a few days. A repeat brain CT scan before the

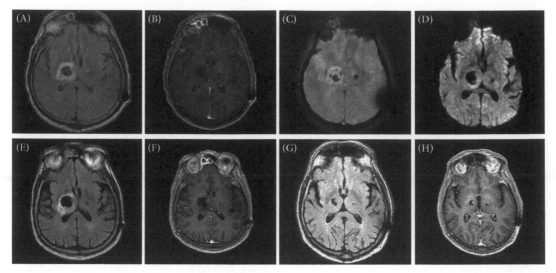

FIGURE 6.1. Brain magnetic resonance imaging (MRI) showing a cystic lesion with surrounding edema on a fluid-attenuated inversion recovery (FLAIR) image (A), no contrast enhancement on T1 (B), susceptibility-weighted imaging (SWI) (C), and diffusion-weighted imaging with no restricted diffusion (D). Follow-up MRI studies at 2 weeks showing enlargement (E and F) and at 6 months after lead removal showing involution of cyst (G and H).

discharge showed no change in the lesion. He was discharged home with a follow-up appointment in the neurology movement disorder clinic. Two weeks after discharge, he continued to have mild gait difficulty and left foot weakness. The tremor in his left hand remained suppressed even in the off-stimulation state. Repeat brain MRI was performed to follow up on the cystic lesion because patient had residual symptoms. The follow-up imaging revealed enlargement of the cystic lesion (2.2 × 2.8 cm) without restricted diffusion or contrast enhancement. Because of persistent gait difficulty and enlargement of the cyst, it was decided to explant the right DBS lead. He underwent successful removal of right thalamic lead. Repeat MRI 6 months after his admission to the hospital showed marked reduction in size of the cyst (0.1 × 0.4 cm) with resolution of the increased FLAIR signal.

OUTCOME

The patient's gait difficulty improved over time. He had slight re-emergence of left hand tremor but continued to have reasonable function in his hand.

DISCUSSION

Although DBS surgery is considered reasonably safe, complications related to the surgical procedure or implanted hardware can occur. Most

severe adverse events are reported immediately following the surgical procedure. Hemorrhage or infarct has an estimated risk of about 1 to 3%.[1,2] Common hardware-related complications include infection, lead fracture, lead migration or misplacement, and skin erosion.[2,3] In some cases, delayed symptomatic intraparenchymal edema around the DBS lead has been described.[4,5]

In this case, the patient presented with new symptoms several weeks after surgery that were initially concerning for acute infarct or hemorrhage. Initial head CT showed a hypodense region around the DBS lead with mass effect warranting further evaluation with brain MRI, which revealed a cystic lesion at the tip of the DBS lead. Suspicion for central nervous system infection was low because of absence of constitutional symptoms, an intact mental status, and normal laboratory investigations. Lack of MRI contrast enhancement or restricted diffusion argued against a brain abscess. Radiographic signal within the lesion suggested a fluid-filled cavity consistent with noninfectious structural cyst formation.

Cyst formation around an implanted DBS lead has been reported as a rare complication of DBS surgery.[6–9] Patients can have mild or even absence of symptoms. Patients can present with neurologic deficits several weeks to months after DBS lead implantation.[6–9] Cyst formation can occur at the tip or along the length of DBS electrode. Although the reason for cyst formation is not clear, cerebrospinal fluid tracking along the lead or an autoimmune/inflammatory reaction to the lead that may have failed to spontaneously resolve have been suggested as potential mechanisms.[6–8] No specific risk factors for cyst development following DBS surgery have been identified. In a previously reported case, cyst formation was preceded by peri-lead edema, but it is not clear whether postoperative peri-lead edema increases the risk for the formation of a cyst.[8] Management

of the cystic lesion should be guided by the patient's symptoms and results of serial imaging. A patient with no symptoms can be managed conservatively with observation or a short course of steroid therapy after excluding an infectious process. As in our case, removal of the DBS lead should be considered when the patient has symptoms or if there is cystic enlargement on serial imaging. In previously reported cases, removal of the DBS lead in symptomatic patients led to complete resolution of the cyst and improvement in symptoms.

PEARLS

- High index of suspicion after DBS of an evolving issue should prompt imaging.
- Proper programming management is unknown in cyst cases, but most experts turn the device off during the workup. It is possible in some cases that the cyst can be watched and the patient programmed for added benefit.
- Recognition of benign noninfectious cyst versus infection, stroke, or hemorrhage should be based on radiographic characteristics—and this may help to avoid additional tests and antimicrobial therapy.
- Explanation has been suggested as a potential treatment if the cyst is enlarging or symptoms fail to resolve over time.
- Cystic lesion can lead to inadvertent suppression of the tremor (a permanent microlesion effect); in these cases, reimplantation may not be needed, and patients can be reassessed after reoccurrence of tremor.

REFERENCES

1. Fenoy AJ, Simpson RK Jr. Risks of common complications in deep brain stimulation surgery: management and avoidance. *Journal of neurosurgery.* Jan 2014;120(1):132–139.
2. Bronstein JM, Tagliati M, Alterman RL, et al. Deep brain stimulation for Parkinson disease: an expert consensus and review of key issues. *Archives of neurology.* Feb 2011;68(2):165.
3. Fernandez-Pajarin G, Sesar A, Ares B, et al. Delayed complications of deep brain stimulation: 16-year experience in 249 patients. *Acta neurochirurgica.* Jun 24 2017.
4. Deogaonkar M, Nazzaro JM, Machado A, Rezai A. Transient, symptomatic, post-operative, non-infectious hypodensity around the deep brain stimulation (DBS) electrode. *Journal of clinical neuroscience: official journal of the Neurosurgical Society of Australasia.* Jul 2011;18(7):910–915.
5. Lefaucheur R, Derrey S, Borden A, et al. Postoperative edema surrounding the electrode: an

unusual complication of deep brain stimulation. *Brain stimulation.* May 2013;6(3):459–460.
6. Ramirez-Zamora A, Levine D, Sommer DB, Dalfino J, Novak P, Pilitsis JG. Intraparenchymal cyst development after deep brain stimulator placement. *Stereotactic and functional neurosurgery.* 2013;91(5):338–341.
7. Sharma VD, Bona AR, Mantovani A, et al. Cystic lesions as a rare complication of deep brain stimulation. *Movement disorders clinical practice.* 2016;3(1):87–90.
8. Jagid J, Madhavan K, Bregy A, et al. Deep brain stimulation complicated by bilateral large cystic cavitation around the leads in a patient with Parkinson's disease. *BMJ case reports.* Oct 16 2015;2015.
9. Katlowitz K, Pourfar MH, Israel Z, Mogilner AY. Intraparenchymal cysts following deep brain stimulation: variable presentations and clinical courses. *Operative neurosurgery (Hagerstown, Md.).* Oct 01 2017;13(5):576–580.

SECTION 3

Parkinson Disease

Case 7

Patient Selection Criteria for Deep Brain Stimulation for Parkinson Disease

LAURA S. SURILLO DAHDAH, PADRAIG O'SUILLEABHAIN,
HRISHIKESH DADHICH, MAZEN ELKURD, SHILPA CHITNIS,
AND RICHARD B. DEWEY, JR.

CANDIDATE SCREENING AND SELECTION

Potential deep brain stimulation (DBS) candidates should be referred to experienced DBS centers for a complete multidisciplinary screening evaluation. Successful outcomes from surgery usually require a multidisciplinary team approach involving neurologists specializing in movement disorders, stereotactic or functionally trained neurosurgeons, neuropsychologists, psychiatrists, and speech, occupational, and physical therapists.[1] Social workers and nutritionists, as well as financial counselors, can be useful. All surgical candidates should ideally undergo brain magnetic resonance imaging (MRI) as well as neuropsychological testing to screen for cognitive and mood issues (within 1 year of DBS surgery). Scoring of patients using a validated motor scale such as the Movement Disorder Society—Unified Parkinson's Disease Rating Scale (MDS-UPDRS) in both the off and on levodopa conditions should be performed and the difference between the *on* and *off* state motor scores calculated because this will provide important predictor information (minus tremor). UPDRS on/off dopaminergic motor scales do not, however, capture on–off fluctuations, which are important potential benefits from DBS surgery. All data collected should be discussed in a multidisciplinary meeting attended by all members of the DBS program team. Generally, the most suitable candidates have few or no medical comorbidities, few or no cognitive deficits, and no disabling behavioral, thought, or mood disorders. Because DBS may sometimes address intolerable medication-related side effects that preclude optimization of medications for effective treatment of motor symptoms,[2] an ideal candidate for DBS may be a patient who is younger, cognitively intact with fluctuating motor symptoms (wearing off, *on–off*, and/or dyskinesia), yet also known to be high-functioning in the *on* dopaminergic state. It is important to note, however, that there is no specific age cutoff for DBS, nor is there a standard optimal patient. It is important that all members of a multidisciplinary team evaluate the patient and construct a comprehensive risk-to-benefit ratio for each potential candidate.

DIAGNOSIS OF IDIOPATHIC PARKINSON DISEASE

Candidates for PD DBS should have a diagnosis of idiopathic Parkinson disease (iPD). Clinically probable PD is diagnosed when a patient meets the UK Brain Bank or MDS criteria.[3] Imaging with dopamine transporter scan (DaTscan) may be only occasionally necessary for select cases to differentiate iPD from neuroleptic-induced parkinsonism, essential tremor, or psychogenic parkinsonism.

The expert neurologist should be reasonably certain that the diagnosis is correct because atypical or other parkinsonian syndromes have revealed generally unfavorable outcomes from DBS.[4-6] Atypical forms of parkinsonism that are exclusionary for DBS surgery include multiple-system atrophy, progressive supranuclear palsy, cortical or diffuse Lewy body disease, corticobasal syndrome, vascular parkinsonism, normal-pressure hydrocephalus, neuroleptic-induced parkinsonism, and age-related parkinsonism. Red flags suggestive of one of these exclusionary conditions may include early falls, nonresponsiveness to levodopa (except tremor), vertical gaze palsy, slowing of vertical saccades, early or severe autonomic dysfunction, and early cognitive impairment. Many centers will follow patients for 5 years after PD diagnosis to reduce the risk for conversion to atypical syndromes.[7]

MOTOR SYMPTOMS RESPONDING TO DEEP BRAIN STIMULATION

Improvement of disabling or troublesome motor symptoms, which include motor fluctuations or dyskinesias, despite optimized pharmacologic treatment, is the primary reason to pursue DBS surgery. The symptoms that improve with levodopa are generally the symptoms that improve with DBS, which include tremor, rigidity, and bradykinesia.[4,8,9] While DBS would not ordinarily be offered for levodopa-resistant symptoms, resting tremor is an exception to this rule and generally responds well to DBS even when it is levodopa-refractory.[4,10] Symptoms that do not usually respond to DBS, and for which DBS surgery is therefore not indicated, include speech difficulty, postural instability, gait impairment, balance problems, and freezing of gait (especially freezing of gait in the *on* state).[4,11,12] These symptoms may improve in patients for whom the symptoms are levodopa-responsive and occasionally respond in other patients, but the improvement is difficult to predict.[8] The objective of DBS surgery is to provide the patient a more sustainable "best *on* state" by decreasing *off* periods and troublesome dyskinesias, and these symptoms are not addressed by on–off motor UPDRS testing.

DEMONSTRATION OF A ROBUST LEVODOPA RESPONSE

Patients undergoing evaluation for DBS should undergo a dopaminergic *off–on* motor examination.[9] This challenge test is accomplished by performing the MDS-UPDRS Part III scale 12 hours after the last dose of short-acting levodopa formulations and at least 24 hours after longer acting medications.[13] Subjects should then be administered their usual dose, or a supratherapeutic dose (i.e., 1.5×) in those without obvious and robust on motor response to their usual doses, of PD medications and then examined after a "best *on*" dopaminergic state develops. It is highly recommended that the examiner video-record both the *off* and *on*

state examinations for review by DBS team members at the multidisciplinary meeting. Another important use of video recordings is a historical record of the best *on* dopaminergic state for postoperative review, if necessary, by the patient or the examiner to ensure DBS treatment has been optimized. A patient is deemed to be levodopa responsive when exhibiting more than 30% improvement in the MDS-UPDRS Part III score in the *on* versus *off* states (excluding tremor scores in cases of levodopa nonresponsive tremor). For patients who meet other inclusion criteria, the magnitude of the difference between *off* and *on* scores is a predictor of success with surgery (the greater the *on–off* difference, the greater the expected benefit from DBS surgery); however, one does not always require a 30% on–off improvement threshold to proceed to DBS surgery.[13] Most important, *on–off* testing does not capture motor fluctuations and dyskinesia, which robustly respond to DBS.

RISKS AND EXPECTATIONS OF DEEP BRAIN STIMULATION

Patients and families must have a clear understanding of both the risks and benefits of DBS. They must have well-formed goals for DBS for the patient, and they must appreciate that DBS is not a cure. Their expectations must be in line with what DBS is capable of achieving, and this issue must be discussed thoroughly before making a final decision about whether to proceed with surgery. Unrealistic expectations in patients or family members can constitute common reasons for DBS failures.[14,15] It is sometimes useful to have patients write out their expectations preoperatively and to discuss them with their physician. Risks inherent to DBS surgery include infection (in the leads or implantable pulse generator [IPG]), bleeding in the brain or subcutaneous tissue, worsening of speech, decline in cognition, and exacerbation of preexisting mood or gait/motor problems.[12,16] Most surgeons will quote a risk for serious adverse events in the 1 to 5% range, although this rate may differ among surgeons and among institutions. Patients should also be counseled that DBS surgery requires a recovery period of several days to weeks after surgery, and that benefits from the procedure may only be realized after many programming sessions. Depending on the patient's response to stimulation, DBS programming visits typically occur four to eight times in the first 6 months after surgery, followed by subsequent sessions every 3 to 6 months thereafter. Challenges with travel or transportation should be discussed in advance. It should also be emphasized in preoperative counseling sessions that reduction or elimination of PD medications is not the primary goal of DBS, although depending on the chosen target and on other factors, this may be accomplished for some individuals.[15,17] In general, the subthalamic nucleus (STN) target is associated with more medication reduction than the globus pallidus internus (GPi) target, and in general bilateral STN is associated with more medication reduction than GPi DBS.[18] However, the GPi target has been shown to be superior in suppressing dyskinesia and in allowing long-term flexibility in the use of dopaminergic therapies. In some cases, for example, STN DBS may exacerbate dyskinesia and make long-term medication management more challenging.

MEDICAL COMORBIDITIES AND DEEP BRAIN STIMULATION

There are no universally agreed-on inclusion or exclusion criteria for the selection of DBS candidates, although larger expert DBS centers agree that a multidisciplinary approach is the safest and can enhance outcomes.[19,20] Certain medical comorbidities may create a relative or absolute contraindication to DBS surgery. Accordingly, medical clearance for the procedure should be routinely obtained before deciding on surgery. Medical comorbidities must be evaluated especially if considering awake versus asleep DBS, and when deciding on whether to employ microelectrode recording (MER). Awake surgery is more favorable if the patient's participation is required (e.g., examination in the operating room). Cardiac, pulmonary, and other conditions such as obesity may increase surgical risk. Patients with hypertension are at an increased risk for hemorrhage during microelectrode recording, and this comorbidity should be managed aggressively before and during the procedure.[21,22] The existence of comorbid diabetes or immunosuppression increases the operative risk for infection and other complications following the DBS surgical procedure. Healthy and cooperative patients are required for a successful awake surgery. There is no specific age above which DBS is contraindicated, although all things being equal, younger patients tend to tolerate DBS surgery better than older patients. Older patients in general have a higher risk for surgical complications compared with younger patients. For example, in one study, patients older than 69 years had an increased risk for adverse cognitive events such as postoperative confusion and cognitive deterioration.[23] The risk-to-benefit ratio should consider age as only one factor in potential DBS outcome.

PSYCHIATRIC ILLNESS AND DEEP BRAIN STIMULATION

Psychiatric comorbidities should be aggressively screened, identified, and treated. These comorbidities have the strong potential to limit the success of DBS therapy.[24] Typically, the screening is performed as part of a battery of neuropsychologic tests done preoperatively, but in complex cases, formal psychiatric consultation and stabilization should ideally occur earlier in the process. Uncontrolled anxiety, depression, impulse control disorders, psychosis, suicidal ideation, and mania may worsen after surgery, particularly when the STN target is chosen.[25,26] Only patients with stable and fully optimized psychiatric disease (depression, anxiety, bipolar disorder, others) should undergo DBS surgery. Impulse control disorders are common in a subset of DBS candidates, and these should be stabilized preoperatively. Uncontrolled impulse control disorders may be a risk factor for postoperative suicide.[27] Impulse control issues may also emerge de novo after DBS, and therefore a postoperative monitoring plan should be employed. Additionally, other psychiatric problems may occur de novo after DBS surgery, even without previous psychiatric history.[28] A wide variety of psychiatric complications have been observed after DBS, including mania, depression, euphoria, irritability, emotional lability, anger, impulsivity, and apathy.[23,26,29]

DEMENTIA

As part of the evaluation of DBS candidacy, neuropsychological testing must be performed and thoughtfully reviewed by the multidisciplinary team. Patients with suboptimal neuropsychological performance, especially in frontal lobe and memory domains, may not be ideal candidates because of the high risk for worsening cognitive function with DBS surgery.[23,30] Medications can also confound the performance on neuropsychological measures, so test administrators should be cognizant of both the disease state (*off* vs.

on) during testing and the potential deleterious effects of medications the patient may be taking such as benzodiazepines or anticonvulsants.[31]

Neuropsychological status is only one area to be considered in constructing a risk-to-benefit profile, and in some cases, DBS may be required for palliation (e.g., can't sit in a chair because of dyskinesia, caregiver burden managing activities of daily living) despite a higher than optimal risk for neuropsychiatric deterioration.

ABNORMAL PREOPERATIVE MAGNETIC RESONANCE IMAGING

Performing brain MRI or reviewing a recent imaging study during the evaluation of a patient's candidacy for DBS can be important not only for confirmation of a treatable diagnosis but also for the assessment of potential surgical risk. Extensive white matter changes may indicate vascular PD or another reason for gait issues, which may, for example, have a suboptimal response to DBS. In addition, patients with major vascular diseases may be at increased risk for brain hemorrhage or stroke. Global cerebral atrophy may increase the risk for subdural hematoma. Preoperative MRI can be useful in some cases for planning the target for lead implantation. Structural lesions such as vascular malformations along the track of lead implantation may be important to identify.[32] Finally, preoperative MRI with contrast enhancement can help to identify blood vessels and particularly venous anatomy, which may be useful in avoiding venous infarction from an unsafe trajectory.[33]

CONCLUSION

The most important aspect of PD DBS surgery is the use of an expert and experienced multidisciplinary team who can construct a risk-to-benefit ratio and also address expectations before and after surgery. It may be useful to put risks and benefits of DBS into context with other interventions, which may include duodenal levodopa gel infusion and high-frequency focused ultrasound treatment. Usually, the primary treating neurologist is in the best position to integrate all considerations, to communicate between the interdisciplinary team and the patient, and also to communicate with family. The input and opinions of the other members of the team provide valuable guidance to the treating neurologist because each discipline can enhance outcomes.

PEARLS

- Candidates for PD DBS should have a diagnosis of iPD.
- Many centers will follow patients for 5 years following PD diagnosis to reduce the risk for conversion to atypical syndromes.
- Potential DBS candidates should be referred to experienced DBS centers for a complete multidisciplinary screening evaluation.
- All surgical candidates should ideally undergo brain MRI as well as neuropsychological testing to screen for cognitive and mood issues (within 1 year of DBS surgery).
- Scoring of patients using a validated motor scale such as the MDS-UPDRS in both the off and on levodopa conditions should be performed and the difference between the *on* and *off* state motor scores calculated because this will provide important predictor information (minus tremor).
- Improvement of disabling or troublesome motor symptoms, which include motor fluctuations or dyskinesias, despite optimized pharmacologic treatment, is the primary reason to pursue DBS surgery.
- The symptoms that improve with levodopa are generally the symptoms that improve with DBS, which include tremor, rigidity, and bradykinesia.
- While DBS would not ordinarily be offered for levodopa-resistant symptoms, resting tremor is an exception to this rule and generally responds well to DBS even when it is levodopa-refractory.

- Risks inherent to DBS surgery include infection (in the leads or IPG), bleeding in the brain or subcutaneous tissue, worsening of speech, decline in cognition, and exacerbation of preexisting mood or gait/motor problems.
- Certain medical comorbidities may create a relative or absolute contraindication to DBS surgery. Accordingly, medical clearance for the procedure should be routinely obtained before deciding on surgery.
- Psychiatric comorbidities should be aggressively screened, identified, and treated. These comorbidities have the strong potential to limit the success of DBS therapy.
- Patients with suboptimal neuropsychological performance, especially in frontal lobe and memory domains, may not be ideal candidates because of the high risk for worsening cognitive function with DBS surgery.
- Patients and families must have a clear understanding of both the risk and benefits of DBS. They must have well-formed goals for DBS for the patient, and they must appreciate that DBS is not a cure.

REFERENCES

1. Stewart, R. M., Desaloms, J. M., & Sanghera, M. K. (2005). Stimulation of the subthalamic nucleus for the treatment of Parkinson's disease: postoperative management, programming, and rehabilitation. *Journal of Neuroscience Nursing: Journal of the American Association of Neuroscience Nurses*, 37(2), 108–114.

2. Deuschl, G., Schade-Brittinger, C., Krack, P., Volkmann, J., Schäfer, H., Bötzel, K., & German Parkinson Study Group, Neurostimulation Section. (2006). A randomized trial of deep-brain stimulation for Parkinson's disease. *New England Journal of Medicine*, 355(9), 896–908.

3. Postuma, R. B., Berg, D., Stern, M., Poewe, W., Olanow, C. W., Oertel, W., & Deuschl, G. (2015). MDS clinical diagnostic criteria for Parkinson's disease. *Movement Disorders: Official Journal of the Movement Disorder Society*, 30(12), 1591–1601.

4. Lang, A. E., Houeto, J.-L., Krack, P., Kubu, C., Lyons, K. E., Moro, E., & Voon, V. (2006). Deep brain stimulation: preoperative issues. *Movement Disorders: Official Journal of the Movement Disorder Society*, 21 Suppl 14, S171–S196.

5. Visser-Vandewalle, V., Temel, Y., Colle, H., & van der Linden, C. (2003). Bilateral high-frequency stimulation of the subthalamic nucleus in patients with multiple system atrophy—parkinsonism. Report of four cases. *Journal of Neurosurgery*, 98(4), 882–887.

6. Tarsy, D., Apetauerova, D., Ryan, P., & Norregaard, T. (2003). Adverse effects of subthalamic nucleus DBS in a patient with multiple system atrophy. *Neurology*, 61, 247–249. https://doi.org/10.1212/01.wnl.0000073986.74883.36

7. Okun, M. S., & Foote, K. D. (2010). Parkinson's disease DBS: what, when, who and why? The time has come to tailor DBS targets. *Expert Review of Neurotherapeutics*, 10(12), 1847–1857.

8. Charles, P. D., Van Blercom, N., Krack, P., Lee, S. L., Xie, J., Besson, G., & Pollak, P. (2002). Predictors of effective bilateral subthalamic nucleus stimulation for PD. *Neurology*, 59(6), 932–934.

9. Welter, M. L., Houeto, J. L., Tezenas du Montcel, S., Mesnage, V., Bonnet, A. M., Pillon, B., & Agid, Y. (2002). Clinical predictive factors of subthalamic stimulation in Parkinson's disease. *Brain: A Journal of Neurology*, 125(Pt 3), 575–583.

10. Kumar, K., Kelly, M., & Toth, C. (1999). Deep brain stimulation of the ventral intermediate nucleus of the thalamus for control of tremors in Parkinson's disease and essential tremor. *Stereotactic and Functional Neurosurgery*, 72(1), 47–61.

11. Krack, P., Batir, A., Van Blercom, N., Chabardes, S., Fraix, V., Ardouin, C., . . . Pollak, P. (2003). Five-year follow-up of bilateral stimulation of the subthalamic nucleus in advanced Parkinson's disease. *New England Journal of Medicine*, 349(20), 1925–1934.

12. Landi, A., Parolin, M., Piolti, R., Antonini, A., Grimaldi, M., Crespi, M., . . . Gaini, S. M. (2003). Deep brain stimulation for the treatment of Parkinson's disease: the experience of the Neurosurgical Department in Monza. *Neurological Sciences: Official Journal of the Italian Neurological Society and of the Italian Society of Clinical Neurophysiology*, 24 Suppl 1, S43–S44.

13. Defer, G. L., Widner, H., Marié, R. M., Rémy, P., & Levivier, M. (1999). Core assessment program for surgical interventional therapies in Parkinson's disease (CAPSIT-PD). *Movement Disorders: Official Journal of the Movement Disorder Society*, 14(4), 572–584.

14. Maier, F., Lewis, C. J., Horstkoetter, N., Eggers, C., Kalbe, E., Maarouf, M., . . . Timmermann, L. (2013). Patients' expectations of deep brain stimulation, and subjective perceived outcome related to clinical measures in Parkinson's disease: a mixed-method approach. *Journal of Neurology, Neurosurgery, and Psychiatry, 84*(11), 1273–1281.

15. Okun, M. S., & Foote, K. D. (2004). A mnemonic for Parkinson disease patients considering DBS: a tool to improve perceived outcome of surgery. *Neurologist, 10*(5), 290.

16. Pandey, S., & Sarma, N. (2015). Deep brain stimulation: current status. *Neurology India, 63*(1),9.

17. Guduru, Z., Schramke, C., Baser, S., & Leichliter, T. (2016). Medication reduction after DBS placement in Parkinson's disease (P6.383). *Neurology, 86*(16 Suppl), P6.383.

18. Liu, Y., Li, W., Liu, X., Wang, X., Gui, Y., Qin, L., Deng, F., Hu, C., & Chen, L. (2014). Meta-analysis comparing deep brain stimulation of the globus pallidus and subthalamic nucleus to treat advanced Parkinson disease. *J Neurosurg, 121*(3), *709–718.*

19. Higuchi, M., Topiol, D., Ahmed, B., et al. (2015). Impact of an interdisciplinary deep brain stimulation screening model on post-surgical complications in esential tremor patients. *PLoS One, 10*(12), e0145623.

20. Higuchi, M., Martinez-Ramirez, D., Morita, H., et al. (2016). Interdisciplinary Parkinson's disease deep brain stimulation screening and the relationship to unintended hospitalizations and quality of life. *PLoS One, 11*(5): e0153785.

21. Gorgulho, A., De Salles, A. A. F., Frighetto, L., & Behnke, E. (2005). Incidence of hemorrhage associated with electrophysiological studies performed using macroelectrodes and microelectrodes in functional neurosurgery. *Journal of Neurosurgery, 102*(5), 888–896.

22. Higuchi, Y., & Iacono, R. P. (2003). Surgical complications in patients with Parkinson's disease after posteroventral pallidotomy. *Neurosurgery, 52*(3), 558–571; discussion 568–571.

23. Saint-Cyr, J. A., Trépanier, L. L., Kumar, R., Lozano, A. M., & Lang, A. E. (2000). Neuropsychological consequences of chronic bilateral stimulation of the subthalamic nucleus in Parkinson's disease. *Brain: A Journal of Neurology, 123*(Pt 10), 2091–2108.

24. Cyron, D. (2016). Mental side effects of deep brain stimulation (DBS) for movement disorders: the futility of denial. *Frontiers in Integrative Neuroscience, 10,* 17.

25. Follett, K. A., Weaver, F. M., Stern, M., Hur, K., Harris, C. L., Luo, P., & CSP 468 Study Group. (2010). Pallidal versus subthalamic deep-brain stimulation for Parkinson's disease. *New England Journal of Medicine, 362*(22), 2077–2091.

26. Rodriguez-Oroz, M. C., Obeso, J. A., Lang, A. E., Houeto, J.-L., Pollak, P., Rehncrona, S., . . . Van Blercom, N. (2005). Bilateral deep brain stimulation in Parkinson's disease: a multicentre study with 4 years follow-up. *Brain: A Journal of Neurology, 128*(Pt 10), 2240–2249.

27. Soulas, T., Gurruchaga, J. M., Palfi, S., Cesaro, P., Nguyen, J. P., & Fenelon, G. (2008). Attempted and completed suicides after subthalamic nucleus stimulation for Parkinson's disease. *J Neurol Neurosurg Psychiatry, 79,* 952–954.

28. Burkhard, P. R., Vingerhoets, F. J. G., Berney, A., Bogousslavsky, J., Villemure, J.-G., & Ghika, J. (2004). Suicide after successful deep brain stimulation for movement disorders. *Neurology, 63*(11), 2170–2172.

29. Voon, V., Kubu, C., Krack, P., Houeto, J.-L., & Tröster, A. I. (2006). Deep brain stimulation: neuropsychological and neuropsychiatric issues. *Movement Disorders: Official Journal of the Movement Disorder Society, 21 Suppl 14,* S305–S327.

30. Rodríguez, R. L., Miller, K., Bowers, D., Crucian, G., Wint, D., Fernandez, H., . . . Okun, M. S. (2005). Mood and cognitive changes with deep brain stimulation: what we know and where we should go. *Minerva Medica, 96*(3), 125–144.

31. Molloy. S., Rowan. E. N., O'Brien. J. T. et al. (2006). The effect of levodopa on cognitive function in Parkinson's disease with and without dementia and dementia with Lewy bodies. *J Neurol Neurosurg Psychiatry, 77*(12), 1323–1328.

32. Lang, A. E., Houeto, J. L., Krack, P., Kubu, C., Lyons, K. E., Moro, E., . . . Uitti, R. (2006). Deep brain stimulation: preoperative issues. *Movement disorders: official journal of the Movement Disorder Society, 21*(S14), S171–S196.

33. Morishita, T., Okun, M. S., Burdick, A., Jacobson, C. E., & Foote, K. D. (2013). Cerebral venous infarction: a potentially avoidable complication of deep brain stimulation surgery. *Neuromodulation, 16*(5), 407–413.

Case 8

Deep Brain Stimulation in Parkinson Disease

Basic Programming Pearls

RAJA MEHANNA

INTRODUCTION

Deep brain stimulation (DBS) directed to the sub-thalamic nucleus (STN) and the globus pallidus interna (GPi) has been demonstrated to improve motor control as well as quality of life in patients with Parkinson disease (PD).[1-3] While patient screening is key to ensure that only patients with the most advantageous risk-to-benefit ratios proceed to DBS,[4-6] effective postoperative programming is key to improving cardinal motor symptoms of PD.

In this chapter, we review the basics of DBS programming for PD.

BASIC APPROACH TO PROGRAMMING IN PARKINSON DISEASE

There is no randomized clinical trial proving the superiority of one DBS programming algorithm over another. However, it is important to have a clear plan when commencing programming on a patient. Clinicians should keep an open mind so that any approach can be modified, particularly based on the patient's feedback.

Programming usually commences on the first postsurgical visit, usually 4 weeks after DBS implantation, to allow any potential clinical benefit that is created during implant to resolve, known as a microlesion effect. Patients should present *off* medication for at least 12 hours to fully assess the benefit of stimulation without the confounding factor of motor fluctuations or levodopa-induced dyskinesia (LID). This first visit is also known as a monopolar review because all four monopolar configurations (using the implantable pulse generator [IPG] as an anode and each of the four circular contacts on the electrode as cathodes, successively) are tested. Electrode impedance is checked to rule out any open circuit or short circuit, which would prevent using the contacts involved. A fixed pulse width (usually 60–90 μsec) and frequency (usually 130 Hz) are selected and kept constant throughout the visit.

Starting with a monopolar configuration at the most ventral contact, the impact of stimulation at increasing voltages (or current) is noted on tremor, bradykinesia, and rigidity, with rigidity being the most reliable sign to examine serially because bradykinesia can be effort dependent and tremor can spontaneously fluctuate. Typical increases in voltage would be in increments of 0.1 to 0.5 V (or 0.1–0.5 mA). Two thresholds are recorded: the therapeutic threshold at which clinically significant improvement is seen, and the adverse effect threshold at which persistent clinically significant side effects are detected. It should be noted that patients frequently report paresthesia and other neurologic symptoms right after a voltage increase that are transient and usually resolve within a few seconds. While important to note, these symptoms do not usually define the adverse event threshold because they are transient. The voltage difference between the therapeutic threshold and the adverse event threshold constitutes a therapeutic interval or therapeutic window. Some experts think that a wide interval could be important to long-term issues such as tolerance, but this has never been shown. After the review of one monopolar configuration is complete, the voltage is brought back to zero, which means that stimulation is stopped. The next monopolar configuration is tested by moving the cathode to the most immediate dorsal contact, but not until the residual benefit from the previous configuration is completely worn off in order to accurately gauge the efficacy of each contact.[7] These steps are repeated for all monopolar configurations, leading to four therapeutic intervals corresponding to the four monopolar configurations. The configuration with the largest interval is selected for stimulation. The type of side effect encountered may also affect the choice of the configuration: patients might habituate to subjective side effects (paresthesia or other subjective changes such as dizziness) but not to muscle twitching/contraction or visual changes, making the latter less desirable. Initiating the stimulation will generally require a decrease in total dopamine equivalent dosage, especially in STN DBS, to avoid LID. In GPi, in many cases, there is not a need to decrease medications. However, one should be careful not to decrease medications too low and too fast so as not to worsen symptom control or precipitate depression, apathy, or neuropsychiatric symptoms.

Over successive visits, voltage can be increased as needed to control motor symptoms, but usually not more than 0.4 V per side of stimulation and per encounter, to avoid side effects from excessive stimulation. Indeed, side effects can sometimes take a few days to develop and not be visible in the clinic. If benefits from the best monopolar configuration are not realized despite successive increases in voltage over multiple visits, one should consider increasing the pulse width and/or frequency. Higher frequency might also be necessary for better tremor control. The STN, being a smaller target, rarely requires greater than 90 μsec of pulse width because it will most likely cause side effects by current spreading to unwanted nearby structures. The GPi, being a larger structure, can possibly tolerate higher pulse width, up to 240 μsec, as seen when treating dystonia[8]; however, such high numbers are usually unnecessary in PD.

If the amplitude of 5 V/mA, frequency of 180 Hz, and pulse width of 90 μsec (for the STN) have been reached at one configuration, but previously medication-responsive motor symptoms aren't improving with DBS, then the monopolar configuration with the next largest therapeutic interval should be used. If improvement remains suboptimal, but without persistent side effects at a low threshold, then a double monopolar configuration should be considered to enlarge the stimulation field. In this configuration, the IPG is selected as the anode, and the two best contacts are selected as cathodes. A lower voltage should be used in this configuration to avoid excessive current spread, and the increase at each visit should be limited to 0.1 to 0.2 V at each cathode.

On the other hand, if side effects are persistent and bothersome, then a bipolar stimulation should be considered. In this configuration, the contact with the best symptom control will be selected as the cathode, and the second best contact as anode. This creates a concentrated field of stimulation, preventing current spread to adjacent neuronal structures. Voltage requirements in the bipolar configuration are typically higher than in a monopolar configuration because of the more condensed field. With newer directional leads now being available, using a segmented contact, which stimulates at a 120-degree sector rather than in a conventional circular direction, allows "shaping" the field to direct stimulation toward the target while avoiding unwanted spread to adjacent structures.[9]

If monopolar, double monopolar, or bipolar settings or directional stimulation do not yield satisfactory results, interleaving can be considered.[10] Interleaving allows a clinician to define two programs that alternate stimulation at different times between each configuration. It is most likely to be useful in two clinical scenarios: (1) when independent contacts are beneficial for separate motor symptoms at different stimulation amplitudes in the monopolar configuration, but their use causes side effects when using them together in the double monopolar stimulation[11]; and (2) when symptoms are resolved incompletely and a further voltage increase is limited by side effects. In these situations, interleaving between two partially successful stimulation programs might allow better symptom control without side effects.[12] However, interleaving may drain the neurostimulator battery faster than the conventional settings, and its maximal frequency is limited to 125 Hz, which may be suboptimal for tremor control.[13]

If all of the previous strategies fail to improve symptoms, the possibility of a suboptimally positioned electrode must be considered and appropriate imaging performed. If suboptimal lead position is confirmed, surgical revision should be considered.

The effects of stimulation spreading into an adjacent structure are summarized in Tables 8.1 and 8.2. These are addressed by changing the cathode used, using bipolar stimulation, and using segmented contacts if available or, alternatively, interleaving, as detailed previously.

TABLE 8.1. EFFECTS OF SUBTHALAMIC NUCLEUS STIMULATION SPREADING TO ADJACENT ANATOMIC STRUCTURES

Observed Side Effects*	Structure	Anatomic Relation to the STN
Autonomic dysfunction (sweating, flushing)	Hypothalamus	Anteromedial
Muscle contractions, dysarthria, facial pulling	Corticospinal fibers of the internal capsule	Anterolateral Lateral
Personality changes, impulsivity, mood symptoms	Limbic STN	Medial
Warm sensations, nausea, diaphoresis	Red nucleus	Medial
Dizziness, dysconjugated ipsilateral eye deviation, diplopia, eyelid opening, apraxia	Cranial nerve III root	Medial
Contralateral conjugated gaze deviation	Frontal eye field fibers of the internal capsule	Lateral
Paresthesia	Medial lemniscus	Posterior
Akinesia, mood symptoms	Substantia nigra	Ventral
Muscle contractions	Internal capsule	Ventral

*Side effects are usually seen on the contralateral side of the stimulation. Note that spreading of the stimulation dorsally to the zona incerta does not seem to cause side effects.
STN = subthalamic nucleus
Source: Koeglsperger T, Palleis C, Hell F, Mehrkens JH, Bötzel K. Deep brain stimulation programming for movement disorders: current concepts and evidence-based strategies. Front Neurol 2019;10:410.

TABLE 8.2. EFFECTS OF GLOBUS PALLIDUS INTERNA STIMULATION SPREADING TO ADJACENT ANATOMIC STRUCTURES

Observed Side Effects*	Structure	Anatomic Relation to the GPi
Flashing lights in the contralateral visual field	Optic tract	Ventral
Muscle contractions	Posterior limb of the internal capsule	Posterior Medial
Worsening dyskinesia (rare)	GPe	Anterior Lateral Dorsal

*Side effects are usually seen on the contralateral side of the stimulation.
GPi = globus pallidus interna; GPe = globus pallidus externa.
Source: Koeglsperger T, Palleis C, Hell F, Mehrkens JH, Bötzel K. Deep brain stimulation programming for movement disorders: current concepts and evidence-based strategies. Front Neurol 2019;10:410.

Special considerations
Impact of frequency of Parkinson disease symptoms

Frequency at or above 130 Hz has been reported to control tremor much better than lower frequency below 100 Hz in STN DBS.[14,15] Conversely, lower frequency (60–80Hz) might confer superior bradykinesia improvement compared with higher frequency stimulation (130–150 Hz) on that same target.[16–18] No studies, however, could demonstrate an interindividual reproducible optimal frequency for rigidity improvement in STN DBS, or for any PD motor symptoms in GPi DBS.

Dyskinesia

While LID resistant to GPi DBS may be more optimally controlled by using more ventral contacts, STN DBS can result in dyskinesia through stimulation or a lesion effect.

Subthalamic nucleus stimulation–induced dyskinesia

Stimulation-induced dyskinesia (SID) usually indicates that the DBS lead is well positioned in the motor region of the STN. SID is not necessarily observed immediately following a stimulation change is made and instead may develop hours later. It is best managed by medication adjustment (decreasing the dose of levodopa and other dopaminergic drugs and the use of amantadine) or by the use of more dorsal STN contacts because these can have a direct antidyskinesia effects.[19] In some cases, slow increases in voltage every 1 or 2 weeks (0.1–0.2V) per increase can treat this issue. If all fails, rescue DBS in the GPi might be an option.[20]

Dyskinesia from a subthalamic nucleus lesion effect

This issue can develop before the stimulator is turned on, can persist even in the off-medication state, and can be resistant to amantadine.[21] However, this phenomenon is usually transient and resolves over weeks to months.[22,23] It may be due to a microbleed.

Gait

Switching from high (≥130 Hz) to lower (≤100 Hz) frequency, with an increase in voltage to maintain a similar amount of energy delivered, could possibly improve gait in PD patients who experience severe gait deterioration after high-frequency STN DBS.[24] In most cases, preoperative medication-resistant gait difficulty will not improve with DBS adjustment. One should also remember that low-frequency stimulation has less benefit on tremor than high-frequency stimulation.[14,15] There are no studies assessing programming strategies to improve gait after GPi DBS.

One theory is that post DBS worsening of gait can result from an unfavorable stimulation setting that accentuates lower limb asymmetry and thus interferes with interlimb coordination.[25] Reducing asymmetry by decreasing stimulation of the better controlled side can be attempted, especially with stimulation-resistant gait freezing.[26] In general, patients should be counseled before and after surgery that gait may not improve, although off-medication freezing may improve in 30% or more of cases.

Dysarthria

Dysarthria is typically resistant to DBS, and it is often difficult to distinguish between natural progression of PD and high-frequency STN DBS–induced dysarthria. Temporarily turning off the DBS in the clinic might be necessary to distinguish between the two issues. STN DBS–induced dysarthria tends to improve on a lower (60 Hz) rather than a higher (130 Hz) frequency.[27,28] A trial of lower pulse width (≤60 μsec) might be beneficial. Speech therapy has also been recommended. Studies reporting programming strategies to improve dysarthria after GPi DBS have not been published.

Neuropsychiatric complications

Depression and suicide rates were elevated in earlier DBS studies, but recently these percentages have not been shown to be increased, perhaps because of better monitoring. The emergence of neuropsychiatric issues may be correlated with a decrease in dopaminergic medications; therefore, this may be more likely after STN DBS because decreases in medications are more common.[29,30] Preoperative neuropsychological testing for a mood disorder, appropriate use of antidepressant medications when needed, and careful postoperative monitoring can be useful. STN DBS–induced depression is more related to stimulation through ventral contacts, and the use of dorsal contacts might alleviate the problem.[10] A psychiatrist and neuropsychologist are both important members of the DBS preoperative and postoperative management team.[31]

PEARLS

- A monopolar review is important to select the more useful contact.
- Stimulation can be in monopolar, double monopolar, bipolar, interleaving, or directional mode, depending on each patient's unique needs.
- Higher frequency might confer better tremor control but less bradykinesia improvement in STN DBS.
- STN stimulation–induced dyskinesia can resolve with medication management or with the use of more dorsal stimulation contacts.
- STN lesion–induced dyskinesia resolves over time.
- Lower frequency stimulation might alleviate STN DBS–induced gait difficulty.
- STN DBS–induced dysarthria tends to improve on a lower stimulation frequency.
- Neuropsychiatric complications may be correlated to a decrease in dopaminergic medications or the use of ventral contacts in STN DBS.

CONCLUSION

Applying sound principles of DBS programming can maximize benefits and reduce side effects of DBS. The use of a systematic approach as suggested in this chapter is an excellent strategy. It is unknown at this time whether multiple independent source programming and the use of segmented contacts will reduce side effects, but conventional thought is that in select cases, these will likely prove to be useful strategies.

REFERENCES

1. Deuschl G, Schade-Brittinger C, Krack P, Volkmann J, Schäfer H, Bötzel K, Daniels C, Deutschländer A, Dillmann U, Eisner W, Gruber D, Hamel W, Herzog J, Hilker R, Klebe S, Kloss M, Koy J, Krause M, Kupsch A, Lorenz D, Lorenzl S, Mehdorn HM, Moringlane JR, Oertel W, Pinsker MO, Reichmann H, Reuss A, Schneider GH, Schnitzler A, Steude U, Sturm V, Timmermann L, Tronnier V, Trottenberg T, Wojtecki L, Wolf E, Poewe W, Voges J; German Parkinson Study Group, Neurostimulation Section: A randomized trial of deep-brain stimulation for Parkinson's disease. N Engl J Med 2006;355:896–908.
2. Weaver FM, Follett K, Stern M, Hur K, Harris C, Marks WJ Jr, Rothlind J, Sagher O, Reda D, Moy CS, Pahwa R, Burchiel K, Hogarth P, Lai EC, Duda JE, Holloway K, Samii A, Horn S, Bronstein J, Stoner G, Heemskerk J, Huang GD; CSP 468 Study Group: Bilateral deep brain stimulation vs best medical therapy for patients with advanced Parkinson disease: a randomized controlled trial. JAMA 2009;301:63–73.
3. Williams A, Gill S, Varma T, Jenkinson C, Quinn N, Mitchell R, Scott R, Ives N, Rick C, Daniels J, Patel S, Wheatley K; PD SURG Collaborative Group: Deep brain stimulation plus best medical therapy versus best medical therapy alone for advanced Parkinson's disease (PD SURG trial): a randomized, open-label trial. Lancet Neurol 2010,9:581–591.
4. Okun MS, Fernandez HH, Pedraza O, Misra M, Lyons KE, Pahwa R, Tarsy D, Scollins L, Corapi K, Friehs GM, Grace J, Romrell J, Foote KD: Development and initial validation of a screening tool for Parkinson disease surgical candidates. Neurology 2004;63:161–163.
5. Okun MS, Foote KD. Parkinson's disease DBS: what, when, who and why? The time has come to tailor DBS targets. Expert Rev Neurother 2010;10:1847–1857.
6. Abboud H, Mehanna R, Machado A, Ahmed A, Gostkowski M, Cooper S, Itin I, Sweeney P, Pandya M, Kubu C, Floden D, Ford PJ, Fernandez HH. Comprehensive, multidisciplinary deep brain stimulation screening for Parkinson patients: no room for "short cuts." Mov Disord Clin Pract 2014;1(4).
7. Mehanna R, Machado AG, Oravivattanakul S, Genc G, Cooper SE. Comparing two deep brain stimulation leads to one in refractory tremor. Cerebellum 2014;13:425–432.
8. Coubes P, Cif L, Fertit El H, Hemm S, Vayssiere N, Serrat S, et al. Electrical stimulation of the globus pallidus internus in patients with primary generalized dystonia: long-term results. J Neurosurg 2004;101:189–194.
9. Timmermann L, Jain R, Chen L, Maarouf M, Barbe MT, Allert N, Brücke T, Kaiser I, Beirer S, Sejio F, Suarez E, Lozano B, Haegelen C, Vérin M, Porta M, Servello D, Gill S, Whone A, Van Dyck N, Alesch F. Multiple-source current steering in

subthalamic nucleus deep brain stimulation for Parkinson's disease (the VANTAGE study): a non-randomised, prospective, multicentre, open-label study. Lancet Neurol 2015;14:693–701.

10. Koeglsperger T, Palleis C, Hell F, Mehrkens JH, Bötzel K. Deep brain stimulation programming for movement disorders: current concepts and evidence-based strategies. Front Neurol 2019;10:410.

11. Wojtecki L, Vesper J, Schnitzler A. Interleaving programming of subthalamic deep brain stimulation to reduce side effects with good motor outcome in a patient with Parkinson's disease. Parkinsonism Relat Disord 2011;17:293–294.

12. Montgomery EB. Deep brain stimulation programming, principles and practice. Oxford, UK: Oxford University Press; 2010.

13. Miocinovic S, Khemani P, Whiddon R, Zeilman P, Martinez-Ramirez D, Okun MS, Chitnis S. Outcomes, management, and potential mechanisms of interleaving deep brain stimulation settings. Parkinsonism Relat Disord 2014;20:1434–1437.

14. Stegemöller EL, Vallabhajosula S, Haq I, Hwynn N, Hass CJ, Okun MS. Selective use of low frequency stimulation in Parkinson's disease based on absence of tremor. Neurorehabilitation 2013;33:305–312.

15. Phibbs FT, Arbogast PG, Davis TL. 60-Hz frequency effect on gait in Parkinson's disease with subthalamic nucleus deep brain stimulation. Neuromodulation 2014;17:717–720.

16. Xie T, Bloom L, Padmanaban M, Bertacchi B, Kang W, MacCracken E, Dachman A, Vigil J, Satzer D, Zadikoff C, Markopoulou K, Warnke P, Kang UJ. Long-term effect of low frequency stimulation of STN on dysphagia, freezing of gait and other motor symptoms in PD. J Neurol Neurosurg Psychiatry. 2018;89:989–994.

17. Momin S, Mahlknecht P, Georgiev D, Foltynie T, Zrinzo L, Hariz M, Zacharia A, Limousin P. Impact of subthalamic deep brain stimulation frequency on upper limb motor function in Parkinson's disease. J Parkinsons Dis 2018;8:267–271.

18. Su D, Chen H, Hu W, Liu Y, Wang Z, Wang X, Liu G, Ma H, Zhou J, Feng T. Frequency-dependent effects of subthalamic deep brain stimulation on motor symptoms in Parkinson's disease: a meta-analysis of controlled trials. Sci Rep 2018;8:14456.

19. Herzog J, Pinsker M, Wasner M, Steigerwald F, Wailke S, Deuschl G, Volkmann J. Stimulation of subthalamic fibre tracts reduces dyskinesias in STN-DBS. Mov Disord 2007;22:679–684.

20. Sriram A, Foote KD, Oyama G, Kwak J, Zeilman PR, Okun MS. Brittle dyskinesia following STN but not GPi deep brain stimulation. Tremor Other Hyperkinet Mov (NY) 2014;4:242.

21. Gago MF, Rosas MJ, Linhares P, Ayres-Basto M, Sousa G, Vaz R. Transient disabling dyskinesias: a predictor of good outcome in subthalamic nucleus deep brain stimulation in Parkinson's disease. Eur Neurol. 2009;61(2):94–9.

22. Herzog J, Volkmann J, Krack P, Kopper F, Potter M, Lorenz D, et al. Two-year follow-up of subthalamic deep brain stimulation in Parkinson's disease. Mov Disord 2003;18:1332–1337.

23. Moro E, Esselink RJ, Benabid AL, Pollak P. Response to levodopa in parkinsonian patients with bilateral subthalamic nucleus stimulation. Brain 2002;125:2408–2417.

24. Mehanna R. Deep brain stimulation in Parkinson's disease. In: Mehanna R (ed). Deep brain stimulation. New York: Nova Science; 2015.

25. Fasano A, Herzog J, Seifert E, et al. Modulation of gait coordination by subthalamic stimulation improves freezing of gait. Mov Disord 2009;26:844–851.

26. Pötter-Nerger M, Volkmann J. Deep brain stimulation for gait and postural symptoms in Parkinson's disease. Mov Disord. 2013;28:1609–1615.

27. Moreau C, Pennel-Ployart O, Pinto S, Plachez A, Annic A, Viallet F, Destée A, Defebvre L. Modulation of dysarthropneumophonia by low-frequency STN DBS in advanced Parkinson's disease. Mov Disord 2011;26:659–663.

28. Morello ANDC, Beber BC, Fagundes VC, Cielo CA, Rieder CRM. Dysphonia and dysarthria in people with Parkinson's disease after subthalamic nucleus deep brain stimulation: effect of frequency modulation. J Voice 2018;Nov 16. [Epub ahead of print]. doi:10.1016/j.jvoice.2018.10.012.

29. Follett KA, Weaver FM, Stern M, Hur K, Harris CL, Luo P, Marks WJ Jr, Rothlind J, Sagher O, Moy C, Pahwa R, Burchiel K, Hogarth P, Lai EC, Duda JE, Holloway K, Samii A, Horn S, Bronstein JM, Stoner G, Starr PA, Simpson R, Baltuch G, De Salles A, Huang GD, Reda DJ; CSP 468 Study Group: Pallidal versus subthalamic deep-brain stimulation for Parkinson's disease. N Engl J Med 2010;362:2077–2091.

30. Odekerken VJ, van Laar T, Staal MJ, Mosch A, Hoffmann CF, Nijssen PC, Beute GN, van Vugt JP, Lenders MW, Contarino MF, Mink MS, Bour LJ, van den Munckhof P, Schmand BA, de Haan RJ, Schuurman PR, de Bie RM: Subthalamic nucleus versus globus pallidus bilateral deep brain stimulation for advanced Parkinson's disease (NSTAPS study): a randomised controlled trial. Lancet Neurol. 2013;12:37–44.

31. Weintraub D, Duda JE, Carlson K, Luo P, Sagher O, Stern M, et al. Suicide ideation and behaviours after STN and GPi DBS surgery for Parkinson's disease: results from a randomised, controlled trial. J Neurol Neurosurg Psychiatry 2013;10:1113–1118.

Case 9

Target Selection for Parkinson Disease With Medication-Refractory Unilateral Resting Tremor

FUYUKO SASAKI, GENKO OYAMA, YASUSHI SHIMO, ATSUSHI UMEMURA, AND NOBUTAKA HATTORI

INDICATION FOR DEEP BRAIN STIMULATION

Parkinson disease with unilateral rest tremor

CLINICAL HISTORY AND RELEVANT EXAM

A 67-year-old right-handed man was referred for consideration for surgical therapy. He had a 7-year history of right-dominant severe resting tremor and action-postural tremor. His tremor became significantly worse and progressed to the left hand over 7 years. The patient developed rigidity, bradykinesia, gait disturbance with freezing, and impaired postural reflexes over the most recent few years. Levodopa therapy was started and increased up to levodopa/carbidopa 900/90 mg because of suspected Parkinson disease (PD); however, his tremor and other parkinsonian symptoms did not improve.

COMPLICATIONS

None

TROUBLESHOOTING AND MANAGEMENT

The acute levodopa challenge test performed by infusion of 200 mg levodopa revealed an excellent response with respect to the patient's parkinsonian symptoms, except for tremor. The Unified Parkinson's Disease Rating Scale (UPDRS) Part III scores improved from 44 to 33 (32%). The diagnosis of PD was made based on the UK Parkinson's Disease Society Brain Bank Diagnostic Criteria. Multiple medications such as trihexyphenidyl, primidone, clonazepam, arotinolol, zonisamide, pramipexole, and rotigotine were ineffective in suppressing the tremor. Because his most bothersome symptom was right-hand tremor, we discussed whether to implant a deep brain stimulation (DBS) lead in the left-sided unilateral ventral intermediate (Vim) nucleus of the thalamus or the posterior subthalamic area (PSA). Because he was diagnosed with PD and had already displayed right-dominant parkinsonism other than the tremor, the subthalamic nucleus (STN) could also be a potential target for treatment. However, the response rate of tremor to STN DBS is thought to be slightly lower than DBS in the Vim or the PSA, although the available case series reporting these outcomes are small. After a long discussion, we decided to perform an implantation of a left STN DBS lead after preparing for reimplantation of the PSA DBS lead intraoperatively if the tremor suppression by STN DBS was not sufficient.

OUTCOME

The left STN DBS lead provided reasonable tremor suppression intraoperatively. A left STN DBS resulted in reduced contralateral resting and action-postural tremor and improved bradykinesia and rigidity. The patient continued taking dopamine agonists and zonisamide with a reduced dose of levodopa. Arotinolol hydrochloride was discontinued.

DISCUSSION

It is established that STN and globus pallidus internus (GPi) DBS are effective treatment options in patients with motor complications in PD.[1] The STN is the most commonly selected target for DBS in PD because of its powerful effect on motor complications and on reduction of medication; however, GPi is just as effective for the motor symptoms. Some studies have focused on the effects in patients with severe tremor, but tremor does not always improve on STN stimulation,[2] and an improvement of the contralateral tremor by unilateral STN DBS has been reported to occur in 86 to 88% of cases.[2-5]

In medication-refractory tremor, historically, Vim DBS is an alternative target because of the effectiveness on parkinsonian tremor as well as essential tremor.[4] A multicenter study reported improvements of 75% for tremor in PD after unilateral Vim DBS. Vim DBS is particularly useful if there is action-postural tremor associated with PD. However, rigidity and bradykinesia were only slightly improved.[4] Additionally, Vim DBS may be associated with gait and balance disturbances.[6]

In recent years, an increasing number of publications investigated DBS in the PSA for treatment of various tremors, including essential tremor, parkinsonian tremor, and other tremors.[7] The PSA is primarily composed of the zona incerta (Zi) and prelemniscal radiation. In particular, the caudal Zi has been shown to be a more effective target for tremor treatment than the STN.[8] Although the mechanism of tremor suppression by PSA stimulation remains unclear, it has been suggested that interruptions of the connections of cerebellothalamic fibers in the PSA have been implicated.[7,8] Previous studies have reported that PSA DBS improved contralateral tremor by 78 to 93%. This improvement was regardless of levodopa responsiveness, although the effects on rigidity and bradykinesia were variable.[7] Furthermore, a comprehensive quantitative literature review showed a significant advantage of PSA/Zi stimulation for tremor compared with stimulation of STN and Vim DBS,[9] although the sample size of the study was small.

In this patient, STN DBS successfully improved the tremor and other parkinsonism symptoms without switching to the PSA target. This case demonstrates that careful target selection is important in unilateral tremor-dominant cases without motor fluctuation. It is also helpful to test intraoperative macrostimulation to decide on the final target. There is one case in the literature demonstrating that STN DBS with a more posterior target within STN may alleviate both essential tremor and PD tremor.[6] If postural action tremor is present, it is important to possibly consider Vim or other targets.

PEARLS

- Unilateral STN DBS is a reasonable indication for medication-refractory parkinsonian tremor with significant laterality. Recent studies, however, have not shown any difference in tremor outcome between GPi and STN DBS.
- The PSA can be an alternative target for DBS for parkinsonian tremor symptoms instead of the Vim or STN.
- Intraoperative macrostimulation may be useful for selecting a better target for DBS in medication-refractory parkinsonian tremor, although sometimes there is a delay in benefit in the intraoperative setting.
- Vim DBS and other options should be considered if there is a significant action-postural component.

REFERENCES

1. Okun MS. Deep-brain stimulation for Parkinson's disease. N Engl J Med 2012;367:1529–1538.
2. Parihar R, Alterman R, Papavassiliou E, Tarsy D, Shih LC. Comparison of VIM and STN DBS for Parkinsonian resting and postural/action tremor. Tremor Other Hyperkinet Mov 2015;5:321.
3. Krack P, Benazzouz A, Pollak P, et al. Treatment of tremor in Parkinson's disease by subthalamic nucleus stimulation. Mov Disord 1998;13:907–914.
4. Kumar R, Lozano AM, Sime E, Halket E, Lang AE. Comparative effects of unilateral and bilateral subthalamic nucleus deep brain stimulation. Neurology 1999;53:561–561.
5. Slowinski JL, Putzke JD, Uitti RJ, et al. Unilateral deep brain stimulation of the subthalamic nucleus for Parkinson disease. J Neurosurg 2007;106:626–632.
6. Stover NP, Okun MS, Evatt ML, Raju DV, Bakay RA, Vitek JL. Stimulation of the subthalamic nucleus in a patient with Parkinson disease and essential tremor. Arch Neurol 2005;62:141–143.
7. Blomstedt P, Fytagoridis A, Astrom M, Linder J, Forsgren L, Hariz MI. Unilateral caudal zona incerta deep brain stimulation for Parkinsonian tremor. Parkinsonism Relat Disord 2012;18:1062–1066.
8. Plaha P, Ben-Shlomo Y, Patel NK, Gill SS. Stimulation of the caudal zona incerta is superior to stimulation of the subthalamic nucleus in improving contralateral parkinsonism. Brain 2006;129:1732–1747.
9. Ramirez-Zamora A, Smith H, Kumar V, Prusik J, Phookan S, Pilitsis JG. Evolving concepts in posterior subthalamic area deep brain stimulation for treatment of tremor: surgical neuroanatomy and practical considerations. Stereotact Funct Neurosurg 2016;94:283–297.

Case 10

Genetic Mutations and Deep Brain Stimulation

JARED HINKLE, ANKUR BUTALA, VALERIY PARFENOV,
KELLY A. MILLS, AND ZOLTAN MARI

INDICATIONS FOR DEEP BRAIN STIMULATION

Medication-responsive, juvenile-onset disease, dyskinesias, dystonia, motor fluctuations

CLINICAL HISTORY AND RELEVANT EXAM

The patient is a Qatari gentleman aged 33 years at the time of initial writing. He is without family history and carries a presumptive diagnosis—made before presentation at our facility—of a levodopa-responsive dystonia syndrome. Initial onset of symptoms began at the age of 10 years with dystonic inverted and plantar-flexed posturing of the left lower extremity, with symptoms subsequently spreading to the contralateral limb. By age 14 years, he was nonambulatory and wheelchair-dependent and required assistance with activities of daily living. It was around this time that he first underwent a levodopa trial (100 mg three times daily); this produced functional restoration to near-normal levels. Over the years, however, his disease progressed. The initially exceptional levodopa response attenuated; by the time we evaluated him he had been taking 100 to 200 mg levodopa every 30 to 60 minutes, averaging well over 3,000 mg daily (peak daily levodopa dose of 4,500 mg).

His condition continued to deteriorate. Most troublesome were dystonic "seizures" with severe, sustained flexion posturing of the extremities, trunk, and face lasting up to 2 hours at a time. These episodes were variably responsive to 100 to 200 mg of levodopa within 30 to 90 minutes, with improvement lasting approximately 45 to 60 minutes. The high levodopa dosing led to prominent *on* dyskinesias, starting by age 16 years. Eventually, these became severe enough to cause postural instability and trauma risk.

Over the years, medication trials have included amantadine (up to 400 mg daily), subcutaneous apomorphine, Rytary (245-mg capsule five times daily), cyclobenzaprine (30 mg daily), pramipexole (4.5 mg daily), and baclofen. Prior diagnostic evaluation was limited and included negative structural analysis by magnetic resonance imaging (MRI) and cerebrospinal fluid analysis.

Aside from the symptoms described previously, the patient's preconsultation history was unremarkable with the exception of a significant anxiety component exacerbated by the fear of recurrent *off* dystonias. It was determined that this resulted in dopamine dysregulation syndrome, that is, levodopa overuse in an attempt to prevent the onset of dystonia. The patient's family history was unremarkable, with no relatives, including his biologic parents and younger brothers, being affected by a similar syndrome or having any neurologic abnormalities. No genetic testing of family members was available.

The neurologic exam, aside from generalized dyskinesias and dystonia, was consistent with parkinsonism with decrementing bradykinesia, mild cogwheel rigidity, intermittent mild resting tremor, diminished arm-swing, and postural instability. Of note, his rigidity scores remained disproportionately low even in the *off* levodopa state. Cranial nerves, sensory exam, muscle strength, muscle stretch reflexes, and cerebellar evaluation were all unremarkable.

We concluded that the initial diagnosis of dopa-responsive dystonia (DRD) had to be revised. Juvenile Parkinson disease (PD), dystonic juvenile parkinsonism (DJP), autosomal recessive early-onset parkinsonism with diurnal fluctuation (AREPDF), and Wilson disease were all considered. Since there was no diurnal fluctuation of symptoms (such as in AREPDF), age of onset was earlier than typical for DJP, and dramatic levodopa response would not be expected in Wilson disease, we felt that the more appropriate diagnosis was juvenile PD. Genetic testing to support a diagnosis of juvenile PD was pursued and revealed homozygous, disease-associated deletions in exon 4 of Parkin with an additional finding of a single c.434 C>T (p.Thr145Met) transition in PINK1. While the c.434 C>T mutation is considered a variant of unknown significance (VUS) with only moderate likelihood of pathogenicity, SIFT and PolyPhen-2.2.2 prediction algorithms disagree on pathogenicity. Concurrent testing of *GCH1* and *TH* did not reveal any mutations that would support a diagnosis of DRD.

Given the severity of motor fluctuations, high levodopa dose burden, severe *off* generalized dystonia, *on* dyskinesias, and consistent response to levodopa, the patient underwent bilateral GPi DBS implantation in December 2008. Before surgery, a routine pre-DBS screening was done, including neurosurgical, neuropsychological, neuropsychiatric, and physical therapy evaluations.

COMPLICATIONS

Because the procedure was performed before our adaptation of the Clearpoint system and an intraoperative MRI suite for DBS under anesthesia, the implantation procedure was complicated by severe anxiety and panic attacks, prompting a reschedule and conscious sedation. The patient also refused to go *off* levodopa for the surgery, a routine measure that improves intraoperative identification of the most effective targets for symptomatic control.

TROUBLESHOOTING AND MANAGEMENT

In general, programming proved to be exceptionally challenging because both the patient and his caretakers considered his condition to be completely intolerable when in the *off* state. His dopamine dysregulation syndrome also generally led to noncompliance with any attempts to shift toward an *off* state. Therefore, initial programming (4 weeks after the operation) had to be conducted largely in the *on* state, and we focused on identifying contacts with the highest threshold of side effects (e.g., visual changes and other sensory disturbances such as "tingling"). At this time, electrode configurations were monopolar (left GPi: C+/3−; right GPi: C+/4−). For both sides, pulse width was 90 μsec, frequency was 185 Hz, and voltage was 3.5 V.

Since the patient's neurologic examination in the clinic was quite variable depending on his levodopa intake, we had instructed the family on how to assess the frequency and severity of dystonic and dyskinetic episodes at home to better characterize his DBS response. During follow-up, the patient and his family reported some initial benefit. Unfortunately, within 1 week, this effect was lost, and the patient subsequently worsened. At an evaluation 6 weeks after surgery, it was noted that the severity of his dyskinesias and dystonias were comparable to those before surgery, although not uniformly throughout the body. For example, his upper extremities were not affected as dramatically as the axial musculature.

We therefore determined that higher stimulation with lower contacts could be beneficial. On the left side, we shifted to contact 0 in monopolar mode, but because of a tactile "shock" sensation as low as 1.6 V, we also changed to a bipolar configuration (0−/1+). He tolerated an increased pulse width on both sides (150 μsec) and an increased right-lead voltage (4.2 V). Two weeks after this adjustment (8 weeks after surgery), physical exam demonstrated substantial improvement in his overall condition, and discussion with the family verified this conclusion.

OUTCOME

Further minor tweaks were made to his programming; by 12 weeks after surgery, final electrode polarities and voltages were 0−/1+, 4 V (left) and 4−/5+, 5 V (right). Bilaterally, pulse width and frequency were maintained at 150 μsec and 185 Hz, respectively. As of 10 months after the initial surgery, we were able to achieve marked improvement of his symptoms with 90% reduction of dyskinesias and 70% reduction of dystonias. Furthermore, at this time he experienced no specific side effects, such as capsular motor symptoms, sensory disturbances, visual or extraocular dysfunction, dizziness, or lightheadedness. However, concurrent with this evaluation, he was undergoing consultations with a neuropsychologist on staff to discuss ongoing dopamine dysregulation syndrome because he was continuing to take preoperative doses of carbidopa/levodopa despite there being no clear medical reason to do so.

DISCUSSION

Several monogenic forms of PD have been identified, and these are often of early onset (<50 years of age) or juvenile onset (<21 years of age).

Examples of associated genes include those coding for a-synuclein (*SNCA*), Parkin (*PRKN*, previously *PARK2*), PTEN-induced kinase 1 (PINK1, *PARK6*), DJ-1 (*PARK7*), and leucine-rich repeat kinase 2 (*LRRK2*). Pathogenic variants in *PRKN* may be responsible for nearly 50% of familial PD cases and present in 15% to 20% of apparently sporadic early-onset Parkinson disease (EOPD) cases.[1] Disease-associated *PARK6* variants are the second most common known genetic cause of early-onset parkinsonism. Certain *GBA* variants are also causatively linked to PD and may result in a more severe disease progression.[2] This course can include an increased risk for cognitive impairment and psychiatric comorbidities, which may be important to consider when evaluating candidates for DBS.[2,3]

The mean age of onset for *PRKN*-associated PD (PRKN-PD) is approximately 32 years, although presentations as young as 7 years old have been reported.[1] Consistent with our case, PRKN-PD cases tend to have higher rates of dystonia than sporadic PD. Generally, levodopa responsivity is more favorable over time than sporadic PD, but the incidence of levodopa-induced dyskinesias may be higher.[1] The mean age at onset for *PARK6*-associated parkinsonism (PARK6-PD, affecting PINK1) is reportedly similar at approximately 33 years, with a similar expected range as monogenic PRKN-PD.[4] Although asymmetric rigidity, tremor, and bradykinesia remain the dominant initial parkinsonian symptoms, early hyperreflexia and lower-limb dystonic onset may lead to a misdiagnosis of a DRD.[5]

We identified another case report describing successful use of DBS in an individual with homozygous *PRKN* and heterozygous *PARK6* variants causing digenic PD of juvenile onset.[6] In that case, bilateral subthalamic nucleus (STN) DBS was performed instead of GPi DBS and not until 45 years after diagnosis (compared with 15 years in our case). Clearly, such cases are rare, and we can only speculate as to whether these digenic cases usually present so early in life. Parkin and PINK1 are cooperative partners in mitochondrial quality control; this connection partly grounds the theory that mitochondrial dysfunction and bioenergetics collapse lead to dopamine cell loss in *PRKN* and *PARK6* monogenic PD.[7] While one could argue that the *PARK6* variant in our patient is likely to be biochemically hypostatic or otherwise inconsequential to mitochondrial quality control, these genes are active in other cellular functions as well, which may contribute to a positive epistatic effect.

Confirming mutations in PD-linked genes can be diagnostically informative in cases of suspected EOPD cases. By extension, this approach can inform the appropriateness of a DBS intervention because EOPD cases are often very responsive to levodopa and amenable to long-term management with DBS. In the case we presented, genetic testing confirmed the diagnosis of juvenile-onset PD, now managed in part by bilateral GPi DBS. Homozygosity for several *PRKN* variants, including those in our patient, are a clear cause of monogenic PD, whereas our patient's heterozygous *PARK6* mutation was a VUS with moderate likelihood of pathogenicity. Nonetheless, it is probably not unreasonable to speculate that having a mutation in an additional PD-linked gene in addition to *PRKN* could have exacerbated his clinical presentation and may partly explain his below-average age of presentation. A large review of publicly available cases suggests a higher preponderance of heterozygosity of pathogenic *parkin* or *PINK1* in persons with EOPD.[8] Anxiety and depression are also common comorbidities in *PARK6*-associated PD, suggesting that it could have contributed to his anxiety and panic attacks as well.[9]

The presence of prominent dyskinesias and dystonias largely informed our decision to perform GPi DBS placement rather than STN DBS.[10] If our patient had prominent tremors, we may have considered bilateral STN DBS instead; however, over the years, the assumption that STN DBS is preferable to GPi DBS for controlling tremor has been challenged by the results of several randomized trials and resultant meta-analyses.[11] The other case report described previously of a patient with digenic juvenile-onset PD—for whom STN DBS was performed—featured tremor as the earliest disease manifestation, although the authors do not discuss other possible rationales for STN DBS in their case.[6] Future work may shed more light on whether STN or GPi DBS is preferable in genetically proven PD, or if a patient's particular phenomenology should retain priority in these decisions. Our case was also complicated by dopamine dysregulation syndrome, which remains a somewhat understudied phenomenon in PD, partly owing to its low prevalence. While STN DBS is generally superior to GPi DBS for reducing levodopa dosage, it is not currently established whether STN DBS is a more effective treatment for this syndrome when present preoperatively.

Conducting research to evaluate the outcomes of DBS in cases of sporadic versus genetic PD is complicated by the fact that multiple predictors of excellent DBS outcome in sporadic PD are overrepresented in certain types of genetic PD. This makes it difficult to dissociate the predictive values of the genotype from those of the correlated phenotypes. Examples of such factors include levodopa-responsive motor symptoms, a tremor-dominant presentation, and lack of cognitive impairment. Nonetheless, a number of studies have compared cohorts of DBS recipients with sporadic and monogenic PD, with mutation carriers generally receiving similar benefits to noncarriers. This was the essential conclusion of a recently published systematic review of DBS outcomes in cases of genetically proven PD.[12] The review addressed 30 relevant studies; while several of these did suggest statistically significant differences in DBS efficacy between carriers and noncarriers of mutations in *PRKN* and *LRRK2*—in both favorable and unfavorable

directions between studies—most reported comparable responses. Given the natural bias to publish papers showing groupwise differences over "negative" findings, we consider it likely that this reflects a lack of real difference between *PRKN* or *LRRK2* mutation carriers and noncarriers in terms of DBS outcome. Only a few publications have examined variants in other genes. For example, a single study of *SCNA* variants found that two tagging single-nucleotide polymorphisms (SNPs) linked to PD-associated haplotypes were correlated with more favorable outcomes,[13] but no cohort studies have examined the effect of *SNCA* gene duplications. Conversely, existing evidence on DBS in *GBA*-associated PD is somewhat more cautionary. Only two studies have analyzed DBS in this population, but both evinced problems associated with severe cognitive decline during follow-up.[14,15] Thus, in our opinion, clinical presentation and cognitive function may be more practically useful for predicting DBS efficacy than genetic status. However, the more aggressive course of *GBA*-associated PD is worth considering.

PEARLS

- PD-associated gene variants can provide critical diagnostic clues in cases of suspected early-onset or juvenile-onset PD, but may not be routinely used to prognosticate the response to DBS.
- Genotype–phenotype interactions may contribute to earlier onset and more severe PD clinical presentations. This necessitates periodic triage of the most predominant and disabling symptoms informing DBS site selection and operative and nonoperative management.
- Effectiveness and outcomes research evaluating the differential effect of stimulation of GPi versus STN in genetically proven PD may inform future management but remains an open subject of research.
- In some patients with dopamine dysregulation syndrome, DBS may not eliminate the compulsion to continue taking dopamine replacement therapy. Neuropsychiatric assessment and consultation are therefore essential to both preoperative and postoperative management in such cases.
- Preoperative cognitive function may be more important than genetic status, but more studies will be needed. The predominance of the evidence suggests that PD patients with genetic abnormalities do well with DBS.

REFERENCES

1. Lucking CB, Durr A, Bonifati V, et al. Association between early-onset Parkinson's disease and mutations in the parkin gene. N Engl J Med 2000;342:1560–1567.
2. Sidransky E, Lopez G. The link between the GBA gene and parkinsonism. Lancet Neurol 2012;11:986–998.
3. Liu G, Boot B, Locascio JJ, et al. Specifically neuropathic Gaucher's mutations accelerate cognitive decline in Parkinson's. Ann Neurol 2016;80:674–685.
4. Hatano Y, Li Y, Sato K, et al. Novel PINK1 mutations in early-onset parkinsonism. Ann Neurol 2004;56:424–427.
5. Ishihara-Paul L, Hulihan MM, Kachergus J, et al. PINK1 mutations and parkinsonism. Neurology 2008;71:896–902.
6. Nakahara K, Ueda M, Yamada K, et al. Juvenile-onset parkinsonism with digenic parkin and PINK1 mutations treated with subthalamic nucleus stimulation at 45 years after disease onset. J Neurol Sci 2014;345:276–277.
7. Pickrell AM, Youle RJ. The roles of PINK1, parkin, and mitochondrial fidelity in Parkinson's disease. Neuron 2015;85:257–273.
8. Brooks J, Ding J, Simon-Sanchez J, Paisan-Ruiz C, Singleton AB, Scholz SW. Parkin and PINK1 mutations in early-onset Parkinson's disease: comprehensive screening in publicly available cases and control. J Med Genet 2009;46:375–381.
9. Marongiu R, Ferraris A, Ialongo T, et al. PINK1 heterozygous rare variants: prevalence, significance and phenotypic spectrum. Hum Mutat 2008;29:565.
10. Williams NR, Foote KD, Okun MS. STN vs. GPi deep brain stimulation: translating the rematch into clinical practice. Mov Disord Clin Pract 2014;1:24–35.
11. Wong JK, Cauraugh JH, Ho KWD, et al. STN vs. GPi deep brain stimulation for tremor suppression in Parkinson disease: a systematic review and meta-analysis. Parkinsonism Relat Disord 2019;58:56–62.
12. Rizzone MG, Martone T, Balestrino R, Lopiano L. Genetic background and outcome of deep brain stimulation in Parkinson's disease. Parkinsonism Relat Disord 2019;64:8–19.
13. Weiss D, Herrmann S, Wang L, et al. Alpha-synuclein gene variants may predict neurostimulation outcome. Mov Disord 2016;31:601–603.
14. Angeli A, Mencacci NE, Duran R, et al. Genotype and phenotype in Parkinson's disease: lessons in heterogeneity from deep brain stimulation. Mov Disord 2013;28:1370–1375.
15. Lythe V, Athauda D, Foley J, et al. GBA-associated Parkinson's disease: progression in a deep brain stimulation cohort. J Parkinsons Dis 2017;7:635–644.

Case 11

Issues to Consider When Mild Cognitive Impairment Is Revealed in Preoperative Screening

SUSHMA KOLA AND ANHAR HASSAN

INDICATIONS FOR DEEP BRAIN STIMULATION

Medication-refractory motor fluctuations and dyskinesia

CLINICAL HISTORY AND RELEVANT EXAM

A 72-year-old man with Parkinson disease (PD) of 7 years' duration complicated by motor fluctuations and dyskinesia was evaluated in the deep brain stimulation (DBS) clinic. He had previously been treated with immediate-release levodopa at regular intervals, then switched to controlled-release levodopa without noticeable improvement. In the *off* state, he reported bradykinesia, impaired dexterity, gait shuffling, freezing, and falls. In the *on* state, there was improved gait shuffling and freezing, accompanied by mild dyskinesias. He reported being a little forgetful when recalling names and was using lists more than he used to. Nonetheless he denied significant change in memory and continued to manage his farm and budget without difficulty. Baseline examination while on medication was remarkable for asymmetric mild bradykinetic rigid parkinsonism, generalized mild dyskinesia, and a multifactorial gait disorder with components of a sensory ataxic gait, orthopedic antalgic gait, and parkinsonian features with a positive pull test. The patient was counseled that DBS should improve the levodopa-responsive symptoms and dyskinesia, but not the antalgic and ataxic components of the gait. The patient proceeded to undergo a multidisciplinary DBS evaluation with a DBS neurologist, DBS neurosurgeon, psychiatrist, neuropsychologist, speech pathologist, and nurse educator. Videos were obtained of the UPDRS examination in the on-medication state (score of 30) and off-medication state (score of 12). These data were presented to the DBS committee.

COMPLICATIONS

It was the opinion of the DBS review committee that the patient's symptoms would likely benefit from either bilateral subthalamic nucleus (STN) or globus pallidus interna (GPi) DBS. However, neuropsychometric testing revealed an abnormal neurocognitive profile consistent with multidomain mild cognitive impairment (MCI). Learning and memory were impaired across all modalities. There were deficits in aspects of spatial organization, semantic fluency, and executive functioning (including mental flexibility, complex problem-solving, and maintaining cognitive set). Other aspects of language, executive functioning, and perceptual processing were normal. It was the opinion of the DBS review committee that the cognitive findings could place the patient at higher risk for future progression to dementia and immediate postoperative issues.

TROUBLESHOOTING AND MANAGEMENT

The DBS committee recommended to defer DBS and to repeat the neuropsychological evaluation in 6 months in order to assess the trajectory of the cognitive impairment. This is based on the natural history of mild cognitive impairment, which may improve, remain stable, or progress to dementia, and thus informs our practice. This is performed after identifying and correcting any treatable causes of cognitive impairment (e.g., removing sedatives, treating sleep apnea, treating B_{12} deficiency), and without starting cognitive-enhancing medications. After 6 months, if the cognitive profile is stable or improved, it is our experience that the patient is less likely to develop postoperative cognitive complications or dementia. However, if the patient progresses to worsening MCI or dementia, then the risk of DBS is deemed unfavorable. This is independent of selecting STN or GPi targets because both targets involve trajectories through the frontal lobes. We also select a 6-month delay because repeating the neuropsychometric testing sooner may confer a learning advantage and make test interpretation unreliable.

The 6-month repeat neuropsychometric test showed the patient's cognition was stable, with mild improvement on measures of delayed verbal memory, visual memory, semantic fluency, basic visual perception, and cognitive speed and flexibility. There was no significant decline in any domains. He was still considered to have MCI, however. The patient was further counseled on risks and benefits of DBS and underwent bilateral STN DBS implantation.

OUTCOME

There was improvement in dyskinesia. The patient continued to experience motor fluctuations despite optimization of programming parameters and additional medication trials of entacapone, pramipexole, and extended-release carbidopa-levodopa (Rytary). Because of ongoing mobility issues of imbalance, freezing, and falling, he reported increasing trouble with self-care at home, and plans were made for him to move into an assisted living facility. The patient felt that his cognitive functioning had not really changed, and if anything was somewhat improved. Nine months after surgery, he underwent repeat neuropsychometric assessment. Unfortunately, this revealed further slowing of mentation and new impairment in learning retention of an unorganized word list and visuospatial information. Compared with psychometric testing before the DBS procedure, this represented a concerning decline in performance. Difficulty was also observed on some measures of executive functioning, including mental flexibility and visuospatial integration skills. The patient showed some variability and possible decline in areas of executive functioning, including mental flexibility. His reading score declined approximately one standard deviation, although that may have been due to separate issues with vision. The progression in memory difficulties was concerning for possible worsening of MCI secondary to DBS. Repeat testing in the next 12 to 18 months was suggested, but the patient did not return for follow-up. His

assisted living facility contacted our DBS clinic about 1 year later to report that the patient was experiencing significant psychosis with daily hallucinations, delusions, and paranoia. With cessation of entacapone, these symptoms decreased from daily to once to twice weekly. However, he continued to struggle with debilitating paranoia. Pimavanserin or quetiapine was suggested, and follow-up is pending.

DISCUSSION

This case demonstrates worsening of preexisting mild cognitive decline following DBS. While it is widely accepted that dementia constitutes an absolute contraindication to DBS, the risk is less well-defined for patients displaying only minor abnormalities on neurocognitive testing. If patients decline neurocognitively on serial follow-up assessments before DBS, there is a presumed increased risk for acceleration to dementia following DBS, and thus it is typically not offered. However, for patients with a stable or improved natural history of MCI, the risk for cognitive decline after DBS is less clear.

It is well-established that cognitive performance may decline after DBS. Meta-analysis and clinical reviews of bilateral STN DBS have concluded that there is a small but measurable decrease in global cognition, memory, verbal fluency, and executive function after STN DBS compared with PD controls on medical therapy.[1,2] Despite improved motor outcomes, patients with borderline global cognitive impairment may report negative quality of life after DBS.[3] In addition to preoperative risk factors such as older age and cognitive impairment, intraoperative factors (surgical trajectories through the frontal lobe and head of the caudate) and postoperative factors (electrode location, stimulation parameters, and medication changes) may affect cognitive outcomes.[2,4-6] When comparing STN with GPi targets, the latter may result in fewer neurocognitive declines.[7,8] Nevertheless, there is not yet sufficient unequivocal evidence to support selection of GPi over STN for patients with preoperative MCI. There is, however, a notion that unilateral DBS may be more appropriate in these cases.

Physicians should therefore exercise caution before performing DBS on patients with preoperative mild cognitive impairment, even if the pattern is improving, and also counsel patients and family members on the potential for postoperative cognitive decline.

PEARLS

- DBS is possible even if MCI is present, but a risk-to-benefit profile must be conducted and shared with the patient and family.
- Serial pre-operative neuropsychological testing to assess cognitive trajectory may be useful. However, as in our case, this did not ensure a better outcome.
- There is some emerging evidence that GPi may be a better target in these cases, although the evidence is not overwhelming.
- Unilateral DBS could be considered because the risk-to-benefit ratio is better for this procedure when preoperative cognitive issues are uncovered.

REFERENCES

1. Xie Y, Meng X, Xiao J, Zhang J, Zhang J. Cognitive changes following bilateral deep brain stimulation of subthalamic nucleus in Parkinson's disease: a meta-analysis. Biomed Res Int 2016;2016:3596415.
2. Massano J, Garrett C. Deep brain stimulation and cognitive decline in Parkinson's disease: a clinical review. Front Neurol 2012;3:66.
3. Witt K, Daniels C, Krack P, Volkmann J, Pinsker MO, Kloss M, Tronnier V, Schnitzler A, Wojtecki L, Bötzel K, Danek A, Hilker R, Sturm V, Kupsch A, Karner E, Deuschl G. Negative impact of borderline global cognitive scores on quality of life after subthalamic nucleus stimulation in Parkinson's disease. J Neurol Sci 2011;310:261–266.
4. Witt K, Granert O, Daniels C, Volkmann J, Falk D, van Eimeren T, Deuschl G. Relation of lead trajectory and electrode position to neuropsychological outcomes of subthalamic neurostimulation in Parkinson's disease: results from a randomized trial. Brain 2013;136:2109–2119.
5. Kurtis M, Rajah T, Delgado L, Dafsari H. The effect of deep brain stimulation on the non-motor symptoms of Parkinson's disease: a critical review of the current evidence. NPJ Parkinsons Dis 2017;3:16024.
6. Volkmann J, Daniels C, Witt K. Neuropsychiatric effects of subthalamic neurostimulation in Parkinson disease. Nat Rev Neurol 2010;6:487–498.
7. Combs H, Folley B, Berry D, Segerstrom S, Han D, Anderson-Mooney A, Walls B, van Horne C. Cognition and depression following deep brain stimulation of the subthalamic nucleus and globus pallidus pars internus in Parkinson's disease: a meta-analysis. Neuropsychol Rev 2015;25:439–454.
8. Wang J, Zhang Y, Zhang X, Wang Y, Li J, Li Y. Cognitive and psychiatric effects of STN versus GPi deep brain stimulation in Parkinson's disease: a meta-analysis of randomized controlled trials. PLoS One 2016;11:0156721.

Case 12

Use of Subthalamic Nucleus and Globus Pallidus Interna Deep Brain Stimulation Targets in the Same Patient With Parkinson's Disease

SHABBIR HUSSAIN I. MERCHANT AND NORA VANEGAS-ARROYAVE

INDICATION FOR DEEP BRAIN STIMULATION

Parkinson disease (PD) with levodopa-refractory tremor and contralateral hemidystonia

CLINICAL HISTORY AND RELEVANT EXAM

A 54-year-old right-handed man with history of PD since age 48 years was referred for deep brain stimulation (DBS) evaluation at our institution for levodopa-refractory tremor and hemidystonia. His motor symptoms included progressive bilateral tremors, worse on the left side, and severe right hemidystonia with comorbid depression and anxiety. There was partial improvement of dystonia with high doses of levodopa and dopaminergic medications, but tremor remained refractory to treatment. Motor fluctuations developed and consisted of worsening dystonia during the off-medication state and during off–on transitional clinical states. Right foot dystonia was not fully responsive to dopaminergic medications or to chemodenervation, it persisted throughout the day and interfered with gait and balance.

His depression and anxiety significantly improved with medical treatment. There were no reports of freezing of gait or speech or swallowing difficulties. *OFF* (off PD medications) Unified Parkinson's Disease Rating Scale (UPDRS) Part III score was 46, and examination was significant for severe bilateral hand and leg tremors, more prominent on the left side, at rest and with posture, and painful dystonic posturing of his right hand and foot, limiting ambulation. *ON* (on PD medications) UPDRS Part III score was 22, and examination revealed marked improvement of rigidity and bradykinesia but minimal improvement of tremor and right foot dystonia.

He was considered to be a suitable candidate for DBS given motor fluctuations and overall levodopa responsiveness. Right subthalamic nucleus (STN) for refractory tremor and left globus pallidus interna (GPi) for right hemidystonia were the proposed targets for implantation. Lead placement was successfully achieved using stereotactic techniques and microelectrode recording (MER). The lead tip coordinates for the right STN were 11 mm lateral, 3 mm posterior, and 4 mm inferior to the mid-commissural point. The coordinates for the left GPi were 19 mm lateral, 3 mm anterior, and 2 mm inferior to the mid-commissural point. Two Medtronic Activa PC implantable pulse generators (IPGs) were placed, one for each side, to allow the independent selection of frequency parameters during DBS programming.

COMPLICATIONS

No complications were noted. The patient's postoperative course was unremarkable, and he experienced a prominent beneficial microlesion effect. During his initial programming, significant tremor control was achieved bilaterally, and his dystonia was markedly reduced. Both leads were initially programmed using a monopolar configuration.

TROUBLESHOOTING AND MANAGEMENT

During subsequent programming optimization, the right DBS electrode was switched to a double bipolar configuration, using high frequency to further improve tremor control. To improve

TABLE 12.1. DEEP BRAIN STIMULATION PROGRAMMING

	Configuration	Pulse Width	Frequency	Voltage
Right	3– 2+ 1–	60	185	2.4
Left	C+ 2–	90	130	2.7

right-sided dystonia, the left DBS electrode was programmed using a higher pulse width (90 μsec) at a frequency of 130 Hz. His *ON/ON* UPDRS Part III score was 11, and benefits were sustained. His current DBS settings are described in Table 12.1.

OUTCOME

DBS benefits have remained sustained three years later, with excellent tremor, relief of transitional dyskinesias, and near-complete resolution of dystonia. There were only occasional feelings of right foot tightness that were experienced primarily in the off-medication state. In addition, his doses of dopaminergic agents were significantly reduced.

DISCUSSION

We present a case of a patient with relatively early onset of PD with a complex phenotype of refractory tremor on one side and hemidystonia on the other, who was successfully treated with DBS using a combination of right STN and left GPi targets. The case highlights the potential benefits of selecting specific DBS targets based on the primary motor impairment in PD. Although

no clear benefits have been demonstrated when comparing GPi and STN targets in terms of tremor, STN DBS has been observed to result in lowering total doses of levodopa.[1–6] GPi is the historically preferred target for treating dystonia, but most of this literature is on primary dystonia and not PD-related dystonia.[7,8] The literature is limited about the relative efficacy of these targets in levodopa-refractory *off* dystonia.[6,9,10] In addition, in cases with severe dystonia associated with concomitant tremor, painful dystonic symptoms may remain refractory despite optimal control of tremor using the bilateral STN target.[10] Postoperative programming and stimulation parameters may also have target-specific effects[11,12]; specifically, stimulation of the STN can induce dystonic dyskinesias.[13]

Considering these observations, we implanted a combined target of STN (contralateral to the tremor predominant side) and GPi (contralateral to the dystonia predominant side) which resulted in significant medication reduction, tremor resolution, and treatment of dystonia and dystonic dyskinesias.

PEARLS

- DBS target selection in PD based on the phenomenologic characteristics and consideration of postoperative programming challenges can lead to optimal outcomes, specifically in the case of refractory hemidystonia and contralateral tremors.
- There are few data showing that PD dystonia would be better treated with a GPi target; however, it is a reasonable choice.
- It is possible to successfully mix conventional DBS targets in an individual PD patient, based on disease phenomenology.

REFERENCES

1. Williams NR, Foote KD, Okun MS. STN vs. GPi deep brain stimulation: translating the rematch into clinical practice. Mov Disord Clin Pract 2014;1:24–35.
2. Sidiropoulos C, LeWitt PA, Odekerken VJ, Schuurman PR, de Bie RM. GPi vs STN deep brain stimulation for Parkinson disease: three-year follow-up. Neurology 2016;87:745–746.
3. Vitek JL. Deep brain stimulation for Parkinson's disease: a critical re-evaluation of STN versus GPi DBS. Stereotact Funct Neurosurg 2002;78:119–131.
4. Martinez-Martinez AM, Aguilar OM, Acevedo-Triana CA. Meta-analysis of the relationship between deep brain stimulation in patients with Parkinson's disease and performance in evaluation tests for executive brain functions. Parkinsons Dis 2017;2017:9641392.
5. Mansouri A, Taslimi S, Badhiwala JH, et al. Deep brain stimulation for Parkinson's disease: meta-analysis of results of randomized trials at varying lengths of follow-up. J Neurosurg 2018;128(4):1199–1213.
6. Krack P, Pollak P, Limousin P, et al. Subthalamic nucleus or internal pallidal stimulation in young onset Parkinson's disease. Brain 1998;121(Pt 3):451–457.
7. Pauls KAM, Krauss JK, Kampfer CE, et al. Causes of failure of pallidal deep brain stimulation in cases with pre-operative diagnosis of isolated dystonia. Parkinsonism Relat Disord 2017;43:38–48.
8. Okun MS, Foote KD. Subthalamic nucleus vs globus pallidus interna deep brain stimulation, the rematch: will pallidal deep brain stimulation make a triumphant return? Arch Neurol 2005;62:533–536.
9. Loher TJ, Burgunder JM, Weber S, Sommerhalder R, Krauss JK. Effect of chronic pallidal deep brain stimulation on off period dystonia and sensory symptoms in advanced Parkinson's disease. J Neurol Neurosurg Psychiatry 2002;73:395–399.
10. Hedera P, Phibbs FT, Dolhun R, et al. Surgical targets for dystonic tremor: considerations between the globus pallidus and ventral intermediate thalamic nucleus. Parkinsonism Relat Disord 2013;19:684–686.
11. Volkmann J, Moro E, Pahwa R. Basic algorithms for the programming of deep brain stimulation in Parkinson's disease. Mov Disord 2006;21(Suppl 14):S284–289.
12. Picillo M, Lozano AM, Kou N, Puppi Munhoz R, Fasano A. Programming deep brain stimulation for Parkinson's disease: the Toronto Western Hospital Algorithms. Brain Stimul 2016;9:425–437.
13. Krack P, Pollak P, Limousin P, Benazzouz A, Deuschl G, Benabid AL. From off-period dystonia to peak-dose chorea: the clinical spectrum of varying subthalamic nucleus activity. Brain 1999;122(Pt 6):1133–1146.

Case 13

Medication-Refractory Parkinsonian Tremor Requiring Dual Lead Implantation for Tremor Control

ANHAR HASSAN

INDICATION FOR DEEP BRAIN STIMULATION

Parkinson disease (PD) with medication-refractory severe unilateral tremor

CLINICAL HISTORY AND RELEVANT EXAM

A 52-year-old man with tremor-predominant PD of 9 years' duration was evaluated in the DBS clinic for severe medication-refractory unilateral tremor and motor fluctuations. At age 43 years, he developed a right-hand pill-rolling tremor and was diagnosed with PD. He was initiated on ropinirole, but this was limited by side effects of aggressive behavior. He next tried pramipexole, which was helpful for tremor but limited by expense. He was switched to levodopa with excellent response. Two to 3 years before presentation, he developed increasingly frequent motor fluctuations. These were managed with carbidopa/levodopa/entacapone 37/150/200 seven times a day, approximately every 2 hours and 45 minutes. Very rarely, he took an extra 0.25 tablet of immediate-release carbidopa/levodopa 25/100 to supplement this. More recently, he noticed that the tremor worsened, particularly when falling asleep. Therefore, pramipexole 0.25 mg was added at bedtime to help him fall asleep. Medication took up to 1 hour to kick in, and mostly connected dose to dose. When medication was on, he reported good symptom control without dyskinesias. When medication wore off, he developed right arm tremor, jaw tremor, and nonmotor off symptoms of throat and chest tightness. His main complaint was bothersome tremor. Preoperative evaluation in the on-medication state was notable for severe right upper limb rest and re-emergent tremor, mild jaw tremor, mild rigidity in the right arm and right leg, and mild bradykinesia in the left hand. Furthermore, there was mild right dyskinetic arm posturing while walking. Gait was otherwise normal-appearing, with a negative retropulsion test. The Unified Parkinson's Disease Rating Scale (UPDRS) Part III motor scores were 15 off-medication and 11 on-medication, weighted for tremor. The UPDRS tremor scores were 4 for both rest and postural/action tremor in the right arm, in both on- and off-medication states. It was the opinion of the DBS committee that the patient would benefit from DBS to treat both medication-refractory tremor and motor fluctuations. There was discussion about the optimal target to best capture tremor and treat fluctuations, and whether to perform unilateral versus bilateral implantation. The committee recommended unilateral subthalamic nucleus (STN) DBS implantation to treat tremor and to address the motor fluctuations. If there was suboptimal tremor capture intraoperatively, then unilateral ventral intermediate (Vim) thalamic DBS could be added concurrently. An experienced functional neurosurgery team, tea, utilizing intraoperative electrophysiology recording, performed the DBS surgery.

COMPLICATIONS

During placement of the left-sided STN-stimulating electrode, there was a microlesional effect of right shoulder tremor, but jaw and face tremor were still present. Test stimulation produced excellent improvement in shoulder and jaw tremor at amplitudes greater than 1 V, but hand tremor did not satisfactorily resolve. The patient experienced transient right lower lip paresthesias

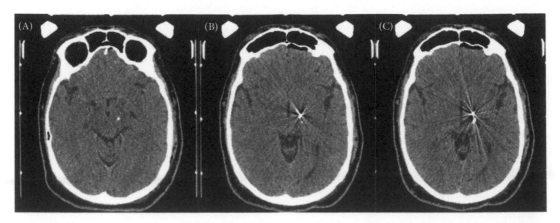

FIGURE 13.1.   (A) Tip of left subthalamic nucleus (STN) lead. (B) Tip of left Vim beside left STN lead (most ventral view). (C) Tip of left Vim beside left STN lead (slightly more dorsal view).

at 1.4 V, mild dysarthria at 2 V, and pulling on his right lower lip at 2.5 V. He tolerated amplitude increase to 3 V without persistent side effects.

TROUBLESHOOTING AND MANAGEMENT

It was decided that the patient would benefit from a second lead targeting the left Vim thalamic nucleus. Surgery continued with placement of the left-sided Vim stimulating electrode along the intended trajectory. The patient had an excellent microlesional reduction of right hand tremor. Test stimulation proceeded, and the amplitude was gradually increased from 0 to 2.5 V. Hand tremor symptoms abated, and facial tremor was significantly reduced at approximately 1 V. The patient experienced right lip numbness and tingling at 0.8 V. He tolerated voltage increase to 1.5 V but had persistent paresthesias in his right thumb. A tighter bipolar configuration was tried without resolution of paraesthesias. It was decided to leave the lead in place given the excellent therapeutic tremor response and because the lip paresthesias were tolerable.

The microlesional effect lasted 4 days. The patient underwent implantation of the pulse generator 2 weeks later. The following day, he returned to clinic for initial DBS programming. (See Table 13.1 for thresholds). He reported his tremor had returned to preoperative baseline. Monopolar review of the STN lead was performed first, and tremor reduction was noted at all contacts. The patient reported jaw tightness and pulling at low to medium voltages. A bipolar configuration reduced tremor, with minimal side effects.

During monopolar review of the thalamic lead, he reported face and hand tingling at low voltages with less improvement with tremor. Thus, a bipolar electrode configuration was selected at very low voltage. (See Table 13.2 for programming parameters). The patient reported sustained tremor control and improvement in motor fluctuations for the following 2 months and could go 15 hours before taking medication. One week before our second visit, the DBS system was interrogated at the local neurologist's office without any changes made, although tremors worsened afterward, and the patient required medication every 3 hours. Programming in our clinic at the second visit assessed a number of alternate settings. A new bipolar electrode configuration was selected for both the STN and Vim leads with suppression of tremor. At the 6-month visit, he continued to have tremor suppression. However, he reported a new shocking and tingling sensation in his neck and jaw when turning his head in either direction or when touching the pulse generator incision site. Impedance checks showed all contact pairs using contact 8 were more than 40,000. Contact 8 was taken out of the active configuration. The tremor remained well-controlled, and the shocking sensations, which were presumably a short circuit, resolved.

OUTCOME

The patient continued to report excellent tremor suppression at the 1-year and 2-year annual follow-up visits. The most recent UPDRS score was 5 (on-stimulation and off-medication) at the 2-year annual visit.

TABLE 13.1. THRESHOLDS TABLE

Side	Electrode	Pulse Width (µsec)	Frequency (Hz)	Amplitude (V)	Therapeutic Effects	Adverse Effects	Setting
Left STN	+C–0	60	130	2.0 V max	1.0 V jaw tremor quieter, tongue movement less	2.0 V felt lightheaded, mouth-pulling, improved at 1.5 V, at 1.8 V "hard to swallow"	Threshold
Left STN	+C–1	60	130	2.3 V max	1.0 V reduced jaw tremor; 1.5 V decreased rigidity arm, leg; less right arm tremor, intermittent increase leg tremor; 2.0 V heaviness in jaw	2.3 V felt tightening in bilateral lower face, difficulty speaking	Threshold
Left STN	+C–2	60	130	3.0 V max	1.0 V reduced arm, leg and jaw tremor	1.0 V jaw feels heavy; 1.5 V jaw squeezing; 2.0 V feels like a rubber band pulling chin back; 3.0 V harder to speak; speech better when returned to 0 V	Threshold
Left STN	+C–3	60	130	2.5 V max	2.0 V reduced mouth and arm tremor, but leg tremor increased to 2+	2.0 V hard to get words out; 2.5 V bilateral jaw tightness	Threshold
Left Vim	+C–8	60	130	1.0 V max		0.8 tongue, upper and lower lip tingling and numbness, 1.0 V persists	Threshold
Left Vim	+C–9	60	130	1.4V max	1.0 V reduced mouth, arm, and leg tremor; arm tremor re-emerges at posture +4	1.0 V neck muscles pulling; 1.3 V tingling fingertips right hand, lower lip; felt weight lift when voltage zeroed	Threshold
Left Vim	+C–10	60	130	1.5 V max	1.0 V mild reduction rest tremor, present with posture	1.0 V lower lip numb, 1.4 V lightheaded	Threshold
Left Vim	+C–11	60	130	0.8 V max	0.7 V reduced jaw tremor	0.7 V lower lip tingling, 0.8 V nausea	Threshold
Left STN	–1+2	60	130	3.0 V max	1.5 V jaw tremor less, no arm tremor, intermittent right leg tremor	3.0 V slight pulling jaw	Final
Left Vim	–9+10	60	130				Final

STN = subthalamic nucleus; Vim = ventral intermediate (thalamus).

TABLE 13.2. PROGRAMMING PARAMETERS AT BASELINE AND SUBSEQUENT VISITS

Programming Session	Left STN	Left Vim
1	−1, + 2; 1.00 V; PW 60 μsec; 130 Hz	−9, +10; 0.50 V; PW 60 μsec; 130 Hz
2 (Arrival)	−1, +2; 1.55V; PW 60 μsec; 130 Hz	−9, +10;1.00 V; PW 60 μsec; 130 Hz
2 (Final)	+0, −1, −2, +3;1.30 V; PW 60 μsec;130 Hz	+8, −9, −10, +11;1.00 V ;PW 60 μsec; 130 Hz
3	+0, −1, −2, +3;1.80 V; PW 60 μsec;130 Hz	−9, −10,+11; 2.00 V; PW 60 μsec;130 Hz
4 (First annual visit)	+0, −1, −2, +3;1.90 V;PW 60 μsec; 130 Hz	−9, −10, +11; 2.50 V; PW 60 μsec;130 Hz
5 (Second annual visit)	+0, −1, −2, +3;1.90 V; PW 60 μsec;130 Hz	−9, −10, +11; 2.50 V; PW 60 μsec;130 Hz

PW = pulse width; STN = subthalamic nucleus; Vim = ventral intermediate (thalamus).

DISCUSSION

This case illustrates a common scenario encountered when planning the optimal DBS target to relieve both medication-refractory tremor and motor fluctuations in PD, particularly when tremor is the main concern. Vim thalamus, STN, and globus pallidus interna (GPi) are all targets reported to improve PD tremor, while the latter two also address PD motor complications.[1,2] Vim was the original target of choice approved for medication-refractory PD tremor.[3] However, this target does not treat bradykinesia or motor fluctuations of PD,[4] and it may worsen speech, especially if used bilaterally.[5] On the other hand, STN and GPi DBS targets provide effective treatment of tremor associated with PD, in addition to other parkinsonian motor features.[2,6] It has been debated which of the targets is superior for PD tremor. Fraix and colleagues concluded that STN was more favorable for tremor, even in PD patients with prior Vim thalamic DBS.[7] While STN, GPi, and Vim thalamus help PD tremor in the short term, it is unclear which is optimal long term. Recently, Vim DBS was reported to be an effective long-term treatment for PD tremor lasting more than 10 years.[8]

There are limited data on implanting two targets simultaneously to suppress PD tremor, as illustrated by our case. Most cases in the literature report staged surgeries, following unsuccessful outcomes with the first target.[7,9] In our case, the staging was performed in real-time in the operating room after assessing immediate tremor response. Whether staged or performed simultaneously during a single surgery, combining two targets may have a synergistic effect. Additive effects of dual electrodes have been reported for a combination of targets. Sequential Vim and STN was beneficial in PD tremor in a small case series[7] and a case report,[9] and a combination of Vim and STN targets has been recommended for Holmes tremor.[10] Other combinations include GPi and STN for PD.[11]

Additionally, the effectiveness of tremor suppression by DBS may reflect the pathologic underpinnings of PD tremor. This may be important to consider because PD tremor has different components. It can be divided into rest and re-emergent tremors, which appear to have a dopaminergic basis, and PD postural tremor, which appears to have in some cases a nondopaminergic basis, suggesting two different oscillatory circuits.[12] Vim thalamic DBS is proposed to modulate a network of structural connectivity comprising primary motor, premotor, supplementary motor, pallidal, cerebellar sites, and the brainstem,[13] which may explain its benefit on all PD tremor subtypes. In comparison, STN DBS also shows ability to suppress rest, re-emergent, and postural PD tremor, possibly through the central oscillator in STN (dopaminergic) or other networks (nondopaminergic) but is less well understood.[6,14] It is effective for severe off/on medication tremor as well as for off-medication action tremor in PD.[14]

Thus, in the preoperative assessment, it is important to carefully consider selection of the DBS target, with a second backup target if necessary to adequately suppress tremor.

PEARLS

- For intraoperative stimulation refractory PD tremor, consider adding a second DBS target (dual DBS targets). This was preplanned in our case. There is, however, a disadvantage to making this decision in the operating room because in some cases more detailed programming in the clinic may resolve the tremor.
- The presence of re-emergent tremor may render it hard to separate how much postural tremor exists in a patient. Many expert centers find adding Vim DBS to be useful when more than a mild postural action tremor exists. In our case, one clue was the presence of proximal shoulder tremor.
- Lead location in our cases may have been suboptimal as evidenced by imaging and programming thresholds. It is possible that a slightly better placement of the STN lead may have obviated the need for a second Vim lead. This scenario was previously published by Stover and colleagues.[15]

REFERENCES

1. Hariz MI, Krack P, Alesch F, et al. Multicentre European study of thalamic stimulation for parkinsonian tremor: a 6 year follow-up. J Neurol Neurosurg Psychiatry 2008;79:694–699.
2. Peppe A, Pierantozzi M, Bassi A, et al. Stimulation of the subthalamic nucleus compared with the globus pallidus internus in patients with Parkinson disease. J Neurosurg 2004;101:195–200.
3. Ondo W, Jankovic J, Schwartz K, Almaguer M, Simpson RK. Unilateral thalamic deep brain stimulation for refractory essential tremor and Parkinson's disease tremor. Neurology 1998;51:1063–1069.
4. Limousin P, Speelman JD, Gielen F, Janssens M. Multicentre European study of thalamic stimulation in parkinsonian and essential tremor. J Neurol Neurosurg Psychiatry 1999;66:289–296.
5. Putzke JD, Uitti RJ, Obwegeser AA, Wszolek ZK, Wharen RE. Bilateral thalamic deep brain stimulation: midline tremor control. J Neurol Neurosurg Psychiatry 2005;76:684–690.
6. Diamond A, Shahed J, Jankovic J. The effects of subthalamic nucleus deep brain stimulation on parkinsonian tremor. J Neurol Sci 2007;260:199–203.
7. Fraix V, Pollak P, Moro E, et al. Subthalamic nucleus stimulation in tremor dominant parkinsonian patients with previous thalamic surgery. J Neurol Neurosurg Psychiatry 2005;76:246–248.
8. Cury RG, Fraix V, Castrioto A, et al. Thalamic deep brain stimulation for tremor in Parkinson disease, essential tremor, and dystonia. Neurology 2017;89:1416–1423.
9. Oertel MF, Schupbach WM, Ghika JA, et al. Combined thalamic and subthalamic deep brain stimulation for tremor-dominant Parkinson's disease. Acta Neurochir (Wien) 2017;159:265–269.
10. Romanelli P, Bronte-Stewart H, Courtney T, Heit G. Possible necessity for deep brain stimulation of both the ventralis intermedius and subthalamic nuclei to resolve Holmes tremor: case report. J Neurosurg 2003;99:566–571.
11. Mazzone P, Brown P, Dilazzaro V, et al. Bilateral implantation in globus pallidus internus and in subthalamic nucleus in Parkinson's disease. Neuromodulation 2005;8:1–6.
12. Dirkx MF, Zach H, Bloem BR, Hallett M, Helmich RC. The nature of postural tremor in Parkinson disease. Neurology 2018;90:e1095–e1103.
13. Klein JC, Barbe MT, Seifried C, et al. The tremor network targeted by successful VIM deep brain stimulation in humans. Neurology 2012;78:787–795.
14. Kim HJ, Jeon BS, Paek SH, et al. Bilateral subthalamic deep brain stimulation in Parkinson disease patients with severe tremor. Neurosurgery 2010;67:626–632; discussion 632.
15. Stover NP, Okun MS, Evatt ML, Raju DV, Bakay RA, Vitek JL. Stimulation of the subthalamic nucleus in a patient with Parkinson disease and essential tremor. Arch Neurol 2005;62:141–143.

Case 14

Use of Constant Current Mode to Allow Both Monopolar and Bipolar Interleaving at a Single Contact

MEREDITH SPINDLER AND LANA CHAHINE

INDICATION FOR DEEP BRAIN STIMULATION

Parkinson disease (PD) with rest tremor, motor fluctuations, and dyskinesias

CLINICAL HISTORY AND RELEVANT EXAM

The patient is a 56-year-old woman who was diagnosed with PD in 2006 and over time developed severe tremor, motor fluctuations, and peak-dose dystonic and choreiform dyskinesias requiring treatment with dopaminergic medications every 2 hours. She was evaluated for deep brain stimulation (DBS) surgery and in October 2013 had bilateral subthalamic nucleus (STN) DBS and two single-channel implantable pulse generators (IPGs) (Medtronic Activa SC) placed using a stereotactic frame with magnetic resonance imaging (MRI)-derived targets, microelectrode recording (MER), and intraoperative test stimulation. One left frontal microelectrode tract was performed, and four right frontal microelectrode tracts were performed. Her immediate postoperative course was uncomplicated. She had a prominent but transient microlesion effect lasting 3 days after surgery with nearly complete resolution of her motor symptoms bilaterally.

COMPLICATIONS

Although DBS clearly improved tremor, programming of the right lead was challenging because of the side effect of diplopia at low voltages using ventral contacts and at higher voltages using the third contact. The most dorsal contact provided substantial but insufficient tremor relief and resulted in blepharospasm and dysarthria at higher voltages. Postoperative MRI confirmed ventral placement of the right lead, which terminated in the ventral substantia nigra (Figure 14.1A–C). She ultimately required right STN lead revision surgery in 2015, with resultant placement more dorsal in the right STN (Figure 14.1D–F).

In May 2016, the patient required battery replacement. She opted to change from the two single-channel IPGs to a single dual-channel rechargeable IPG (Medtronic Activa RC). Intraoperatively, her new Activa RC was programmed to interleave the two right lead programs with one program on the left lead, all at 125 Hz (because one IPG cannot stimulate two electrodes at differing frequencies in the interleaving mode). She experienced refractory tremor of her right side soon after IPG replacement.

TROUBLESHOOTING

Before resorting to revision of the R STN lead, several settings on the right lead were trialed. Monopolar stimulation of contact 3 was insufficient for tremor control and at higher voltages caused blepharospasm and dysarthria. Bipolar stimulation, whether with a single or double cathode, was insufficient for tremor control. Double monopolar stimulation using contacts 2 and 3 caused multiple side effects on various trials, including dysarthria, neck tightness, blepharospasm, and diplopia at higher voltages. Interleaving of single monopolar contacts 2 and 3 did not achieve adequate tremor control without causing diplopia. Interleaving of monopolar stimulation of contact 3 with bipolar stimulation of contact 3 (2+ 3–) required use of constant current mode with various amplitude ratios and pulse widths and was inadequate for tremor control and limited by the side effects of blepharospasm

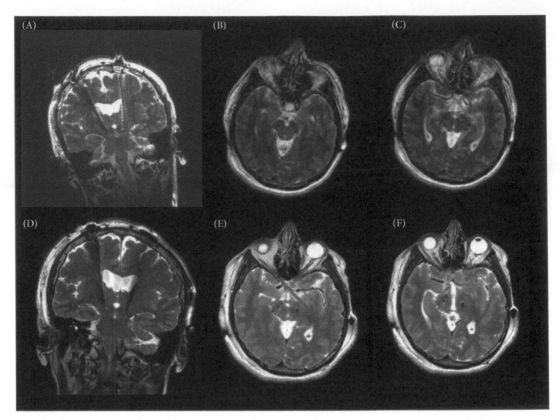

FIGURE 14.1. Postoperative brain magnetic resonance images after initial DBS placement in the (A) coronal and (B, C) axial planes illustrating ventral placement of right lead terminating in ventral substantia nigra; of left lead terminating in dorsal substantia nigra; and after right lead revision in the (D) coronal and (F, F) axial planes illustrating placement of the right lead terminating in the subthalamic nucleus.

and dysarthria. Ventral placement of a right STN lead was suspected based on the side effect of diplopia with multiple contacts, suggesting either stimulation of the oculomotor region of the STN, located ventrolaterally, or stimulation of the oculomotor fibers, located ventrally and medially. Postoperative MRI suggested ventrolateral placement (see Figure 14.1A–C), and right STN electrode was revised in August 2015, using a stereotactic frame with MRI-derived targets, a single microelectrode recording tract, and intraoperative test stimulation. Postoperative MRI revealed placement of the tip of the new lead in the right STN (see Figure 14.1D–F). After the surgical revision, monopolar review was re-performed in constant voltage mode, with significantly improved therapeutic window at all contacts. Contacts 1 and 2 provided the best tremor control. However, with time, titration in single monopolar mode of contact 1 was insufficient for tremor control and of contact 2 caused facial tightness. These were

ultimately interleaved, with successful control of tremor. Her settings for both IPGs in April 2016 are outlined in Table 14.1.

After implantation of a single rechargeable IPG, a shared frequency of 125 Hz of the interleaved programs of the right lead and the single program of the left lead was required. The frequency reduction from 185 to 125 Hz resulted in re-emergence of the previously well-controlled right-sided tremor, despite increasing voltage to compensate. Elimination of interleaving mode on the right lead to enable the higher frequency of 185 Hz bilaterally caused dystonia, dysarthria, and inadequate control of left-sided tremor. Thus, in order to allow adjustment of frequency without compromising the tenuous symptom control of her left side, it was determined that interleaving would be required for her left lead as well, to allow a combined frequency of 250 Hz. Her current setting of monopolar stimulation of contact 3 had been chosen because of exacerbation

TABLE 14.1. PROGRAMMING PARAMETERS

Date	Device	Mode	Side	Contacts Active	Amplitude	Frequency (Hz)	Pulse Width	Impedance (Ohm)	Measured current
April 2016	Right Activa SC	Constant voltage	R1	C+ 1–	2.8 V	125	60	1087	2.417
			R2	C+ 2–	2.5 V	125	60	1046	2.587
	Left Activa SC		Left	C+ 3–	3.2 V	185	90	1104	2.941
May2016	Activa RC	Constant current	R1	C+ 1–	2.8 mA	125	60	877	
			R2	C+ 2–	2.6 mA		60	858	
			L1	C+ 3–	3.1 mA	125	100	985	
			L2	2+ 3–	4.7 mA		100	1339	
October 2017	Activa RC	Constant Current	R1	C+ 0–	2.5 mA	125	90	828	
			R2	C+ 2–	1.8 mA		90	986	
			L1	C+ 3–	3.5 mA	125	100	769	
			L2	2+ 3–	4.7 mA		100	875	

R1 = right STN1; R2 = right STN2; L1 = left STN1; L2 = left STN2.

of on-dystonia with the more ventral contacts. Interleaving of contacts 2 and 3 in monopolar mode did not achieve tremor control without the side effect of being painful on dystonia. Thus, it was determined that the best results would likely be achieved by interleaving two programs (allowing 250 Hz stim) that both employed contact 3 as cathode; that is, monopolar stimulation of contact 3 interleaved with bipolar mode using contact 3 as cathode and contact 2 as anode (see Table 14.1, May 2016). Such a setting is prohibited in constant voltage mode; thus, both electrodes were reprogrammed in constant current mode. The current amplitude was adjusted gradually in the office and at home until tremor control was achieved. Over the same time period, tremor control on her left side waned, and this side was reprogrammed to interleave monopolar stimulation of contacts 0 and 2 (instead of 1 and 2), using a wider pulse width due to the larger span between contacts, with improved tremor control (see Table 14, 1, October 2017).

OUTCOME

The patient had good control of motor fluctuations and tremor with minimal dyskinesias at final settings (see Table 14.1, October 2017). Side effects from stimulation consisted of very mild blepharospasm. Final levodopa equivalent daily dose (LEDD) was 420 mg.

DISCUSSION

Most PD patients who undergo bilateral STN DBS achieve significant benefit with minimal side effects using conventional programming approaches. However, in a subset, symptom control is not possible below the side-effect threshold using conventional settings. In such patients, as our case highlights, electrode placement needs to be confirmed and lead revision surgery considered if symptom control is suboptimal despite best programming techniques to troubleshoot a suboptimally positioned electrode. Additionally, our case also illustrates the successful use of interleaved programs in both the constant voltage and constant current modes.

Interleaving stimulation was first introduced in Activa SC, PC, and RC models of the Medtronic DBS stimulator (Medtronic, Minneapolis, MN). With interleaving, done primarily in the constant voltage mode, stimulation rapidly "toggles" between two programs in an alternating fashion on the same lead. Each of the two programs may apply different amplitudes, pulse widths, and electrode contacts in monopolar or bipolar configuration (Figure 14.2). The active contact

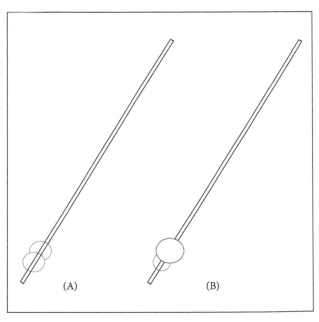

(A)   (B)

FIGURE 14.2. (A) Conventional double monopolar mode, in which each stimulus delivers current through both contacts with the same amplitude and pulse width, thus with the same volume of tissue activated. (B) Interleaving, in which stimuli alternate between contacts, can be programmed with differing amplitudes and pulse widths and thus with differing volumes of tissue activated.

(cathode) is stimulated at a *net* maximum frequency of 250 Hz, or 125 Hz for each program. Interleaving has been purported to achieve "current shaping," wherein the individualized current fields are directed to minimize stimulation of off-target anatomic regions in and around the STN. For example, interleaving an adjacent dorsal contact can steer current dorsally and thus away from ventral structures that may be causing side effects.

As with all DBS programming approaches, the application of interleaving stimulation is individualized to the specific patient. There are, however, several situations in which it is important to consider application of interleaving.[1] For example, in some instances, conventional programming to achieve motor control is limited due to corticobulbar and corticospinal side effects. Typically, two adjacent contacts have slightly different thresholds for benefit and side effects. In such cases, interleaving those two contacts, each programmed just under its threshold for side effects, can achieve greater motor control with fewer side effects than conventional double monopolar or double bipolar mode.[2] More specifically, applying higher stimulation amplitude at a more dorsal contact and lower amplitude at a more ventral contact may achieve tremor control while minimizing dysarthria.[1,2] Applying different programming settings to more dorsal versus more ventral contacts may also allow for the treatment of different PD manifestations[1] (e.g., targeting tremor vs. hypokinesia and/or rigidity,[3] or targeting parkinsonism vs. dyskinesia[4]). A third application of interleaving is in the treatment of patients with PD and comorbid essential tremor (ET). Strategic lead implantation and subsequent interleaving programming may achieve PD and ET symptom control potentially with stimulation of both the dorsolateral STN and ventrolateral anterior thalamic region near the ventral intermediate (Vim) nucleus of the thalamus.[5]

The constant current mode is also a relatively recent introduction in the United States, first available in the Activa SC, PC, and RC models of the Medtronic DBS stimulator, although it had been available previously in devices manufactured by St. Jude Medical in other parts of the world. Older Medtronic models (R, TM, or C superscripts) delivered stimulation only in constant voltage mode. To understand the implications of this, consider the characteristics that govern how much electrical stimulation is ultimately applied at the neuronal level. Ohm's law ($I = V/R$) dictates that the delivered current (I) is a function of the voltage (V) divided by the resistance (R), also known as impedance. Impedance is determined by stimulation frequency as well as electrode characteristics, the interface between the electrode and brain tissue, and properties/activity of the brain tissue itself.[6] Impedance is not constant over time but varies as a result of several factors. For example, in the immediate postoperative period, impedance slowly increases as the mild edema in the area surrounding the recently placed electrode resolves. In the constant voltage mode, the current that is ultimately delivered will vary based on the impedance. However, fluctuations in impedance continue to occur even with chronic stimulation.[7] On the other hand, in the constant current mode, a constant current is maintained through a built-in mechanism that adjusts the voltage as the impedance changes. This ensures stability of the size of the current field over time. What little data are available suggest that there are not significant differences in clinical outcomes in the application of constant current versus constant voltage stimulation.[8] Constant current stimulation may increase battery drain, a consideration in patients who do not have rechargeable IPGs. However, there are some cases in which constant current stimulation is required for practical reasons, as is depicted in our case. In constant voltage mode, not all charge delivered with each pulse is fully recovered when the pulse is completed, leaving residual charge on the electrodes being used. This accumulated charge can affect the total charge delivered with a second interleaved pulse using the same contact. To avoid this, programs interleaved in constant voltage mode are prohibited from using the same active contact in certain configurations (Medtronic Inc., personal communication), again as illustrated in our case. On the other hand, constant current mode more directly controls the amount of charge delivered and thus is not affected by residual charge, allowing interleaved programs to have shared cathodes.

PEARLS

- DBS lead placement should be investigated and revision surgery should be considered if symptom control remains suboptimal despite best programming techniques.
- Replacement of two single-channel IPGs with one dual-channel IPG can disrupt therapeutic efficacy if different stimulation frequencies were used for optimal symptom control, with one side being conventionally programmed and the other requiring interleaved programs.
- Interleaving should be considered if differential and near simultaneous stimulation of two active contacts affords better symptom control than conventional programming (monopolar, bipolar, or double monopolar).
- Constant current mode, but not constant voltage mode, allows for interleaving two programs using the same active contact.

REFERENCES

1. Miocinovic S, Khemani P, Whiddon R, Zeilman P, Martinez-Ramirez D, Okun MS, Chitnis S. Outcomes, management, and potential mechanisms of interleaving deep brain stimulation settings. *Parkinsonism Relat Disord.* 2014;20:1434–1437.
2. Barbe MT, Dembek TA, Becker J, Raethjen J, Hartinger M, Meister IG, Runge M, Maarouf M, Fink GR, Timmermann L. Individualized current-shaping reduces DBS-induced dysarthria in patients with essential tremor. *Neurology.* 2014;82:614–619.
3. Ramirez-Zamora A, Kahn M, Campbell J, DeLaCruz P, Pilitsis JG. Interleaved programming of subthalamic deep brain stimulation to avoid adverse effects and preserve motor benefit in Parkinson's disease. *J Neurol.* 2015;262:578–584.
4. Wojtecki L, Vesper J, Schnitzler A. Interleaving programming of subthalamic deep brain stimulation to reduce side effects with good motor outcome in a patient with Parkinson's disease. *Parkinsonism Relat Disord.* 2011;17:293–294.
5. Baumann CR, Imbach LL, Baumann-Vogel H, Uhl M, Sarnthein J, Surucu O. Interleaving deep brain stimulation for a patient with both Parkinson's disease and essential tremor. *Mov Disord.* 2012;27:1700–1701.
6. Bronstein JM, Tagliati M, McIntyre C, Chen R, Cheung T, Hargreaves EL, Israel Z, Moffitt M, Montgomery EB, Stypulkowski P, Shils J, Denison T, Vitek J, Volkman J, Wertheimer J, Okun MS. The rationale driving the evolution of deep brain stimulation to constant-current devices. *Neuromodulation.* 2015;18:85–88; discussion 88–89.
7. Cheung T, Nuno M, Hoffman M, Katz M, Kilbane C, Alterman R, Tagliati M. Longitudinal impedance variability in patients with chronically implanted DBS devices. *Brain Stimul.* 2013;6:746–751.
8. Preda F, Cavandoli C, Lettieri C, Pilleri M, Antonini A, Eleopra R, Mondani M, Martinuzzi A, Sarubbo S, Ghisellini G, Trezza A, Cavallo MA, Landi A, Sensi M. Switching from constant voltage to constant current in deep brain stimulation: a multicenter experience of mixed implants for movement disorders. *Eur J Neurol.* 2016;23:190–195.

Case 15

Subthalamic Nucleus Deep Brain Stimulation May Improve Pain in the Setting of Parkinson Disease

ANJALI GERA AND GIAN PAL

INDICATION FOR DEEP BRAIN STIMULATION

Parkinson disease (PD) with motor fluctuations, dyskinesia, and levodopa-responsive pain

CLINICAL HISTORY AND RELEVANT EXAM

A 45-year-old man with PD presented with intermittent left arm resting tremor. Approximately 1 year after symptom onset he developed constant pain in his proximal and distal left arm, which gradually worsened over time. This pain was exacerbated by the tremor. He initially declined dopaminergic therapy but after approximately 5 years he began carbidopa/levodopa 25/100 mg, one tablet three times a day. Carbidopa/levodopa completely alleviated both his left arm tremor and his pain.

Over the next several years, he gradually developed motor fluctuations and dyskinesia. His *off* periods were associated with bothersome tremor and pain, and his *on* periods were associated with prominent neck and left arm dyskinesias, which resulted in significant pain. His medication regimen was modified to carbidopa/levodopa 25/100 mg tablets (five tablets per day) and amantadine 100 mg three times a day. Dyskinesia was only minimally reduced by the addition of amantadine. Eventually, his maximum levodopa equivalent daily dose (LEDD) was 800 mg per day. At age 60 years, after 15 years of PD, he underwent bilateral subthalamic nuclei (STN) deep brain stimulation (DBS) implantation with the goal of reducing prominent motor fluctuations and dyskinesia.

COMPLICATIONS

There were no complications during or after surgery.

TROUBLESHOOTING AND MANAGEMENT

One month after surgery, the patient presented for his initial DBS programming. During monopolar stimulation, his left upper extremity tremor, rigidity, motor fluctuations, and pain significantly improved. This improvement persisted during the subsequent 4-week period. Over the next 6 months, he experienced a 70% reduction in his LEDD, and he reported complete resolution of dyskinesia and neck pain.

OUTCOME

Bilateral STN DBS implantation resulted in significant improvement in motor fluctuations, dyskinesia, neck pain, and left arm pain.

DISCUSSION

This case illustrates an example of chronic limb pain that resolved following bilateral STN DBS surgery for PD. Our patient had musculoskeletal pain related to both his *off* and *on* states, and this was a significant and meaningful response to DBS. It has been reported that more than 50% of PD patients may experience chronic pain, and this pain may affect quality of life.[1–3] Pain is a heterogeneous symptom and has many causes in PD patients. Additionally, the intensity and the duration of pain can widely vary. The current subclassification of pain in PD is complicated by a lack of standardized assessments. There can be confusion in determining whether a particular source of pain may be considered possibly related to PD.[4] As a result, pain in PD is often described as directly related, indirectly related, or unrelated to PD, and this assessment is based on clinical judgment. This convention of reporting PD pain has led to variations in descriptions.[4,5] Musculoskeletal pain is the most common source of PD pain and may be experienced as rigidity, cramps, shoulder issues, spinal or hand and foot deformities, dystonic pain, or nonradicular back pain.[4,6] Other sources of PD pain to consider include neuropathic pain (peripheral or central) or pain related to akathisia, restless legs syndrome, or depression.[6,7]

Although pain related to PD is not fully understood, it is thought to be related to dysfunction of the cortical-basal ganglia-thalamic circuit. Studies have suggested that the basal ganglia circuit is involved in the processing of nociceptive inputs and in the formation of complex motor responses to pain.[8,9] For example, in rats trained in a conditioned avoidance response task, more than 80% of the neural recording sites demonstrated task-related activity in the caudate-putamen and nucleus accumbens.[10] Also, it has been shown that the medial striatum plays a role in the sensory aspects of avoidance tasks, while the motor aspects of avoidance tasks are processed by the lateral striatum, suggesting that distinct striatal regions are involved in pain processing.[10] Furthermore, bilateral striatal lesions in rats result in impaired avoidance responses.[11]

STN DBS is thought to exert an antinociceptive effect by modulating descending pain pathways in the anterior cingulate cortex and periaqueductal gray.[12] In a 6-hydroxydopamine (6-OHDA) rat model of PD, high-frequency (150 Hz) STN stimulation attenuated the firing frequency in the anterior cingulate cortex and increased neuronal activity in the periaqueductal gray, suggesting that STN DBS may decrease excitatory projections from the anterior cingulate cortex to the periaqueductal gray, resulting in modulation of descending pain pathways within the spinal cord.[13]

STN DBS has been shown to have a beneficial effect on pain (especially *off* pain[14]) in PD, and this improvement may be independent of motor function or mood.[1] In a prospective cohort study, 17 of 18 subjects (94%) had improvement in pain associated with motor fluctuations when comparing preoperative and postoperative STN DBS pain scores at 6 months. In this study, dystonic pain was the most responsive to STN DBS (100%), followed by central (92%), radicular (63%), and musculoskeletal pain (61%). Another prospective observational study examined the effects of STN DBS on pain scores in a group of 58 moderate to advanced PD patients using the McGill Pain Questionnaire (MPQ).[1] Comparing preoperative and postoperative MPQ scores, subjects had a significant reduction in total scores (pre-DBS: 13.8 ± 11.3 vs. post-DBS: 7.6 ± 6.9; $p < 0.0001$). Additionally, both affective (7.3 ± 6.8 vs. 3.0 ± 4.1; $p < 0.0001$) and sensory (6.5 ± 5.9 vs. 4.6 ± 3.7; $p = 0.03$) subscores of the MPQ were significantly reduced after surgery.[1] The improvement in pain did not correlate with motor improvement, changes to depression rating scales, or reduction in the LEDD, suggesting that STN DBS may play a role in improving both the sensory and affective components of pain. Finally, STN DBS has been observed to raise the threshold of pain in PD subjects.[14] In PD subjects with and without neuropathic pain, Dellapina and colleagues determined (1) the thresholds of subjective heat pain in STN DBS *on* and *off* conditions and (2) changes in positron emission tomography (PET) imaging in response to painful stimuli. STN DBS (*on* condition only) significantly increased the threshold of subjective heat pain and reduced pain-induced activity in the primary somatosensory cortex and insula in PD subjects with pain, but not in those without pain.

STN DBS has been associated with improvement in dystonic, musculoskeletal, and neuropathic pain, and these features may prove to be independent of motor function or status of mood.[1] Additional work will be required to determine the mechanisms by which STN DBS modulates pain pathways and pain thresholds in PD patients.

PEARLS

- Musculoskeletal pain is the most common source of PD pain and may be experienced as rigidity, cramps, shoulder disturbances, spinal or hand and foot deformities, dystonic pain, or nonradicular back pain. Other sources of pain to consider include neuropathic pain (peripheral or central) or pain related to akathisia, restless legs syndrome, or depression.
- STND BS may produce an antinociceptive effect by raising the threshold of pain and by modulating analgesia systems in the anterior cingulate cortex and periaqueductal gray, thereby altering descending pain pathways within the spinal cord.
- STN DBS for PD may be beneficial for dystonic, musculoskeletal, and neuropathic pain, and this improvement may be independent of motor function or status of mood. There are, however, cases of PD pain that may not respond to STN or GPi DBS, and when counseling patients it is important not to overestimate the potential benefits.
- STN DBS may improve pain by relieving rigidity or dystonia, and there are also reports of GPi DBS similarly improving pain.

REFERENCES

1. Pellaprat J, Ory-Magne F, Canivet C, Simonetta-Moreau M, Lotterie JA, Radji F, et al. Deep brain stimulation of the subthalamic nucleus improves pain in Parkinson's disease. Parkinsonism Relat Disord 2014;20:662–664.
2. Beiske AG, Loge JH, Ronningen A, Svensson E. Pain in Parkinson's disease: prevalence and characteristics. Pain 2009;141:173–177.
3. Broen MP, Braaksma MM, Patijn J, Weber WE. Prevalence of pain in Parkinson's disease: a systematic review using the modified QUADAS tool. Mov Disord 2012;27:480–484.
4. Lee MA, Walker RW, Hildreth TJ, Prentice WM. A survey of pain in idiopathic Parkinson's disease. J Pain Symptom Manage 2006;32:462–469.
5. Negre-Pages L, Regragui W, Bouhassira D, Grandjean H, Rascol O, DoPaMiP Study Group. Chronic pain in Parkinson's disease: the cross-sectional French DoPaMiP survey. Mov Disord 2008;23:1361–1369.
6. Blanchet PJ, Brefel-Courbon C. Chronic pain and pain processing in Parkinson's disease. Prog Neuropsychopharmacol Biol Psychiatry 2017;17:30599.
7. Ha AD, Jankovic J. Pain in Parkinson's disease. Mov Disord 2012;27:485–491.
8. Chudler EH, Dong WK. The role of the basal ganglia in nociception and pain. Pain 1995;60:3–38.
9. Borsook D, Upadhyay J, Chudler EH, Becerra L. A key role of the basal ganglia in pain and analgesia: insights gained through human functional imaging. Mol Pain 2010;6:27.
10. White IM, Rebec GV. Responses of rat striatal neurons during performance of a lever-release version of the conditioned avoidance response task. Brain Res 1993;616:71–82.
11. Kirkby RJ, Kimble DP. Avoidance and escape behavior following striatal lesions in the rat. Exp Neurol 1968;20:215–227.
12. Gee LE, Walling I, Ramirez-Zamora A, Shin DS, Pilitsis JG. Subthalamic deep brain stimulation alters neuronal firing in canonical pain nuclei in a 6-hydroxydopamine lesioned rat model of Parkinson's disease. Exp Neurol 2016;283:298–307.
13. Dellapina E, Ory-Magne F, Regragui W, Thalamas C, Lazorthes Y, Rascol O, et al. Effect of subthalamic deep brain stimulation on pain in Parkinson's disease. Pain 2012;153:2267–2273.
14. Kim HJ, Paek SH, Kim JY, Lee JY, Lim YH, Kim MR, et al. Chronic subthalamic deep brain stimulation improves pain in Parkinson disease. J Neurol 2008;255:1889–1894.

Case 16

Deep Brain Stimulation–Responsive Camptocormia in Parkinson Disease

ELENA CALL AND HELEN BRONTE-STEWART

INDICATIONS FOR DEEP BRAIN STIMULATION

Medication-responsive, positional camptocormia, motor fluctuations, and dyskinesia

CLINICAL HISTORY AND RELEVANT EXAM

A 66-year-old man with history of Parkinson disease (PD), primary biliary cirrhosis, gout, osteoarthritis, and chronic hyponatremia presented to the Stanford Movement Disorders Clinic for consideration of deep brain stimulation (DBS) surgery. The onset of his PD was 5 years prior with resting tremor of the left hand, bradykinesia left greater than right, decreased left arm swing, and a truncal tilt to the right. His symptoms progressed over the next several years to include imbalance, freezing of gait, slurred speech, hypophonia, and progressive flexion of the thoracic trunk with rightward tilt, and we diagnosed camptocormia. The camptocormia was not evident when he was supine; there was progressive involuntary flexion of the thoracic trunk to about 30 degrees when he sat up, which increased to 70 to 90 degrees as he stood up and resulted in profound gait impairment. He exhibited an approximately 20-degree tilt to the right. He also demonstrated severe freezing of gait (FOG), on gait initiation, when walking through doorways, along a straight corridor, and when turning but was able to ambulate unassisted for short periods, although he required the use of a cane during normal daily function. He had severe retropulsion but was able to stand unassisted for short periods of time.

The patient's medication regimen consisted of immediate-release carbidopa/levodopa; the onset of medication effect was approximately 30 to 40 minutes after administration, and its effects wore off 2 hours later. He reported feeling in the *on*-state about 50% of the day, although the *on*-state was complicated by dyskinesias. His goals for DBS surgery included improvement of his posture, gait, balance, and dyskinesias. His Unified Parkinson's Disease Rating Scale (UPDRS) score was 23 on and 35 off dopaminergic medication, with improvement in resting tremor, bradykinesia, posture, gait, and FOG. There was partial improvement of the camptocormia: upon standing his truncal flexion was about 10 degrees, but as he walked the thoracic flexion increased to about 30 degrees; his gait speed and FOG also improved, and the issue was present only when turning. However, his lateral tilt was similar to the off state. He underwent formal neuropsychiatric testing, which was notable for no significant executive function or word-finding deficits. Since his postural abnormalities resolved in a recumbent position, it appeared his camptocormia was related to PD/dystonia rather than to a fixed skeletal deformity. This and the partial improvement in camptocormia on medication were discussed in detail at the DBS surgical review board and swayed the decision to approve his candidacy for DBS; he had no other exclusion criteria. He underwent bilateral subthalamic nuclei (STN) DBS lead implantation using frameless functional stereotaxy and intraoperative microelectrode recording, microstimulation, and macrostimulation.

COMPLICATIONS

Severe camptocormia, dyskinesias, freezing of gait, postural instability.

TROUBLESHOOTING AND MANAGEMENT

At the time of initial programming, the patient reported improvement of his tremor and

TABLE 16.1. SUBTHALAMIC NUCLEUS DEEP BRAIN STIMULATION PARAMETERS
AFTER INITIAL PROGRAMMING

	Electrode Configuration	Voltage (V)	Pulse Width (microsec)	Frequency (Hz)
Left STN	2–	1.5	60	130
Right STN	9–	2.0	60	130

STN = subthalamic nucleus.

camptocormia after the DBS procedure, suggesting a microlesion effect. His initial UPDRS III score off medication and before turning on his DBS stimulator was 37. After initial DBS programming (Table 16.1), his UPDRS III score off medication, on high frequency (130 Hz) STN DBS improved to 16, representing a 57% improvement from STN DBS alone. At his second programming session, his R STN settings (Table 16.2) were changed to a double monopolar configuration with great improvement of his posture, gait, and rigidity on the left and a reduction in his UPDRS III score to 13. After 14 months of STN DBS, off medication, his camptocormia had resolved completely, and his FOG was limited to some hesitation when turning; he had no retropulsion and no dyskinesia.

OUTCOME

This case presented a possible option for consideration of STN DBS in a PD patient with camptocormia: the camptocormia was responsive to dopaminergic medication and satisfied standard DBS inclusion criteria; it also resolved in the supine position, suggesting a functional not skeletal disorder, which would not be amenable to DBS. However, the camptocormia was not expected to completely resolve after STN DBS because medication only resulted in partial improvement and was associated with dyskinesia. The time course of the improvement in camptocormia was similar to dystonia because there was progressive improvement over several months to a year. The patient continues to follow up in our clinic, and the effect of DBS on his camptocormia has been sustained for more than 5 years.

DISCUSSION

Camptocormia is defined as an involuntary flexion of the spine and is observed in approximately 3 to 17% of PD patients[1,2] after 7 to 8 years of disease.[1] Clinically, camptocormia is aggravated by action, particularly walking and standing, and improves when patients are in a recumbent position. There are multiple theories for the pathophysiology of camptocormia, with many attributing the phenomenon to dystonia of the muscles involved in flexion of the spine. Others believe that it may result from myopathy affecting muscles involved in spinal extension.[3]

Unfortunately, camptocormia in PD is frequently refractory to treatment with dopaminergic medications. Studies have shown that a low percentage of patients can gain some relief from Botox injections of the rectus abdominus and external oblique muscles, although the majority of patients received no benefit.[3] This case illustrates that, in carefully selected patients, camptocormia can be treated effectively with DBS. In our patient's case, his camptocormia was positional and not fixed, which is an important distinction because postural abnormalities that are fixed in nature are unlikely to improve with DBS stimulation.

TABLE 16.2. SUBTHALAMIC NUCLEUS DEEP BRAIN STIMULATION PARAMETERS
AFTER 3 MONTHS OF TREATMENT

	Electrode Configuration	Voltage (V)	Pulse Width (microsec)	Frequency (Hz)
Left STN	2–	1.8	60	130
Right STN	9–, 10–	2.4	60	130

STN = subthalamic nucleus.

DBS has been used to treat severe, medication-refractory camptocormia in a total of 47 patients in the literature according to a review of 361 published articles by Chieng and colleagues in 2015.[4] In 93% of these DBS surgeries, groups targeted the STN bilaterally, with the remaining 7% targeting the globus pallidus interna (GPi) bilaterally. Among these patients, there was a range of outcomes, with 68% reporting marked improvement in their symptoms and 32% reporting no improvement in their camptocormia.[4] Few studies have quantified this improvement with measurements of flexion angle of the spine, but a small study of 17 patients by Yamada and colleagues showed that the thoracolumbar angle improved by greater than 50% in half of their patients after bilateral STN DBS implantation.[5] The other half of their cohort responded poorly, with less than 20% improvement of their thoracolumbar angle.

Because response to DBS surgery is variable, it is important to identify clinical features that may predict whether individual patients are likely to have camptocormia that may be responsive to DBS. In the previously mentioned study by Yamada, improvement of camptocormia was negatively correlated with the preoperative severity of the camptocormia in the on state. Additionally, camptocormia was less likely to respond if the symptoms were of longer duration, particularly if onset was greater than 1.5 years.[5] Our patient's camptocormia responded better to DBS than to dopaminergic medication, as has been observed in other reported cases in the literature.

Overall, DBS can be an excellent treatment option for patients with severe camptocormia that is medically refractory in carefully selected candidates. Further research is needed to help define criteria to predict its efficacy and to clarify whether response to dopaminergic medication is clearly associated with positive outcomes.

PEARLS

- Severe camptocormia partially responsive to dopaminergic medication, if not associated with a fixed skeletal deformity, might respond to bilateral high-frequency STN DBS.
- There are fewer cases using GPi DBS, but this also be a brain target option.
- The available literature suggests that camptocormia may be more likely to respond to DBS earlier in its clinical presentation (in the first 1.5 years) than later, although further research is needed.
- Our case suggests that a combination of resolution of camptocormia in the supine position and improvement on dopaminergic medication may predict a good response of camptocormia to STN DBS. Further research with a larger number of well-characterized PD camptocormia subjects will help to support and refine these predictive features.
- There is suspicion in some cases that the camptocormia may be a DBS-responsive dystonic symptom; however, this remains unknown.

REFERENCES

1. Margraf NG, Wrede A, Deuschl G, Schulz-Schaeffer WJ. Pathophysiological concepts and treatment of camptocormia. *J Parkinsons Dis* 2016;6:485–501.
2. Tiple D, Fabbrini G, Colosimo C, Ottaviani D, Camerota F, Defazio G, Berardelli A. Camptocormia in Parkinson disease: an epidemiological and clinical study. *J Neurol Neurosurg Psychiatry* 2009;80:145–148.
3. Srivanitchapoom P, Hallet M. Camptocormia in Parkinson's disease: definition, epidemiology, pathogenesis and treatment modalities. *J Neurol Neurosurg Psychiatry* 2015;87:75–85.
4. Chieng LO, Madhavan K, Wang MY. Deep brain stimulation as a treatment for Parkinson's disease related camptocormia. *J Clin Neurosci* 2015;22:1555–1561.
5. Yamada K, Shinojima N, Hamasaki T, Kuratsu J. Subthalamic nucleus stimulation improves Parkinson's disease-associated camptocormia in parallel to its preoperative levodopa responsiveness. *J Neurol Neurosurg Psychiatry* 2015;87:703–709.

Case 17

Deactivation of One Subthalamic Nucleus Deep Brain Stimulation Device to Address Brittle Ipsilateral Dyskinesia in a Patient With Tremor-Dominant Parkinson Disease

JULIA KROTH, SUSANNE SCHNEIDER, AND SERGIU GROPPA

INDICATION FOR DEEP BRAIN STIMULATION

Parkinson disease (PD) with left-sided resting tremor, rigidity, bradykinesia, and gait freezing

CLINICAL HISTORY AND RELEVANT EXAM

A 78-year-old right handed woman with a 10-year history of tremor-dominant PD was evaluated for possible deep brain stimulation (DBS) therapy. At the time of presentation, a left-sided low-frequency resting tremor with associated rigidity, bradykinesia, fluctuations, and gait freezing was appreciated. These symptoms had worsened over the previous 2 years and did not improve after optimization of the pharmacologic treatment. No cognitive deficits were revealed in the neuropsychological assessment. Magnetic resonance imaging (MRI) attested only a minor symmetric atrophy. The patient had a significant improvement (>35%) in the levodopa challenge. After exclusion of contraindications, bilateral subthalamic nucleus (STN) DBS was discussed and recommended.

COMPLICATIONS

The implantation of STN electrodes (a multiple-source, constant-current, eight-contact omnidirectional DBS system) was performed without complications. The postoperative leads projection on preoperative MRI is shown in Figure 17.1.

Bradykinesia, rigidity, and left-sided tremor improved during surgery; the STN stimulation was started on the third day after implantation. The patient's medication was subsequently reduced. During the first 3 weeks after implantation, most of the motor symptoms improved considerably.

During the postoperative rehabilitation, the left-sided resting tremor re-emerged. With personalized programming and an increase in current to control tremor suppression, the patient developed painful dyskinesia and hemiballism of the right side of the body, mainly in the lower limb. Moreover, gait worsened significantly, and the patient presented unsteadiness. To control the right-sided dyskinesia, the dopaminergic medication was further reduced. Increases in the current amplitude on the right STN slightly improved the left-sided resting tremor, while ipsilateral dyskinesias worsened. The programming for the left STN was kept unchanged, and ipsilateral hemiballism was persistent.

TROUBLESHOOTING AND MANAGEMENT

Programming steps were undertaken by adapting the stimulation from one active contact to current steering over two contacts (most superior and third dorsal), thereby changing the distribution of the current achieved in the tissue between two active contacts for tremor and antiparkinsonian control.[1,2] A further adaptation of medication was also required. Six weeks after implantation, the clinical situation stabilized, and the left-sided tremor was well-controlled under combination DBS plus medication therapy. Right-sided dyskinesia improved but fluctuated during the day. In the next 3 months, the resting tremor was stable,

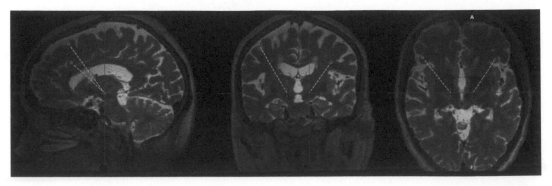

FIGURE 17.1. Postoperative computed tomography coregistration on preoperative magnetic resonance images in sagittal, coronal, and axial (transverse) presentation. The *dashed lines* represent the DBS electrodes trajects with leads position in the subthalamic nucleus. A = anterior, P = posterior.

but the dyskinesia of the right body increased. A further survey of the electrodes was performed, but no definitive control was achieved on omnidirectional lead configurations. During the off phases of stimulation, a considerable direct improvement of hyperkinesia was noted, and the decision to turn off the left STN electrode was made. A rescue lead with left globus pallidus interna (GPi) lead was considered but was declined by the patient, who did not agree on a new surgical intervention. See Table 17.1 for programming parameters.

OUTCOME

After turning off the left STN electrode, the dyskinesia of the right body disappeared completely. In the following weeks, the amperage of the right STN electrode was increased gradually to control the left-sided resting tremor. This was possible without development of ipsilateral dyskinesia. All other motor symptoms were improved at follow-up visits.

DISCUSSION

This case shows the phenomenon of development of contralateral and ipsilateral painful dyskinesia

TABLE 17.1. PROGRAMMING PARAMETERS

Left STN	Right STN
G+ 4– (50%)/3– (50%)	G+ 13– (60%)/9– (40%)
2.2 mA	3 mA
90 μsec	90 μsec
130 Hz	130 Hz

STN = subthalamic nucleus.

and hemiballism 4 weeks after DBS surgery. Previous studies showed that STN DBS, but also GPi and pallidotomy, can ameliorate contralateral and ipsilateral dyskinesia.[2,3] Very often, dyskinesia occurs postoperatively but improves with the reduction of levodopa dosage and adaptation of stimulation parameters. DBS-induced contralateral dyskinesia may indicate optimal electrode placement.[4] In cases of refractory dyskinesia, gradual reduction of the stimulation amplitude to threshold values where dyskinesia is minimal and the optimal clinical benefit occurs is required. A slight worsening of contralateral dyskinesia after the first year and marginal benefit for ipsilateral dyskinesia by the second year have been reported.

The current views of the basal ganglia physiology suggest that modulation of ventral GPi output might induce dyskinesia, while modulation of the dorsal pallidum provides relief of dyskinesia, although this notion remains to be confirmed by large data sources. A recent study suggested an abnormal dopaminergic modulation of striatocortical networks, mainly between presupplementary motor area or primary motor cortex and putamen, may contribute to levodopa-induced dyskinesia.[5] Ipsilateral dyskinesia and hemiballism are rare conditions that might occur with STN DBS or STN lesions. However, the exact pathophysiology is not clear. A bilateral control of the motor networks from the STN might be an explanation.[5] There is no existing evidence of crossed subthalamopallidal projections or interhemispheric subthalamic connections. Another explanation might arise from ipsilateral motor control from motor and premotor cortical area outputs overlapping in the ipsilateral postcommissural putamen. Bilateral connections from premotor areas (mainly supplementary motor area) to primary motor cortex might be involved as well. The influence of bilateral STN on motor control has been documented on visuospatial processing by showing that left-sided STN DBS increased the reaction times of both hands to visual stimuli. This case illustrates the brittle dyskinesia phenomenon, which has been previously described. Slow changes over many months and use of dorsal contacts have been suggested as management options.[6] In severe cases, GPi DBS has been used as a rescue procedure.

PEARLS

- Ipsilateral dyskinesia may occur with STN DBS. Adaptation of the medication and stimulation parameters is often needed to ameliorate symptoms. Advanced programing and current steering options could (but not always will) improve the clinical outcome.
- The knowledge of the involved cerebral circuits and a better understanding of the ipsilateral and contralateral motor networks would be helpful (STN and subthalamopallidal projections or interhemispheric subthalamic connections).
- Use of more dorsal contacts and consideration of GPi DBS are options in severe cases. In our case, we achieved a good outcome by deactivating one device.

REFERENCES

1. Fleury V, Pollak P, Gere J, Tommasi G, Romito L, Combescure C, et al. Subthalamic stimulation may inhibit the beneficial effects of levodopa on akinesia and gait. Movement disorders: official journal of the Movement Disorder Society. 2016;31(9):1389–1397.
2. Fasano A, Appel-Cresswell S, Jog M, Zurowkski M, Duff-Canning S, Cohn M, et al. Medical management of Parkinson's disease after initiation of deep brain stimulation. Canadian Journal of Neurological Sciences/Journal Canadien des Sciences Neurologiques. 2016:1–9.
3. Godinho F, Thobois S, Magnin M, Guenot M, Polo G, Benatru I, et al. Subthalamic nucleus stimulation in Parkinson's disease. J Neurol. 2006;253(10):1347–1355.
4. Herzog J, Fietzek U, Hamel W, Morsnowski A, Steigerwald F, Schrader B, et al. Most effective stimulation site in subthalamic deep brain stimulation for Parkinson's disease. Movement disorders. 2004;19(9):1050–1054.
5. Muthuraman M, Koirala N, Ciolac D, Pintea B, Glaser M, Groppa S, et al. Deep brain stimulation and L-dopa therapy: concepts of action and clinical applications in Parkinson's disease. Front Neurol. 2018;9:711.
6. Allert N, Cheeran B, Deuschl G, Barbe MT, Csoti I, Ebke M, et al. Postoperative rehabilitation after deep brain stimulation surgery for movement disorders. Clin Neurophysiol. 2018 Mar;129(3):592–601.

Case 18

Management of Stimulation-Induced Dyskinesia in Parkinson Disease With Interleaving Programming Settings

VIBHASH D. SHARMA, KELLY E. LYONS, AND RAJESH PAHWA

INDICATION FOR DEEP BRAIN STIMULATION

Parkinson disease (PD) with medication-resistant tremor

CLINICAL HISTORY AND RELEVANT EXAM

A 65-year-old right-handed man with PD for 4 years was evaluated for deep brain stimulation (DBS) surgery. His most bothersome symptom was right hand tremor. He did not exhibit motor fluctuations or dyskinesia at the time of evaluation. His examination revealed marked resting tremor in the right hand, along with mild bradykinesia and rigidity. He also had mild postural and kinetic tremor in the right hand. There was no tremor in the left hand. His tremor did not respond to multiple medications, including carbidopa/levodopa (up to 1,200 mg/day), pramipexole, ropinirole, rotigotine patch, amantadine, or trihexyphenidyl—all tried at therapeutic doses. All the medications were slowly discontinued because of poor tremor response and tolerability issues. After careful evaluation, he was determined to be a reasonable candidate for unilateral DBS for tremor control. While awake, he underwent a left subthalamic nucleus (STN) DBS lead implantation (Medtronic type 3389, Medtronic, Minneapolis, MN) with the assistance of intraoperative microelectrode recording. There were no abnormalities noted on the postoperative brain computed tomography (CT) scan and the lead appeared reasonably well placed.

COMPLICATIONS

When the patient presented 1 week following his surgery for placement of the implantable pulse generator (IPG), the patient and family reported new onset of headache for 2 to 3 days, which was progressively worsening. There was no nausea, vomiting, fever, or focal weakness. His neurologic examination did not differ from the presurgical examination. A head CT showed a small amount of hypodensity surrounding the lead in the left frontal lobe that was consistent with mild edema. He was treated with dexamethasone and levetiracetam tapered over 10 days. His headache resolved within a week. A follow-up head CT 3 weeks after surgery showed nearly complete resolution of the edema. He underwent placement of the IPG 4 weeks after the initial lead placement.

The patient presented for initial monopolar DBS programming 6 weeks after DBS lead implantation. During the screening visit, he did not report any new bothersome symptoms. His neurologic examination showed marked resting tremor in the right hand. After extensive screening of contacts at pulse width 60 µsec and a frequency of 130 Hz, contact 1 was determined to be most therapeutic for tremor control. There were no motor or sensory side effects at any contact up to a maximum of 4 V. At the initial visit, he had adequate tremor control with stimulation at contact 1 (case +, 1–, 2 V, 60 µsec, 150 Hz). After a few days, the patient reported worsening of tremor. At the follow-up programming visit, the stimulation parameters were adjusted, and he was switched to double monopolar programming (case +, 1– 2–, 3 V, 60 µsec, 130 Hz), which resulted in excellent tremor suppression; however, within a few days, he developed bothersome right foot dyskinesia.

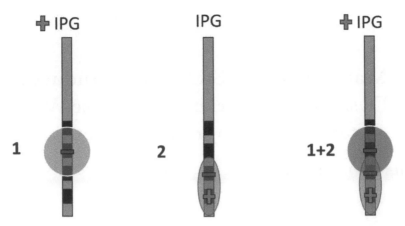

FIGURE 18.1. Representation of interleaving settings on DBS lead: 1—monopolar stimulation at contact 2; 2—bipolar stimulation with stimulation at most therapeutic contact 1; 1+2—interleaving settings. IPG = implantable pulse generator.

TROUBLESHOOTING AND MANAGEMENT

The patient was evaluated for a follow-up programming visit due to onset of stimulation-induced right foot dyskinesia. Because he was not taking dopaminergic medications, management was focused on adjusting stimulation. On reducing the voltage to 2 V, dyskinesia improved, but his tremor worsened. Switching him to contacts 2 and 3 did not provide adequate tremor control. He was switched to a different bipolar configuration with stimulation at contact 1 (3+ 1–, 90 μsec, 130 Hz; 2+ 1–, 90 to 120 μsec, 130 Hz; 0+ 1– to 2–, 120 μsec, 130 Hz), which improved dyskinesia but did not provide adequate tremor control up to 3.5 to 4 V. His symptoms were bothersome so interleaved settings were explored. He was switched to an interleaved setting and multiple parameters with stimulation at different contacts were tested.

OUTCOME

Interleaved settings with stimulation at contacts 1 and 2 (C+ 2–, 3.5 V, 60 μsec; 0+ 1–, 3 V, 90 μsec, 125 Hz) improved his tremor significantly without inducing stimulation-induced dyskinesia (Figure 18.1).

DISCUSSION

STN DBS can induce dyskinesia, including choreiform, ballistic, or dystonic movements resembling levodopa-induced dyskinesia.[1,2] Stimulation-induced dyskinesia typically occurs during the postoperative programming period; however, dyskinesia can occur intraoperatively during lead placement and is considered as a good predictor of motor outcome.[3] Dyskinesia can present immediately or after several hours of stimulation.[1] In the majority of cases, dyskinesias are managed by adjusting medications and stimulation parameters; however, in some cases, the dyskinesias are challenging to control and are described as brittle STN DBS–induced dyskinesia.[4] The predictors and risk factors for the development of stimulation-induced dyskinesia are not clear. It has been suggested that patients with preoperative dyskinesia and early-onset PD are at an increased risk.[5]

Different strategies are recommended for the management of stimulation-induced dyskinesia (Table 18.1). These include reducing stimulation parameters and gradually increasing stimulation in smaller increments (0.1 or 0.05 V); reducing dopaminergic medications to avoid worsening of stimulation-induced dyskinesia and/or peak dose dyskinesia[6]; and switching to a less effective contact and narrowing the electric field by lowering stimulation or switching to a bipolar configuration. These strategies, however, can lead to suboptimal control of motor symptoms. When stimulation-induced dyskinesias pose a challenge in achieving good control, adding dorsal contacts to stimulate the zona incerta region can provide an antidyskinetic effect presumably by activating pallidofugal fibers.[7] In cases in which dyskinesia is resistant to the previous strategies and interferes with optimal control of motor symptoms, a rescue DBS lead in the globus pallidus interna (GPi) can be considered.[4]

TABLE 18.1. STRATEGIES TO MANAGEMENT OF STIMULATION-INDUCED DYSKINESIA

- Reducing voltage/current at the most therapeutic contact
- Reducing dopaminergic medications
- Switching to less effective contact or to bipolar configuration
- Adding or activating dorsal contacts (monopolar, double monopolar, bipolar, or interleaving)
- Slowly ramping up the voltage over many months to control tremor without inducing dyskinesia
- Using rescue deep brain stimulation lead in globus pallidus interna

This patient underwent DBS surgery for medication-refractory tremor. Before the surgery, dopaminergic therapy was stopped because of limited benefit and side effects. He did not develop levodopa-induced dyskinesia when on dopaminergic therapy. His tremor responded well to initial programming with stimulation at the most therapeutic contact, but tremor re-emerged within a few days. Adjusting stimulation parameters to double monopolar settings improved his tremor, but these parameters induced dyskinesia. Multiple configurations, including using bipolar settings and activating dorsal contacts, improved dyskinesia, but did not provide good tremor suppression. Interleaving with stimulation at the most therapeutic contact and a dorsal contact (see Figure 18.1) provided tremor resolution without stimulation-induced dyskinesia. It is possible that if we had given the stimulation more time and slowly ramped up over several months, we may have controlled tremor without dyskinesia. However, as symptoms were bothersome to the patient, we explored interleaved programming.

Interleaving stimulation allows activation of two different contacts at varying amplitudes and/or pulse widths, but at the same or reduced frequency of 125 Hz. The two interleaved programs create a different field and provide stimulation alternating with each other.[8] Interleaving can be considered when conventional programming does not provide optimal results, but it may deplete the battery faster. The exact mechanism of how interleaving stimulation modulates neuronal pathways is not clear, and potential synergistic effects of the overlapping fields of two programs have been suggested.[8] In our case, the potential explanations for the overall beneficial effect include (1) reduction of the electrical field at the most effective electrode, which typically induces dyskinesia; (2) activation of a relatively dorsal electrode, which likely induces an antidyskinetic effect; and (3) potential synergistic effect of interleaving on tremor control from overlapping electrical fields.[8]

In summary, interleaving programming is a potential option for maximizing DBS benefit in PD, minimizing stimulation-induced dyskinesia, and potentially avoiding another DBS surgery for rescue GPi leads.

PEARLS

- Stimulation-induced dyskinesias are an infrequent complication of STN DBS and typically occur during the postoperative programming period.
- Although stimulation-induced dyskinesias are considered a good predictor of motor outcome, they can interfere with effective control of motor symptoms with DBS programming.
- Reducing dopaminergic medications, lowering stimulation at the most therapeutic contact, or switching to a less effective contact (with monopolar or bipolar configuration) can alleviate stimulation-induced dyskinesia; however, motor symptoms can worsen.
- Adding a dorsal contact to stimulate pallidofugal fibers can have an antidyskinetic effect.
- Interleaving programming settings with stimulation at both the dorsal and therapeutic contacts can be a potential option, but it can more quickly drain the battery.
- A rescue DBS lead in the GPi can be considered in refractory cases.

REFERENCES

1. Limousin P, Pollak P, Hoffmann D, Benazzouz A, Perret JE, Benabid AL. Abnormal involuntary movements induced by subthalamic nucleus stimulation in parkinsonian patients. *Movement disorders: official journal of the Movement Disorder Society.* 1996;11(3):231–235.
2. Zheng Z, Li Y, Li J, Zhang Y, Zhang X, Zhuang P. Stimulation-induced dyskinesia in the early stage after subthalamic deep brain stimulation. *Stereotactic and functional neurosurgery.* 2010; 88(1):29–34.
3. Houeto JL, Welter ML, Bejjani PB, et al. Subthalamic stimulation in Parkinson disease: intraoperative predictive factors. *Archives of neurology.* 2003;60(5):690–694.
4. Sriram A, Foote KD, Oyama G, Kwak J, Zeilman PR, Okun MS. Brittle dyskinesia following STN but not GPi deep brain stimulation. *Tremor and other hyperkinetic movements (NY).* 2014;4:242.
5. Baizabal-Carvallo JF, Jankovic J. Movement disorders induced by deep brain stimulation. *Parkinsonism and related disorders.* 2016;25:1–9.
6. Picillo M, Lozano AM, Kou N, Puppi Munhoz R, Fasano A. Programming deep brain stimulation for Parkinson's disease: The Toronto Western Hospital algorithms. *Brain stimulation.* 2016;9(3):425–437.
7. Herzog J, Pinsker M, Wasner M, et al. Stimulation of subthalamic fibre tracts reduces dyskinesias in STN-DBS. *Movement disorders: official journal of the Movement Disorder Society.* 2007;22(5):679–684.
8. Miocinovic S, Khemani P, Whiddon R, et al. Outcomes, management, and potential mechanisms of interleaving deep brain stimulation settings. *Parkinsonism and related disorders.* 2014;20(12):1434–1437.

Case 19

Management of Brittle Dyskinesia and Dopamine Dysregulation Syndrome in Subthalamic Deep Brain Stimulation

JUNAID SIDDIQUI, RAJA MEHANNA, AND JAWAD A. BAJWA

INDICATION FOR DEEP BRAIN STIMULATION

Parkinson disease (PD) with motor complications including wearing off and dyskinesia

CLINICAL HISTORY AND RELEVANT EXAM

A 66-year-old right-handed man was referred for evaluation of PD and candidacy for deep brain stimulation (DBS) surgery. He first developed a right-hand rest tremor, followed by bradykinesia and rigidity. He was subsequently diagnosed with PD at the age of 60 years. In the early stages of the disease, he reported a very good response to carbidopa/levodopa, and his regimen is shown in Table 19.1.

He was not taking his prescribed entacapone, which was scheduled to be taken three times a day with each dose of carbidopa/levodopa, 25/250 mg.

He later started to experience wearing off every 3.5 hours, requiring frequent dosing, but he did not agree to the idea of taking more medications. He also had mild left upper extremity wearing-off dyskinesia. In our clinic, his carbidopa/levodopa on/off evaluation showed a robust 65% improvement in the motor section of the Movement Disorder Society Unified Parkinson's Disease Rating Scale (MDS UPDRS) Part III. He was considered to be a good DBS candidate after neuropsychological testing and was offered DBS surgery. Preoperative brain magnetic resonance imaging (MRI) (Figure 19.1) was unremarkable.

He subsequently had bilateral subthalamic nucleus (STN) DBS performed in a single stage.

COMPLICATIONS

Immediately after surgery, even before the impulse generator (IPG) was activated, the patient developed a left upper extremity continuous dyskinesia, which was resistant to amantadine, probably from a microlesion effect. Although the spontaneous dyskinesia resolved on its own within 2 to 3 weeks, it recurred at the slightest stimulation or the smallest dose of carbidopa/levodopa, a phenomenon known as *brittle dyskinesia*.

Over the 6 months following his DBS implant, there was excellent control of the motor PD symptoms on the right side of the body, while the left upper extremity dyskinesia continued to be resistant to amantadine, limiting control of the left-sided motor parkinsonian symptoms. To complicate his clinical course, the patient overmedicated himself with carbidopa/levodopa (dopamine dysregulation syndrome, or DDS). At that time, his DBS settings were as recorded in Table 19.2.

The patient was offered the possibility to switch to an alternative program at home with the following settings as indicated in Table 19.3.

The patient was subsequently lost to follow-up for a year. He pursued a nonmovement disorders neurologist for DBS programming because one was not available close to his home. He returned to our clinic after 14 months, when he had unintelligible speech and was unable to walk without

TABLE 19.1. DOPAMINERGIC REGIMEN AT FIRST VISIT

	7 AM	Noon	4 PM	5:30 PM	10 PM
Carbidopa/levodopa 25/250 mg	1	1	½	1	½

a walker. He had severe freezing of gait and was having daily falls. In addition, his cardinal motor parkinsonian symptoms were not controlled. His settings at that time were as recorded in Table 19.4

TROUBLESHOOTING AND MANAGEMENT

The pulse width on the patient's device was decreased from 150 to 90 μsec, with marked improvement in speech and gait, but worsening of tremor, bradykinesia, and rigidity. The amplitude was increased and resulted in better control of his PD symptoms. At the end of the visit, his settings were as indicated in Table 19.5.

OUTCOME

The addition of one tablet of carbidopa/levodopa 25/100 mg yielded a complete control of his tremor and markedly improved rigidity and bradykinesia. There was no dyskinesia despite use of higher voltages and higher doses of carbidopa/levodopa.

DISCUSSION

Development of dyskinesia intraoperatively during STN DBS surgery generally indicates good placement. However, occasionally troublesome dyskinesias, called *brittle dyskinesias*, can develop shortly after STN DBS implantation even before turning the IPG on, which may cause them to become even worse. These gradually improve with time and may be troublesome in terms of management, requiring a close follow-up, transient reduction of dopaminergic medications, and even delay in activation of DBS while trying complex programming with or without anti-dyskinetic medications. Planning programming over multiple sessions and reduction in dopaminergic medications may be helpful, although coexistent DDS can make the situation difficult to manage.

High pulse width can worsen speech and gait in STN DBS. This is important to recognize because these parameters are readily adjustable.

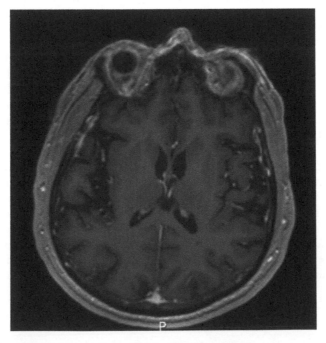

FIGURE 19.1. Axial magnetic resonance image of brain, T1 with contrast.

TABLE 19.2. DEEP BRAIN STIMULATION SETTINGS AT
6-MONTH FOLLOW-UP

Side and Target	Contacts	Amplitude	Pulse Width	Frequency
Right STN	1+ 2–	3 V	60 μsec	130 Hz
Left STN	C+ 11–	5 V	60 μsec	130 Hz

STN = subthalamic nucleus.

TABLE 19.3. ALTERNATE DEEP BRAIN STIMULATION PROGRAM
PROVIDED TO THE PATIENT

Side and Target	Contacts	Amplitude	Pulse Width	Frequency
Right STN	1+ 2–	2.5 V	60 μsec	180 Hz
Left STN	C+ 11–	5 V	60 μsec	180 Hz

STN = subthalamic nucleus.

TABLE 19.4. DEEP BRAIN STIMULATION SETTINGS WHEN
PATIENT RETURNED WITH SEVERE FREEZING OF GAIT

Side and Target	Contacts	Amplitude	Pulse Width	Frequency
Right STN	2+ 3–	3.9 V	150 μsec	180 Hz
Left STN	C+ 11–	4 V	150 μsec	180 Hz

STN = subthalamic nucleus.

TABLE 19.5. NEW DEEP BRAIN STIMULATION SETTINGS IN
CLINIC WITH IMPROVEMENT OF SPEECH AND PARKINSONISM

Side and Target	Contacts	Amplitude	Pulse Width	Frequency
Right STN	2+ 3–	4.4 V	90 μsec	180 Hz
Left STN	C+ 11–	4.5 V	90 μsec	180 Hz

STN = subthalamic nucleus.

PEARLS

- LID can develop after DBS implantation from a microlesion effect even before activation of the device.
- Improvement may take time and several sessions of programming together with reduction of dopaminergic medications.
- High pulse width can worsen speech and gait in STN DBS. A trial of lower pulse width and frequency should be tried in patients with prominent freezing of gait after STN DBS placement.
- Strategies to manage brittle dyskinesia and DDS are important to improving outcome.

REFERENCES

1. Farris SM, Giroux ML. Rapid assessment of gait and speech after subthalamic deep brain stimulation. *Surg Neurol Int*. 2016;7(Suppl 19):S545–550.
2. Gago M, Rosas M, Linhares P, Ayres-Basto M, Sousa G, Vaz R. Transient disabling dyskinesias: a predictor of good outcome in subthalamic nucleus deep brain stimulation in Parkinson's disease. *Eur Neurol*. 2009;61(2):94–99.
3. Herzog J, Pinsker M, Wasner M, et al. Stimulation of subthalamic fibre tracts reduces dyskinesias in STN-DBS. *Mov Disord*. 2007;22(5):679–684.
4. Houeto J-L, Welter M-L, Bejjani P-B, et al. Subthalamic stimulation in Parkinson disease: intraoperative predictive factors. *Arch Neurol*. 2003;60(5):690–694.
5. Reich MM, Steigerwald F, Sawalhe AD, et al. Short pulse width widens the therapeutic window of subthalamic neurostimulation. *Annals Clin Translat Neurol*. 2015;2(4):427–432.
6. Volkmann J, Herzog J, Kopper F, Deuschl G. Introduction to the programming of deep brain stimulators. *Mov Disord*. 2002;17(S3):S181–S187.
7. Martinez-Ramirez D, Giugni J, Vedam-Mai V, et al. The "brittle response" to Parkinson's disease medications: characterization and response to deep brain stimulation. *PLoS One*. 2014;9:e94856.
8. Sriram A, Foote KD, Oyama G, *et al*. Brittle dyskinesia following STN but not GPi deep brain stimulation. *Tremor Other Hyperkinet Mov*. 2014;4:242.

Case 20

Freezing of Gait After Bilateral Globus Pallidus Interna Deep Brain Stimulation in Generalized Dystonia

MARIANA MOSCOVICH

INDICATION FOR DEEP BRAIN STIMULATION

Medication-refractory generalized dystonia

CLINICAL HISTORY AND RELEVANT EXAM

Our patient, aged 49 years, had generalized dystonia and noticed reduced right hand dexterity at age 15 years, followed 1 year later by clumsiness of his right arm. He was initially diagnosed with focal dystonia. Brain magnetic resonance imaging (MRI) was normal, and a DYT1 test for early-onset autosomal dominant dystonia was negative. He responded well to botulinum toxin injections for 10 years, but there was slowly progressive worsening of dystonia despite the use of numerous medications, including levodopa, baclofen, trihexyphenidyl, biperiden, and lithium. The dystonia progressed to involve his neck, and in the same year he developed severe status dystonicus. No gait disorder or lower limb involvement was observed. He underwent stereotactic implantation of bilateral globus pallidus interna (GPi) deep brain stimulation (DBS) leads in 2008 at age 39 years. There were some technical difficulties placing the right-sided lead due to intraoperative capsular responses, so the lead had to be repositioned. A quadripolar DBS electrode (model 3387, Medtronic Inc., Minneapolis, MN) was implanted. Microelectrode recording (MER) was not performed during surgery, but macrostimulation (130 Hz, 210 µsec) was used to assess thresholds for visual phosphenes and capsular responses. After the surgery, the patient experienced pronounced improvement in dystonic symptoms lasting approximately 8 months. One year later, his implantable pulse generator (IPG)

had to be replaced, at which point he continued to endorse significant global improvement except for his right hand, which remained dystonic. Two years later, the IPG was switched to a rechargeable model.

COMPLICATIONS

After the last IPG change, the patient noticed worsening of dystonic symptoms and spread of dystonia to his legs. He had moderate difficulty in gait initiation and turning and severe freezing of gait (FOG) that appeared similar to what would be observed in a typical PD patient, although he required no assistance to walk and denied falling. While walking, he presented with worsening cervical dystonia (manifesting as retrocollis and laterocollis to the right) and dystonia of his trunk, arms, and hand. Right foot inversion and toe-curling were also noted.

TROUBLESHOOTING AND MANAGEMENT

When the IPG was turned off, he reported clear worsening of cervical dystonia but also had improvement in FOG. Suboptimal lead placement was evaluated by imaging (using the software Opti-Vise), and the right-sided lead was 3 mm more lateral. He did not have stimulation related capsular side-effects. Increasing voltages improved dystonia but rapidly triggered FOG. No optimal configuration could be uncovered that would alleviate FOG despite extensive testing of various configurations (monopolar, bipolar, interleaved; pulse width 60–210 µsec; frequency 60–180 Hz). Nevertheless, a compromise between optimal stimulation for treatment of dystonia and the minimization of FOG was achieved using two programming groups during the day depending on his activity. The best setting for this patient was decreasing the pulse width and adapting the amplitude. His final settings were: group A left side case +/7–6–, 3.4 V, 240 μsec, 220 Hz and right side case +/2–, 3 V, 240 μsec, 220 Hz; group B left side case +/7–6–, 3.7 V, 180 μsec, 130 Hz and right side case +/2–, 3.4 V, 120 μsec, 130 Hz.

OUTCOME

After 1 month, the patient reported 70% subjective improvement of his gait, especially during gait initiation and walking, and he reported no worsening in his dystonia. This report illustrates that GPi DBS–induced gait disturbance may occur as a delayed phenomenon and can be associated with suboptimal lead placement. We want to draw attention to this side effect, which may be more common than reported. Based on previous reports,[1,2] we are considering "rescue" STN stimulation to treat the residual symptoms of dystonia.

DISCUSSION

Gait disturbance in PD, including FOG, has been associated with falls and injuries.[3,4] In dystonia, FOG can emerge after DBS and can be disabling. Typically, freezing occurs when the patient is turning and lasts for few seconds.

Stimulation-induced FOG and bradykinesia can occur as adverse effects of bilateral GPi DBS and have been reported in patients with generalized dystonia.[5-7] However, these side effects are not restricted to generalized disease and may also occur in patients with segmental dystonia, after chronic GPi stimulation.[6-10] It was shown in previous reports that stimulation-induced bradykinesia is worse when ventral contacts are stimulated and dystonia is worse when stimulating the dorsal contacts, although this has not been systematically confirmed.[11] In our case, we could not replicate the findings in our patient. However, FOG was clearly a stimulation-induced phenomenon that worsened by increasing the pulse width, as has been reported previously.[6] The physiopathology of FOG is still unknown, and it is likely multifactorial. DBS-inducing FOG has been hypothesized as resulting from a general alteration of neuronal activity in striato-pallido-thalamo-cortical motor pathways following chronic stimulation of the posteroventral lateral GPi[9]; however, the hypothesis of selective gamma-aminobutyric acid (GABA) release as the mode of action of high-frequency stimulation is also possible.[7] In our case, it is difficult to disentangle the effects of disease progression from the effects of DBS.

PEARLS

- FOG or gait hypokinesia can occur as a delayed complication of chronic GPi DBS, or it can occur because of disease progression. As in our case, they can be tricky to disentangle.
- Although in other cases the DBS leads have been documented as optimally positioned, in our case the suboptimal lead placement may have contributed to the symptom.
- Reprogramming, reimplanting, and adding a rescue DBS lead are all treatment options.

REFERENCES

1. Fonoff ET, Campos WK, Mandel M, Alho EJ, Teixeira MJ. Bilateral subthalamic nucleus stimulation for generalized dystonia after bilateral pallidotomy. *Mov Disord.* 2012;27:1559–1563.

2. Schjerling L, Hjermind LE, Jespersen B, et al. A randomized double-blind crossover trial comparing subthalamic and pallidal deep brain stimulation for dystonia. *J Neurosurg.* 2013;119:1537–1545.

3. Bloem BR, Hausdorff JM, Visser JE, Giladi N. Falls and freezing of gait in Parkinson's disease: a review of two interconnected, episodic phenomena. *Mov Disord.* 2004;19:871–884.

4. Youn J, Okuma Y, Hwang M, Kim D, Cho JW. Falling direction can predict the mechanism of recurrent falls in advanced Parkinson's disease. *Sci Rep.* 2017;7:3921.

5. Ostrem JL, Marks WJ Jr., Volz MM, Heath SL, Starr PA. Pallidal deep brain stimulation in patients with cranial-cervical dystonia (Meige syndrome). *Mov Disord.* 2007;22:1885–1891.

6. Schrader C, Capelle HH, Kinfe TM, et al. GPi-DBS may induce a hypokinetic gait disorder with freezing of gait in patients with dystonia. *Neurology.* 2011;77:483–488.

7. Amtage F, Feuerstein TJ, Meier S, Prokop T, Piroth T, Pinsker MO. Hypokinesia upon pallidal deep brain stimulation of dystonia: support of a GABAergic mechanism. *Front Neurol.* 2013;4:198.

8. Tisch S, Zrinzo L, Limousin P, et al. Effect of electrode contact location on clinical efficacy of pallidal deep brain stimulation in primary generalised dystonia. *J Neurol Neurosurg Psychiatry.* 2007;78:1314–1319.

9. Wolf ME, Capelle HH, Bazner H, Hennerici MG, Krauss JK, Blahak C. Hypokinetic gait changes induced by bilateral pallidal deep brain stimulation for segmental dystonia. *Gait Posture.* 2016;49:358–363.

10. Zauber SE, Watson N, Comella CL, Bakay RA, Metman LV. Stimulation-induced parkinsonism after posteroventral deep brain stimulation of the globus pallidus internus for craniocervical dystonia. *J Neurosurg.* 2009;110:229–233.

11. Berman BD, Starr PA, Marks WJ Jr., Ostrem JL. Induction of bradykinesia with pallidal deep brain stimulation in patients with cranial-cervical dystonia. *Stereotact Funct Neurosurg.* 2009;87:37–44.

Case 21

Globus Pallidus Interna Stimulation–Induced Gait Disturbance and Management by Reprogramming

DHANYA VIJAYAKUMAR AND JOOHI JIMENEZ-SHAHED

INDICATION FOR DEEP BRAIN STIMULATION

Parkinson disease (PD) with inadequate tremor control, motor fluctuations, and dyskinesia despite optimal medical management

CLINICAL HISTORY AND RELEVANT EXAM

A 55-year-old woman with PD received bilateral globus pallidus interna (GPi) deep brain stimulation (DBS) surgery with intraoperative magnetic resonance imaging (MRI) guidance to treat refractory right-sided rest tremor, motor fluctuations including wearing-off foot dystonia, and medication-induced dyskinesia. Foot dystonia was the major factor affecting gait before surgery, although she also experienced gait shuffling. There was no gait freezing before DBS. An experienced neurosurgical team performed GPi DBS placement under intraoperative MRI guidance. Intraoperative test stimulation and postoperative programming yielded marked improvements in motor symptoms without side effects (Table 21.1) confirmed appropriate electrode positioning, as did the final intraoperative MRI (Figure 21.1).

COMPLICATIONS

DBS programming substantially improved the patients' tremor, dystonia, motor fluctuations, and dyskinesia. After the first renewal of her implantable pulse generator (IPG, Activa PC), the same DBS parameters were reprogrammed (Table 21.2). After about 6 to 8 weeks, she began to experience increased shuffling, falls, freezing, dystonia, and problems with her balance. She was noted to be under stress because of her husband's diagnosis of cancer. Symptoms did not improve with physical therapy.

TROUBLESHOOTING AND MANAGEMENT

During DBS reprogramming 4 months after surgery for IPG renewal, although electrode impedances were normal, the therapy impedance was slightly higher on the right GPi electrode compared with the presurgical reading. The pulse width and frequency were increased, resulting in relief of toe-curling and mild improvement in gait. However, she noted marked gait exacerbation within a few days. DBS parameters were reduced by 0.2 mV, which was the maximum that could be lowered using patient control, followed by medication adjustment, which did not improve gait. Freezing of gait increased significantly, and gait markedly declined to the point of needing a wheelchair. DBS stimulation was turned off, which resulted in an initial reduction of gait freezing in 48 hours, but 1 or 2 days later she experienced right-sided rest tremor, dystonia, and increased gait shuffling. The patient began to use the DBS only at night to alleviate symptoms in order to sleep, while turning it off during the day.

At her follow-up programming visit (see Table 21.2, T + 6 months), her *off/on* examination (off PD medications with DBS turned on) showed 2+ right-sided rest tremor, 1+ right arm and 2+ left arm bradykinesia, normal tone, and a hesitant and shuffling gait with en bloc turning. Her *off/off* examination 20 minutes after stimulation was turned off showed 3+ right-sided rest tremor, no change in bradykinesia or rigidity, but normal stride length and turns. DBS settings were further adjusted (see Table 21.2, T + 6 months) to achieve the optimal treatment of motor symptoms, including gait. On final settings, patient had 2+ right-sided tremor, 1+ bradykinesia right more than left, and minimal shuffling of gait without freezing.

TABLE 21.1. MONOPOLAR REVIEW OF BILATERAL GLOBUS PALLIDUS INTERNA DEEP BRAIN STIMULATION ELECTRODES

	Onset of Clinical Genefit	Onset of Side Effects (Type)	Setting With Most Robust Benefit in Baseline Symptoms
Left GPi			
0	1.0 V	3.0 V (speech slurring)	None
1	1.5 V	4.0 V (none)	2.5 V
2*	1.0 V	4.0 V (none)	1.5 V
3	1.0 V	4.0 V (none)	2.0 V
Right GPi			
8	1.0 V	2.5 V (jaw clenching)	2.0 V
9	1.0 V	4.0 V (none)	3.0 V
10*	1.0 V	4.0 V (speech slower)	2.0 V
11	1.0 V	3.5 V (non-reproducible face pulling)	2.0 V

Note: Monopolar review conducted with standard settings of pulse width at 60 μsec and frequency at 130 Hz. All contacts produced improvement in contralateral tremor and dystonia (when present), bradykinesia, and rigidity.
* Contact selected for chronic stimulation based on optimal combination of benefit and least/no side effects; maximum settings tested clinically during troubleshooting were c+ 2–/4.7 V/110 μsec/200 Hz and c+ 10–/4.2 V/110 μsec/200 Hz, without adverse effects other than worsening gait freezing.
GPi = globus pallidus interna.

OUTCOME

After this reprogramming, only mild further adjustment of settings (see Table 21.2, T + 10 months) was required to maintain a notable sustained improvement in gait and freezing with only residual right-hand rest tremor in the medication off state. This benefit has persisted at additional follow up visits.

DISCUSSION

Gait impairment and postural instability are "axial symptoms" of PD that do not typically improve with DBS.[1,2] The phenomenology and management of gait dysfunction that occurs after DBS surgery have been mostly described in patients following subthalamic nucleus (STN)

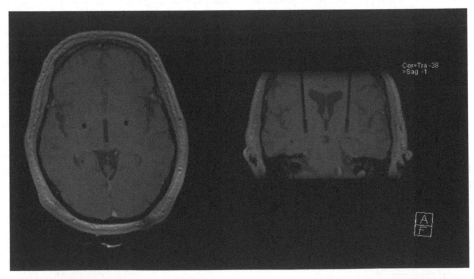

FIGURE 21.1. Intraoperative magnetic resonance image shows appropriate positioning of bilateral globus pallidum interna deep brain stimulation electrodes.

TABLE 21.2. STIMULATION PARAMETERS BEFORE AND AFTER ADJUSTMENT FOR STIMULATION-INDUCED GAIT DISTURBANCE FOLLOWING BILATERAL GLOBUS PALLIDUS INTERNA DEEP BRAIN STIMULATION

Time	Clinical Features	Left GPi Settings	Right GPi Settings
Last programming visit before IPG exchange (T – 4 mo)	Symptoms well-controlled, ambulating without difficulty. Examination *off* meds/*on* stim with short strides and en bloc turning.	C+ 2– 4.7 V/90 μsec/180 Hz 1,169 ohm/3.888 mA TEED = 306	C+10– 3.6 V/70 μsec/180 Hz 1,410 ohm/2.605 mA TEED = 115
T + 4 mo (after IPG exchange), before reprogramming	Onset of worsening gait complaints in interval following IPG exchange: constant gait freezing when *on* and *off* medications. Examination *off* meds/*on* stimulation: bilateral foot dystonia, start hesitation, frequent freezing with walking and turns, and marked shuffling.	C+ 2– 4.7 V/90 μsec/180 Hz 1,175 ohm/4.001 mA TEED = 304	C+ 10– 3.6 V/70 μsec/180 Hz 1,207 ohm/3.007 mA TEED = 135
T + 6 mo, immediately after reprogramming	Examination *off* medications and *on* stimulation, immediately after reprogramming, with normal stride length and turns.	C+ 2– 3.0 V/90 μsec/160 Hz (impedance not checked)	C+ 10– 2.9 V/60 μsec/160 Hz (impedance not checked)
T + 10 mo (stable settings)	Resolution of gait freezing, even when medications wear off. Examination *off* medications/*on* stimulation: gait shuffling without freezing.	C+ 2– 2.8 V/90 μsec/160 Hz 1,256 ohm/2.237 mA TEED = 90	C+10– 3.1 V/60 μsec/160 Hz 1,161 ohm/2.697 mA TEED = 79

GPi = globus pallidus interna; IPG = implantable pulse generator; T = time of IPG exchange; TEED = total electrical energy delivered.

implantation and programming. Although gait and balance impairment may represent disease progression, multiple reports have now established that changing to low-frequency (e.g., 60–80 Hz) STN stimulation can improve axial symptoms, including freezing of gait, in some PD patients.[3] The results of these studies, including the duration of improvement after low-frequency stimulation, have been variable and reproducible only in selected patients.[4,5]

Although fewer data exist regarding response of axial PD symptoms following GPi stimulation, one article describes improvement of worsened gait in three of five PD patients following change to low-frequency GPi stimulation.[6] This is similar to what was observed in our patient, who did better with gait and balance after slight reduction in frequency of GPi stimulation, along with other parameters.

It is also interesting to note that our patient experienced worsening gait symptoms after IPG renewal despite unchanged DBS settings, leading to the observation that a new IPG may result in reduced impedances causing a greater net current flow, and thus a higher total electrical energy delivered (TEED), ultimately accounting for stimulation-related side effects (see Table 21.2). TEED is calculated by the following formula,[7] which is used for constant voltage devices:

TEED = [(volts)2 × pulse width × frequency]/ impedance

Attempts at physical therapy, medication titration, and stimulation titration did not improve symptoms. However, reduction in TEED clearly led to alleviation of side effects in this case.

With GPi DBS, the full effects of stimulation adjustments may be delayed, making it difficult to make a complete determination of the appropriate strategy during the clinic visit. This delay is a well-recognized feature of GPi stimulation, regardless of disease state, although the interval is probably longer with dystonia.[8,9]

If the motor symptoms cannot be optimized despite delivering a similar TEED value, then a contact switch should be considered. Particularly in the case of GPi stimulation, assuming appropriate electrode positioning, stimulating at the most ventral contact can reduce rigidity and dyskinesia, while worsening akinesia and gait.[10] Gait and akinesia could be improved by stimulating the higher, more dorsal contacts, but potentially at the expense of worsened dyskinesia even in the off-medication state.

Regardless, this case illustrates the concept that new or worsened gait dysfunction, which may occur weeks after programming in patients with PD treated with GPi DBS, should prompt investigation for a stimulation-induced problem. Spread of current to unwanted areas or recruitment of unwanted neural elements could be the reason, and reduction in TEED (frequency, pulse with, or amplitude, or combinations of these) can be effective without compromising symptom control.

PEARLS

- Chronic high-frequency GPi DBS could cause freezing of gait and postural instability in patients with PD, similar to what has been described in STN DBS for PD.
- Stimulation-induced gait dysfunction should be considered as a possible etiology in patients otherwise symptomatically well-controlled with DBS who develop newly worsened gait disturbance.
- Reducing TEED could help improve these gait problems, although the long-term sustainability of these settings due to recurrence of other motor symptoms should be continually assessed.
- If gait symptoms are primarily related to wearing off of medication, an adjustment of timing or dosing of dopaminergic medications should be considered. In some patients, postural instability unrelated to medication timing may also improve with levodopa titration, especially considering the likelihood that medications had been reduced postoperatively. A levodopa challenge at a higher dose or trial of medication adjustment should always be considered but may not be helpful when stimulation-induced gait problems are the cause.
- If symptoms are temporally associated with a recent stimulation change, during initial postoperative stimulation optimization period, or occur following a recent DBS procedure such as an IPG exchange, then a stimulation-related phenomenon should be considered. In this case, the patient should be assessed *on* or *off* stimulation and/or with higher or lower stimulation parameters to confirm the appropriate strategy. The effects of higher and lower amplitudes and frequency of stimulation should be assessed. This can be done during the clinic evaluation or may require a longer duration of time to evaluate.
- If medication changes and stimulation alterations are unrevealing, progression of PD, development of other age-related brain changes, or non-PD-related changes should be considered as possibilities. Interventions such as physical therapy or referrals to other specialists (e.g., orthopedics) may be most appropriate in this setting.
- Reduction in stimulation settings may lead to worsening motor symptoms, including gait, highlighting the importance of differentiating between understimulation (emergence of undertreated disease-related symptoms) and overstimulation (emergence of stimulation-related side effects). This could complicate the clinical identification and management of these symptoms.

REFERENCES

1. Moro, Elena, Andres M Lozano, Pierre Pollak, Yves Agid, Stig Rehncrona, Jens Volkmann, Jaime Kulisevsky, et al. 2010. "Long-Term Results of a Multicenter Study on Subthalamic and Pallidal Stimulation in Parkinson's Disease." *Movement Disorders: Official Journal of the Movement Disorder Society* 25 (5): 578–586. doi:10.1002/mds.22735.

2. Fasano, Alfonso, Camila C Aquino, Joachim K Krauss, Christopher R Honey, and Bastiaan R Bloem. 2015. "Axial Disability and Deep Brain Stimulation in Patients with Parkinson Disease." *Nature Reviews: Neurology* 11 (2): 98–110. doi:10.1038/nrneurol.2014.252.

3. Sidiropoulos, Christos, Richard Walsh, Christopher Meaney, Y Y Poon, Melanie Fallis, and Elena Moro. 2013. "Low-Frequency Subthalamic Nucleus Deep Brain Stimulation for Axial Symptoms in Advanced Parkinson's Disease." *Journal of Neurology* 260 (9): 2306–2311. doi:10.1007/s00415-013-6983-2.

4. Xie, Tao, Mahesh Padmanaban, Lisa Bloom, Ellen MacCracken, Breanna Bertacchi, Abraham Dachman, and Peter Warnke. 2017. "Effect of Low versus High Frequency Stimulation on Freezing of Gait and Other Axial Symptoms in Parkinson Patients with Bilateral STN DBS: A Mini-Review." *Translational Neurodegeneration* 6 (1): 13. doi:10.1186/s40035-017-0083-7.

5. Zibetti, Maurizio, Elena Moro, Vibhor Krishna, Francesco Sammartino, Marina Picillo, Renato P Munhoz, Andres M Lozano, and Alfonso Fasano. 2016. "Low-Frequency Subthalamic Stimulation in Parkinson's Disease: Long-Term Outcome and Predictors." *Brain Stimulation* 9 (5): 774–779. doi:10.1016/j.brs.2016.04.017.

6. Zibetti, Maurizio, Andres M. Lozano, Marina Picillo, Renato P. Munhoz, and Alfonso Fasano. 2015. "Low-Frequency Stimulation of Globus Pallidus Internus for Axial Motor Symptoms of Parkinson's Disease." *Movement Disorders Clinical Practice* 2 (4): 445–446. doi:10.1002/mdc3.12215.

7. Koss, Adam M, Ron L Alterman, Michele Tagliati, and Jay L Shils. 2005. "Calculating Total Electrical Energy Delivered by Deep Brain Stimulation Systems." *Annals of Neurology* 58 (1): 168; author reply 168–9. doi:10.1002/ana.20525.

8. Lee, John Y.K., Milind Deogaonkar, and Ali Rezai. 2007. "Deep Brain Stimulation of Globus Pallidus Internus for Dystonia." *Parkinsonism & Related Disorders* 13 (5): 261–265. doi:10.1016/j.parkreldis.2006.07.020.

9. Ruge, Diane, Stephen Tisch, Marwan I Hariz, Ludvic Zrinzo, Kailash P Bhatia, Niall P Quinn, Marjan Jahanshahi, Patricia Limousin, and John C Rothwell. 2011. "Deep Brain Stimulation Effects in Dystonia: Time Course of Electrophysiological Changes in Early Treatment." *Movement Disorders: Official Journal of the Movement Disorder Society* 26 (10): 1913–1921. doi:10.1002/mds.23731.

10. Krack, P, P Pollak, P Limousin, D Hoffmann, A Benazzouz, J F Le Bas, A Koudsie, and A L Benabid. 1998. "Opposite Motor Effects of Pallidal Stimulation in Parkinson's Disease." *Annals of Neurology* 43 (2): 180–192. doi:10.1002/ana.410430208.

Case 22

Rescue Ventral Intermediate Thalamus Deep Brain Stimulation to Address Refractory Tremor Following Subthalamic Nucleus Deep Brain Stimulation With Brittle Dyskinesia

MITRA AFSHARI, JILL L. OSTREM, MARTA SAN LUCIANO, AND PAUL S. LARSON

INDICATION FOR DEEP BRAIN STIMULATION

Medication-refractory upper extremity tremor

CLINICAL HISTORY AND EXAM

A 52-year-old right-handed woman presented with complaints of action tremor in both hands over the previous 7 years, as well as significant voice, head, and lower facial tremor for 3 years, and more recently concerns of slowness in her movements, rigidity, and gait imbalance. She was initially diagnosed with essential tremor (ET) and treated with primidone, propranolol, trihexyphenidyl, and gabapentin. She reported limited improvement. Her examination revealed prominent postural and kinetic tremor in her hands, worse on the left side, and intermittent mild low-amplitude, low-frequency rest tremor in the bilateral hands and right leg. The rest tremor was consistently observed on multiple visits. There was a significant voice tremor and slight hypophonia. There was a mild "no–no" head and chin tremor. Additionally, she had mild hypomimia, significant neck rigidity, slight rigidity in the upper extremities with augmentation, reduced arm swing, and slight postural instability. Given her emerging signs of possible parkinsonism and lack of response to typical medications used for ET, the concern was for an ET "plus" syndrome such as ET-Parkinson disease (PD). She was treated with a high-dose levodopa trial. There was no notable improvement in her tremor, and this was confirmed by examining the patient in the off-levodopa and on-levodopa states. No levodopa-induced dyskinesia was noted. A dopamine transporter scan (DaTscan) was not feasible because this patient presented before US Food and Drug Administration approval of the test in the United States.

Given the patient's progressive disability from her tremor, she was evaluated for deep brain stimulation (DBS) therapy, and the consensus was to proceed with bilateral subthalamic nucleus (STN) DBS. This option was chosen to treat both her tremor and her emerging parkinsonism. She received standard stereotactic microelectrode recording (MER)-guided awake bilateral STN implantation. In the operating room, macrostimulation showed mild improvement in tremor without development of dyskinesia.

COMPLICATIONS

Programming of the patient's STN DBS system aimed at tremor control was limited by stimulation-induced dyskinesia of the left hemibody. Of note, the patient was off levodopa therapy for many days before the programming visit. During the initial programming, the left STN DBS voltage was increased from 1 to 3.2 V using contact 1 in a monopolar configuration, and this resulted in improved right-sided tremor control. However, on the contralateral side, using contact 5 in the monopolar setting, immediate stimulation-induced dyskinesia in the left arm was noted at any voltage above 1 V. The dyskinesia was also observed in the left leg with higher stimulation amplitudes. Adding a dorsal contact

6 to this setting failed to reduce dyskinesia. The pulse width was maintained at 60 μsec, and a range of frequencies were tried (130–155 Hz). The higher frequency of 155 Hz was chosen because it was associated with the best tremor control. Bothersome dyskinesia of the left arm persisted with a monopolar setting using contact 6 alone at 2 V, but it improved with a double monopolar setting using contact 6 and when applying a more dorsal contact 7. This change facilitated a voltage increase to 2.2 V with resultant improvement in left-sided tremor. Unfortunately, the patient developed delayed onset of left arm dyskinesia and poor tremor control. Several more programming iterations were attempted, including triple monopolar settings bilaterally with contacts 1, 2, and 3 on the left STN DBS and 5, 6, and 7 on the right STN DBS, and an increased pulse width of 90 μsec on the right STN DBS; however, these settings failed to resolve tremor. There was a slightly reduced left arm dyskinesia when the patient was switched to a double bipolar setting of 5+, 6–, and 7–; however, tremor control was limited. Head and chin tremor did not benefit from DBS. Rest tremor in the bilateral hands and right leg mildly improved but did not resolve. The postural and kinetic tremor mildly improved but did not resolve.

The patient inadvertently turned her DBS off for a period of several months and experienced worsening bilateral tremor. She did not follow up for programming until 5 years later when she was found to have a depleted battery, which was subsequently replaced. DBS programming of the right STN DBS was again hindered by left-hemibody stimulation-induced dyskinesia, and over time her bilateral postural and kinetic tremor progressed in severity and became the most disabling feature of her syndrome. When the STN DBS system was turned off, she experienced further worsening of all tremor types. Zonisamide, methazolamide, topiramate, and clonazepam were unsuccessful in treating tremor. Over time, her initial parkinsonian signs remained unchanged, and she expressed that her gait imbalance was slightly improved. The team was concerned that the parkinsonian symptoms may not have been idiopathic PD.

TROUBLESHOOTING AND MANAGEMENT

A decision was made to add a unilateral left ventral intermediate (Vim) thalamus "rescue"

electrode to her existing bilateral STN electrodes with the hope of mitigating the patient's disabling and progressive dominant hand tremor. A left Vim electrode was implanted nearly 8 years after her initial STN DBS implantation under standard stereotactic guidance and was performed without the use of MER. In the operating room, macrostimulation at 1.5 V revealed completed tremor suppression of the right arm. There were capsular side effects at 6 V.

OUTCOME

Minimal programming of the left Vim DBS resulted in marked improvement of right hand postural and action tremors (stimulation settings: C+ 0–, 1.8 mA, 60 μsec, 150-Hz). Interestingly, despite these results, she was reluctant to turn off her STN DBS because she felt she had experienced some improvement in her tremor, posture, and gait with STN stimulation, and this was corroborated on examination. The patient's bilateral STN DBS leads were inactivated for approximately 30 days. The STN stimulators were then activated with double bipolar settings bilaterally, and this strategy was used in conjunction with the Vim stimulation. Together, this resulted in improvement in her postural and action tremor and no dyskinesia. Approximately 4 months after left Vim DBS implantation, right Vim DBS surgery was performed and resulted in marked improvement of the left hand postural and action tremor. Bilateral VIM stimulation also resulted in improvement in voice and head tremor.

DISCUSSION

Historically, the Vim thalamic nucleus was one of the first DBS and lesional targets used for PD tremor; however, other parkinsonian signs, including bradykinesia and rigidity, which can in the majority of cases contribute to greater disability as the disease progresses, is not responsive to thalamic stimulation.[1,2] STN and globus pallidus interna (GPi) have been more commonly employed DBS targets for PD because of greater effects on bradykinesia, rigidity, and PD features.[3,4] Vim remains the preferred DBS target for ET and other forms of tremor and is employed in cases of PD-associated severe action tremor. Vim is useful in some cases of ET-PD,[5,6] although the important feature is how much action tremor is present.

First, this case underscores the importance of selecting the DBS target based on a patient's most disabling symptoms. In this case, the most disabling symptom was tremor, and over time the action tremor worsened. Action tremor that is moderate to severe may require Vim DBS, although there are reported cases of STN and GPi DBS. In addition, brittle dyskinesia emerged in our case even without dopaminergic therapy. Thus, ultimately a rescue DBS strategy helped the action tremor and allowed the STN DBS to be programmed at a threshold below dyskinesia.[6] If available, a DaTscan or Fluoro-Dopa brain positron emission tomography scan may or may not have assisted in differentiating ET from PD and may or may not have informed target selection at the time of initial DBS surgery. It is also important to keep in mind that an abnormal DaTscan, while confirming neurodegenerative parkinsonism, does not eliminate the possibility of underlying ET, which can coexist with PD. ET can also be associated with a rest tremor component. Finally, select patients can present with ET initially and develop parkinsonism, dystonia, and balance difficulties as the disease progresses. ET and PD tremor are both possibly unresponsive or partially responsive to medications.[7–10] The dyskinesia in this case would strongly suggest there was both PD and ET.

This case highlights the potential complication of stimulation-induced brittle dyskinesia, a treatment-limiting side effect of STN DBS stimulation. Dyskinesia may in select cases be minimized by using dorsal contacts, by switching to bipolar settings, by increasing stimulation gradually, and by reducing levodopa dose.[11] There are, however, cases in which even slight adjustments result in brittle dyskinesia.[12]

This case demonstrates the feasibility of "salvage" Vim DBS implanted *as a rescue lead*. The Vim was a powerful addition for treatment of action tremor. Action tremor that is moderate to severe may require more than either STN or GPi DBS.[13]

Vim DBS outcomes can also be limited by stimulation-induced dysarthria, paresthesias, ataxia, poor control of proximal tremor, and loss of therapeutic efficacy over time in a proportion of patients.[14,15] Larger studies will be required to establish selection guidelines and to improve the effectiveness of rescue DBS procedures. In our patient, a combination of bilateral STN and Vim DBS ultimately resulted in significant improvement of tremor and resolution of brittle dyskinesia.

PEARLS

- Early and predominant complaints of kinetic/action tremor with mild parkinsonian features could be ET, PD, or ET-PD. DaTscan is not always useful in differentiation.
- Brittle dyskinesia is a possible complication of STN DBS whether the patient is on levodopa therapy or not and, in some cases, cannot be managed with expert programming adjustments without loss of therapeutic benefit. It can be considered a treatment-limiting complication of STN DBS.
- In select cases, rescue Vim DBS implantation may be considered to mitigate refractory kinetic/action tremor persisting after STN or GPi DBS.

REFERENCES

1. Ondo W, Jankovic J, Schwartz K. Unilateral thalamic deep brain stimulation for refractory essential tremor and Parkinson's disease tremor. *Neurology* 1998;51:1063–1069.
2. Hariz MI, Krack P, Alesch F, et al. Multicenter European study of thalamic stimulation for parkinsonian tremor: a 6 year follow-up. *J Neurol Neurosurg Psychiatry* 2008;79:694–699.
3. Krack P, Benazzouz A, Pollak P, et al. Treatment of tremor in Parkinson's disease by subthalamic nucleus stimulation. *Mov Disord* 1998;13:907–914.
4. Follett KA, Weaver FM, Stern M, et al; CSP 468 Study Group. Pallidal versus subthalamic deep-brain stimulation for Parkinson's disease. *N Engl J Med* 2010;362(22):2077–2091.
5. Kim HJ, Jeon BS, Paek SH, et al. Bilateral subthalamic deep brain stimulation in Parkinson disease patients with severe tremor. *Neurosurgery* 2010;67:626–632.
6. Parihar R, Alterman R, Papavassiliou E, et al. Comparison of VIM and STN DBS for Parkinsonian resting and postural/action tremor. *Tremor Other Hyperkinet Mov* 2015;5:321.

7. Algarni M, Fasano A. The overlap between essential tremor and Parkinson disease. *Parkinsonism Relat Disord* 2018:46(Suppl 1):S101–104.

8. Fekete R, Jankovic J. Revisiting the relationship between essential tremor and Parkinson's disease. *Mov Disord* 2011;26:391–398.

9. Jankovic J. Essential tremor: a heterogenous disorder. *Mov Disord* 2002;17:638–644.

10. Jimenez-Jimenez, FJ, Alonso-Navarro H, Garcia-Martin E, et al. The relationship between Parkinson's disease and essential tremor: review of clinical, epidemiologic, genetic, neuroimaging and neuropathological data, and data on the presence of cardinal signs of parkinsonism in essential tremor. *Tremor Other Hyperkinet Mov* 2012;2:8–30.

11. Limousin P, Pollak P, Hoffmann D, et al. Abnormal involuntary movements induced by subthalamic nucleus stimulation on Parkinsonian patients. *Mov Disord* 1996;11:231–235.

12. Sriram A, Foote KD, Oyama G, Kwak J, Zeilman PR, Okun MS. Brittle dyskinesia following STN but not GPi deep brain stimulation. *Tremor Other Hyperkinet Mov (NY)* 2014;4:242.

13. Stover NP, Okun MS, Evatt ML, Raju DV, Bakay RA, Vitek JL. Stimulation of the subthalamic nucleus in a patient with Parkinson disease and essential tremor. *Arch Neurol* 2005;62(1):141–143.

14. Putzke JD, Wharen RE Jr, Wszolek ZK, et al. Thalamic deep brain stimulation for tremor-predominant Parkinson's disease. *Parkinsonism Relat Disord* 2003;10(2):81–88.

15. Favilla CG, Ullman D, Wagle Shukla A, et al. Worsening essential tremor following deep brain stimulation: disease progression versus tolerance. *Brain* 2012;135:1455–1462.

Case 23

Postural Instability and Gait Disorder After Subthalamic Nucleus Deep Brain Stimulation

MÓNICA M. KURTIS AND JAVIER R. PÉREZ-SÁNCHEZ

INDICATION FOR DEEP BRAIN STIMULATION

Parkinson disease (PD) with tremor, dystonia, and motor and nonmotor fluctuations.

CLINICAL HISTORY AND RELEVANT EXAM

A 49-year-old right-handed woman with a high-demand consulting job presented with a 6-month history of progressive limping and occasional tremor in her right leg. She had previously consulted with rheumatology, traumatology, and neurosurgery and had unremarkable results on blood work, brain and lumbar magnetic resonance imaging (MRI), and lower limb electromyography. She had not benefited from treatment with physiotherapy and anti-inflammatory drugs. On exam, she showed mild hypomimia, rigidity, and bradykinesia of the right limbs and intermittent resting right foot tremor and dystonia (toe flexion). Gait was fast, with long strides, mild lagging of the right leg, and decreased arm swing bilaterally (more notably on the right). A diagnosis of PD was made, and she was started on rasagiline, with ropinirole (added early in her therapy and increased progressively to 16 mg). She showed partial response, but after a few months developed hyperphagia and compulsive shopping. The agonist was tapered down, and levodopa was started.

Eighteen months into the disease course, with a total dose of 500 levodopa equivalents (LED) she developed wearing off. Six months later, truncal and craniocervical biphasic dyskinesias and non-motor fluctuations (depression/fatigue) appeared along with punding, which kept her awake into the early morning hours organizing photo albums. She did not tolerate amantadine because of nausea and vomiting, nor apomorphine because of somnolence. Genetic tests for *LRRK2* and *PARK2* were negative. At age 52 years (4 years into the disease course), because of the small therapeutic window with conventional treatments due to side effects, she underwent bilateral subthalamic nucleus (STN) deep brain stimulation (DBS) to better control the debilitating motor and non-motor fluctuations, dyskinesias, impulse control disorder (ICD), punding, and insomnia.

Surgery was performed at another center in her hometown with placement of a rechargeable stimulation system (Versice, Boston Scientific) that had 8 active contacts on each electrode (Figure 23.1). Perioperative results were positive, and she was discharged with no PD treatment (levodopa was also stopped) and left only on clonazepam and trazodone at bedtime. A week later, she developed dysarthria, orobuccal dyskinesias, and unstable gait. She was managed locally, medication was restarted, program adjustments were made, and adequate control of speech and gait problems was attained. She was very satisfied with the surgical results because motor and nonmotor fluctuations, ICDs, and punding improved significantly. She returned to her highly demanding job.

COMPLICATIONS

Two years later, the patient consulted our team again because of festinating gait and propulsion causing forward instability and near falls. PD treatment had been restarted and increased (750 LED: 450 levodopa/entacapone + 300 rotigotine), and she thought it was beneficial. Balance and gait problems had appeared the previous year but had been aggravated 1 to 2 months prior, showing no predictable pattern or apparent relation to levodopa schedule. In an initial evaluation, generator battery, impedances, and history of

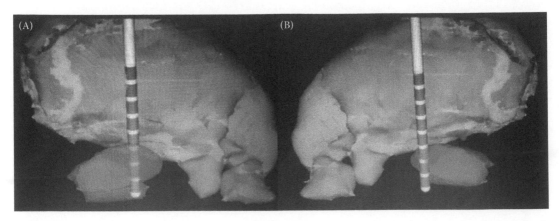

FIGURE 23.1. (A) Left subthalamic nucleus (STN) electrode (contacts 1–8). (B) Right STN electrode (contacts 9–16).

DBS therapy changes were verified, confirming normal limits and no recent changes. She had bilateral bipolar high-frequency stimulation settings (left DBS: 4– 8+, current (I) = 3.5 mA, pulse width = 60 μsec, frequency = 145 Hz; right DBS: 12– 13+, 3.2 mA, 60 μsec, 145 Hz). Concomitant infection and systemic processes were ruled out. After an unsuccessful levodopa challenge, stepwise changes were made without success: (1) current stimulation changes (increases and decreases) were tried, without changing active leads; (2) medication was raised (900 LED, 500 levodopa/entacapone + 400 rotigotine); and (3) she was progressively switched to low-frequency stimulation (left DBS: 4– 8+, 3.5 mA, 60 μsec, 60 Hz; right DBS: 12– 13+, 3.2 mA, 60 μsec, 60 Hz).

Her symptoms worsened, and she developed progressive fluctuations with episodes of dysarthria, strained voice, hypophonia, and festinating gait with propulsion and falls. She began to use a walker. After 3 months of progressive instability, she was finally convinced to take time off work and was admitted for DBS reprogramming and medication adjustments.

TROUBLESHOOTING AND MANAGEMENT

With the existing DBS programming (discussed previously), the patient was tested in four possible clinical settings:

1. Off/off (off medication for 15 hours/ DBS turned off): Exam was remarkable for moderate hypophonia, no dysarthria, mild hypomimia, moderate cervical rigidity and mild limb rigidity, severe bradykinesia in the right arm, moderate

in the right leg and left arm, and mild in the left leg. She showed dystonic posturing in the right arm and toe flexion with accompanying small-amplitude tremor-like jerky movements in the right foot. She arose from the chair without help. Posture was normal. She fell on the examiner during the pull test. Gait was slow, narrow based, with medium-sized steps, no arm swing, and decomposition of turns, without freezing. Motor Unified Parkinson's Disease Rating Scale (UPDRS) = 39, Hoehn and Yahr = 3.

2. Off/on (off medication/DBS on): Speech, bradykinesia, and rigidity clearly improved. She recovered with two steps on the pull test. Gait showed long strides, good heel strike, and decreased right arm swing. Motor UPDRS = 14; Hoehn and Yahr = 2.

3. On/on (on medication/DBS on): Speech was normal, bradykinesia and rigidity remain unchanged (mild), but gait was clearly unstable, showing narrow base, bent knees, extended trunk, no arm swing, and festinating, short jumpy quick steps on toes with progressive whole-body propulsion. She could not stop voluntarily and stopped the forward inertia by bumping into walls or other large objects. She fell on the examiner during the pull test. No clear dyskinesias or chorea were observed, but gait was reminiscent of festinating parkinsonian gait and the hyperkinetic gait of choreic patients (jumpy and stepping on toes). Motor UPDRS = 16, Hoehn and Yahr = 3.

4. On/off (on medication/DBS off): Right arm and leg bradykinesia and dystonia reappeared, but gait clearly improved, showing normal steps, heel strike, and no festination. Motor UPDRS = 24, Hoehn and Yahr = 2

Clinical exam was satisfactory in the off medication/on DBS state (UPDRS = 14, without disabling symptoms) but worsened after 36 hours off medication with the reappearance of disabling limb bradykinesia and dystonia. Thus, a reprogramming session was scheduled.

Monopolar (100%) screening of all the contacts was performed using the following reference parameters; 60 μsec pulse width and 119 Hz (Table 23.1). Both sides revealed a narrow therapeutic window because of the emergence of speech impairment. On the left electrode, contact 3 showed the best results (tremor on the left foot was used as the guiding symptom) but had a low therapeutic window (>1.5 mA current caused dysarthria). On the right side, leads 10 and 11 showed good results, with current higher than 2.5 mA causing dysarthria.

Postsurgery MRI was performed to ensure correct lead placement. The left electrode had a relatively lateral trajectory, with contacts 2 and 3 within the dorsolateral region of the STN, while the right electrode had a more medial and posterior trajectory, with contacts 10 and 11 slightly contacting the dorsolateral region of the STN (see Figure 23.1).

Using imaging guidance and screening results, DBS programming parameters were set to contacts 3 and 11 as anodes, initially in a monopolar configuration (left DBS: 3– C+, 1 mA, 60 μsec, 119 Hz; right DBS: 11– C+, 1 mA, 60 μsec, 119 Hz) with immediate motor improvement, but after 1 tablet of carbidopa/levodopa 25/100, mild craniocervical dyskinesias appeared that were intolerable to the patient. Stimulation was switched to a bipolar configuration bilaterally (left DBS: 3– 4+, 1 mA, 60 μsec, 119 Hz; right DBS 11– 12+, 1 mA, 60 μsec, 119 Hz).

Medication was decreased to carbidopa/levodopa 25/100 alternating 1 tablet and ½ tablet every 4 hours (five times a day) with unchanged rotigotine (from 900 to 800 LED). After these adjustments, postural instability and abnormal gait were resolved, but the patient complained of generalized slowness, particularly in the early morning and later in the afternoon (close to levodopa doses). Because of better positioning of the left electrode, stimulation was adjusted to monopolar only on the left side (contact 3) to better control her more parkinsonian side, while right-sided stimulation was kept in a bipolar configuration (left DBS 3– C+, 1 mA, 60 μsec, 119 Hz; right DBS 11– 12+ 1 mA, 60 μsec, 119 Hz). She was discharged understanding that we were probably understimulating and undermedicating to avoid disturbing dyskinesias, postural instability, and abnormal gait. The plan was to increase parameters and medication over the next weeks.

OUTCOME

At follow-up, the patient still complained of slowness, especially in her right limbs. Initially, intensity was increased bilaterally, +0.5 mA in the left STN and +0.2 in the right STN without pole configuration changes (left DBS: 3– C+, 1.5 mA, 60 μsec, 119 Hz; right DBS: 11– 12+ 1.2 mA, 60 μsec, 119 Hz). Over the next weeks, levodopa was also increased (+100 LED, 900 total). With these changes, she recuperated upper body mobility without troublesome dyskinesias, and her gait showed long strides and heel-strike without forward falling. In the following 6 months, she benefited from a further small increase in stimulation (+0.2 mA) and medication (+100, 1,000 LED) to control gait problems and forward falling. Currently, she no longer needs a walker and continues working.

DISCUSSION

Because usual troubleshooting for gait impairment,[1] including low-frequency stimulation, which may improve gait after DBS,[2] was unsuccessful, admission for reprogramming was recommended. Based on the clinical history, festinating gait with propulsion fluctuated erratically; thus, our main objective was to characterize the gait disturbance and evaluate the effect of DBS and medication.

We hypothesized that DBS could be aggravating postural instability and causing a gait disturbance leading to falls because this has been described in the past.[3] Stimulation was seemingly causing an anterior shift of the patient's center of gravity, leading to toe-walking.[4] Another possible explanation was that the natural progression of PD, 7 years into disease course, was resulting in refractory axial symptoms.[5,6] A recent meta-regression of the long-term effects of DBS on balance and gait in PD concluded that DBS initially improves both cardinal and postural instability and gait disturbance (PIGD) symptoms; however,

TABLE 23.1. MONOPOLAR (100%) SCREENING FOR EVERY CONTACT

Left DBS STN On/Right DBS STN Off

Contact	Current	Outcome
1 (–) C (+)	0.5 mA	No improvement
	1.0 mA	Worse bradykinesia
	1.5 mA	Worse bradykinesia and dysarthria
2 (–) C (+)	0.5 mA	Mild motor improvement, resting tremor right foot
	1.0 mA	Moderate motor improvement, mild resting tremor right foot
	1.5 mA	Moderate motor improvement, resting tremor disappears, mild dysarthria
	2.0 mA	Moderate motor improvement, resting tremor disappears, dysarthria worsens
3 (–) C (+)	0.5 mA	Mild motor improvement, resting tremor right lower limb
	1.0 mA	Moderate motor improvement, no resting tremor, no speech impairment, speaking, gait shows long strides
	1.5 mA	Notable motor improvement, no resting tremor, mild dysarthria
	2.0 mA	Notable motor improvement, no resting tremor, dysarthria
4 (–) C (+)	0.5 mA	No improvement, speech impairment
	1.0 mA	No improvement, speech worsens, resting tremor right foot
	1.5 mA	Worse dysarthria, mild tremor improvement

Right DBS STN On/Left DBS STN Off

Contact	Current	Outcome
9 (–) C (+)	0.5 mA	No changes
	1.0 mA	No changes
	1.5 mA	Bradykinesia and dysarthria become worse
10 (–) C (+)	0.5 mA	Bradykinesia and hypophonia improve
	1.0 mA	Bradykinesia and speaking improve
	1.5 mA	Bradykinesia, speaking, and gait improve
	2.0 mA	Bradykinesia, speaking, and gait improve
	2.5 mA	Dysarthria
11 (–) C (+)	0.5 mA	Bradykinesia and hypophonia improve
	1.0 mA	Notable motor improvement, including left foot, good speech
	1.5 mA	Notable improvement, good speech
	2.0 mA	Notable improvement, good speech
	2.5 mA	Speech worsens, dysarthria
12 (–) C (+)	0.5 mA	No changes
	1.0 mA	Bradykinesia improves, including left foot, good speech
	1.5 mA	Dysarthria
	2.0 mA	Dysarthria
13 (–) C (+)	0.5 mA	No changes
	1.0 mA	No changes
	1.5 mA	Dysarthria

DBS = deep brain stimulation; STN = subthalamic nucleus.

the benefit to PIGD is lost after the first 2 years, especially for patients with STN DBS compared with globus pallidus interna DBS.[7] The initial benefit to PIGD symptoms is probably due to improvement of limb rigidity and bradykinesia, with subsequent benefit of posture and stride length.

In this patient, neurologic exam in the off-medication/off-stimulation state and after DBS was switched on clearly demonstrated that stimulation improved hypophonia, limb rigidity, bradykinesia, and gait, decreasing the UPDRS motor score by 25 points. In fact, the UPDRS Part III score was best in the off-medication (12 hours) and on-stimulation state but not maintained over time, thus requiring levodopa reintroduction. Freezing of gait was not really an issue, in the on[8] or off state. We noted that postural instability appeared in the on-medication/on stimulation and off-medication/off-stimulation settings, but not in the off-medication/on-stimulation nor the on-medication/off-stimulation state. These findings suggested that stimulation in isolation was not the cause of imbalance but that the combination of STN DBS and dopaminergic treatment was leading to postural instability and falls.

This phenomenon has not been extensively described. Numerous studies have investigated the effect of STN on stance and gait, and results are conflicting.[4,9,10] A classic study based on posturography identified a synergistic increase in postural sway during quiet stance in the on-medication/on-stimulation conditions.[11] Other studies have described the synergistic effect of levodopa and STN on gait velocity.[12,13] Phenomenologically, the patient's gait was hyperkinetic, with elements reminiscent of dystonia because gait was much more impaired than other tasks such as climbing stairs. We thus postulated that exacerbated postural sway and velocity, combined with a lower limb dystonic component, may have explained the patient's problems in the on/on state.

After analysis of DBS and levodopa effects with the initial programming, contact screening, and imaging results, the more dorsal contacts in the STN territory were chosen as anodess to better control dyskinesias[1] and to increase stride length.[14] Her programming up to then had used contacts that were practically outside the STN. After adjustments and good tolerance, a low constant monopolar current (1.5 mA) was set in the left electrode to control the more parkinsonian side, while a low bipolar current (1.2 mA) was used in the posteromedially placed right electrode to minimize spread. These new stimulation parameters, along with small medication changes (COMT inhibitor suppression, levodopa increase, and agonist reduction) were successful in managing the gait and balance problems for this patient. Further investigation is needed to disentangle the pathophysiology of gait and balance networks in order improve our understanding of the mechanisms of DBS and evolving changes relative to stimulation time and disease progression.

PEARLS

- The relative resistance of postural instability and gait disturbances to both dopaminergic medication and STN stimulation is well-established in PD. However, careful analysis of a patient's axial problems may open the door to therapeutic improvement in a small number of cases.
- If a PD patient who has undergone DBS develops refractory postural instability and gait disorder, hospitalization or extensive outpatient workup for complete DBS programming and medication adjustments should be considered.
- DBS of the STN added to standard medication may cause worsening of postural instability and gait in PD, as seen in this patient. Electrode location and stimulation programing may be partially resposible. This cause must be identified because it can be improved with adequate stimulation and medication adjustments.
- DBS adjustments should be made considering the location of electrodes and the more symptomatic side.
- Disease progression, stimulation settings, and medication adjustments can all affect gait and balance issues.

REFERENCES

1. Picillo M, Lozano AM, Kou N, Puppi Munhoz R, Fasano A. Programming deep brain stimulation for Parkinson's disease: the Toronto Western Hospital Algorithms. Brain Stimul 2016;9:425–437.

2. Moreau C, Defebvre L, Devos D, Marchetti F, Destée A, Stefani A, Peppe A. STN versus PPN-DBS for alleviating freezing of gait: toward a frequency modulation approach? Mov Disord 2009;24:2164–2166.

3. Follett KA, Weaver FM, Stern M, Hur K, Harris CL, Luo P, et al. Pallidal versus subthalamic deep-brain stimulation for Parkinson's disease. N Engl J Med 2010;362:2077–2091.

4. Collomb-Clerc A, Welter M-L. Effects of deep brain stimulation on balance and gait in patients with Parkinson's disease: a systematic neurophysiological review. Neurophysiol Clin Neurophysiol 2015;45:371–388.

5. Fasano A, Romito LM, Daniele A, Piano C, Zinno M, Bentivoglio AR, Albanese A. Motor and cognitive outcome in patients with Parkinson's disease 8 years after subthalamic implants. Brain 2010;133:2664–2676.

6. Merola A, Zibetti M, Angrisano S, Rizzi L, Ricchi V, Artusi CA, et al. Parkinson's disease progression at 30 years: a study of subthalamic deep brain-stimulated patients. Brain 2011;134:2074–2084.

7. St George RJ, Nutt JG, Burchiel KJ, Horak FB. A meta-regression of the long-term effects of deep brain stimulation on balance and gait in PD. Neurology 2010;75:1292–1299.

8. Espay AJ, Fasano A, van Nuenen BFL, Payne MM, Snijders AH, Bloem BR. "On" state freezing of gait in Parkinson disease: a paradoxical levodopa-induced complication. Neurology 2012;78:454–457.

9. Bakker M, Esselink RA, Munneke M, Limousin-Dowsey P, Speelman HD, Bloem BR. Effects of stereotactic neurosurgery on postural instability and gait in Parkinson's disease. Mov Disord 2004;19:1092–1099.

10. Fasano A, Aquino CC, Krauss JK, Honey CR, Bloem BR. Axial disability and deep brain stimulation in patients with Parkinson disease. Nat Rev Neurol 2015;11:98–110.

11. Maurer C, Mergner T, Xie J, Faist M, Pollak P, Lücking CH. Effect of chronic bilateral subthalamic nucleus (STN) stimulation on postural control in Parkinson's disease. Brain 2003;126:1146–1163.

12. Faist M, Xie J, Kurz D, Berger W, Maurer C, Pollak P, et al. Effect of bilateral subthalamic nucleus stimulation on gait in Parkinson's disease. Brain 2001;124:1590–1600.

13. Ferrarin M, Rizzone M, Bergamasco B, Lanotte M, Recalcati M, Pedotti A, Lopiano L. Effects of bilateral subthalamic stimulation on gait kinematics and kinetics in Parkinson's disease. Exp Brain Res 2005;160:517–527.

14. McNeely ME, Hershey T, Campbell MC, Tabbal SD, Karimi M, Hartlein JM, et al. Effects of deep brain stimulation of dorsal versus ventral subthalamic nucleus regions on gait and balance in Parkinson's disease. J Neurol Neurosurg Psychiatry 2011;82:1250–1255.

Case 24

Nonsurgical Management of an Exposed Deep Brain Stimulation Lead

ETHAN G. BROWN, MONICA VOLZ, SUSAN HEATH,
NICHOLAS B. GALIFIANAKIS, AND JILL L. OSTREM

INDICATION FOR DEEP BRAIN STIMULATION

Parkinson disease (PD) complicated by motor fluctuations, freezing of gait, and dyskinesia

CLINICAL HISTORY AND RELEVANT EXAM

A 55-year-old man with a history of PD for 8 years underwent bilateral subthalamic nucleus (STN) deep brain stimulation (DBS) implantation to improve motor fluctuations and dyskinesia. His surgery and initial management were performed at an outside center. He had bilateral STN leads placed using microelectrode recording (MER), and bilateral internal pulse generators (IPGs) were placed several weeks later. When his neurostimulators were turned on, he developed diplopia, which was sensitive to adjustment of the right STN stimulation amplitude. Still at an outside center, his DBS parameters were adjusted, and magnetic resonance imaging (MRI) was performed to confirm lead location. His diplopia was thought to be related to medial and deep placement of his right lead, with spread of stimulation to oculomotor fibers. He returned for surgical revision; his original lead was removed, and a new lead was implanted in a position that was lateral to the prior lead, again using MER.

COMPLICATIONS

Despite revision, the stimulation settings resulted in side effects, including dyskinesia, instability, and mild diplopia, likely from persistent medial stimulation of oculomotor fibers. For the first several years, a therapeutic programming setting could not be found, and the patient usually kept the stimulation turned off. Over time, it became increasingly difficult to manage his parkinsonism on medication alone because of severe impulse control behaviors and dyskinesia.

Up until this time, his management and workup had been performed at an outside center; he then transferred care to our center, where his DBS system was evaluated and reprogrammed. His MRI was reviewed, and the leads did appear slightly more medial than usual, which may have explained his oculomotor side effects. He was in a bipolar setting on the right (7+, 6–) and a monopolar setting on the left (case positive, 3–). A new tripolar setting was identified, using contacts (3+, 2–, 1+) at 3 V, 80 μsec, and 100 Hz on the left and contacts (7+, 6–, 4+) at 3.7 V, 80 μsec, and 100 Hz on the right. This setting was established in an attempt to focus the stimulation even more within a therapeutic contact, preventing any spread to neighboring structures. Stimulation at the new setting eliminated diplopia and improved his PD symptoms substantially. He reported improvement in medication-induced dyskinesia and freezing of gait as well as rigidity (~60–70%), and his bradykinesia and gait improved on exam. He was able to slowly titrate down his PD medications.

Unfortunately, he subsequently developed scalp irritation over his right DBS lead. Over the course of several months, the lead eroded through the skin and was exposed (Figure 24.1). The DBS system was still electrically intact with normal impedances, and the area surrounding the lead did not appear infected, but the exposed lead was clearly a high infection risk.

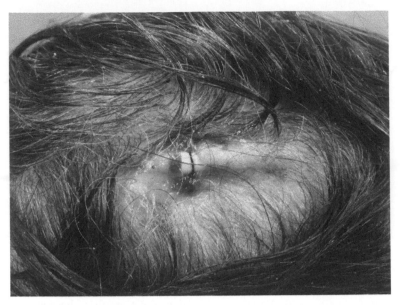

FIGURE 24.1. Deep brain stimulation lead erosion through the scalp, without significant signs of infection.

TROUBLESHOOTING AND MANAGEMENT

As is recommended in such cases, full explanation of the device, including the neurostimulator and lead, was considered to avoid development of infection. However, given his prior complicated surgical course, intolerance of PD medication, and significant benefit from DBS after recent reprogramming, other management options were considered.

In an attempt to reduce infection risk, a reconstructive scalp flap was surgically placed over the lesion, transposed from an area lower in the neck. The graft was successful in covering the lead; however, several months later, the lead eroded again (this time more anterior to the previous location). This lesion also developed slowly without any drainage, redness, or pain. We decided to regularly monitor the wound region for any sign of infection and leave the DBS system in place. He was told to apply daily prophylactic topical antibiotics over the wound.

OUTCOME

The patient's follow-up continued for 3 years with visits for monitoring confirming no sign of infection. Finally, at a recent follow-up, his lesion did show evidence of hardware infection, with purulent material surrounding the lead, without any systemic or intracranial signs of infection (Figure 24.2). He was therefore taken back to surgery for his lead and hardware to be explanted and given intravenous antibiotics.

DISCUSSION

This case offers several teaching points. First, DBS therapy can only be effective if the electrode is implanted accurately into the target nucleus. Even extensive programming strategies may not prevent repositioning of a lead if it is misplaced. In our case, stimulation caused diplopia, potentially from too medial of a position and inadvertent stimulation of oculomotor tracts. After revision surgery, stimulation was able to provide benefit without side effects, albeit with a very focused field and with expert programming.

The other major teaching point of this case involves strategies for management of a chronically eroded lead, potentially a more common clinical scenario as the number of patients with long-standing implanted hardware increases. Delayed erosion of skin overlying DBS hardware is an increasingly recognized long-term complication of DBS therapy, occurring in anywhere from 1 to 10% of a retrospective series.[1] While erosion is a strong risk factor for infection,[2] a meta-analysis found that on average 1.3% of patients developed erosion without infection.[3]

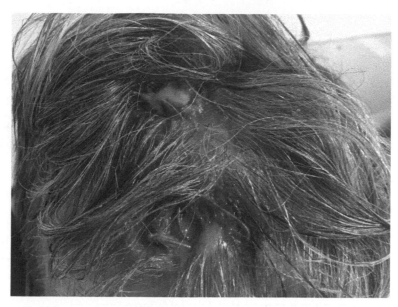

FIGURE 24.2. Development of superficial infection around an exposed lead. Given the evidence of infection, the lead was urgently explanted.

Skin erosion most often occurs over the connector site, especially if the connector is placed low around the mastoid process, but can also occur in frontal areas over the DBS cap.[3] Surgical technique may alter the risk for subsequent scalp erosion. In one institution, no erosions occurred in a group of patients who underwent countersinking of the DBS cap and connector lead during surgery, whereas erosions occurred in 2.9% of patients who did not receive countersinking surgery.[4]

If erosion does develop, the risk for subsequent infection is high, and surgical management is often mandatory. No consensus on management exists, and treatment may be specific to each patient's clinical presentation. In most cases of hardware erosion, especially when signs of local inflammation or infection are notable, immediate initiation of antibiotics and explantation of the device are necessary to avoid intracranial spread of infection. After completing a course of antibiotics and wound healing, replacement of the lead can be considered. In some cases, removal of the internal pulse generator and lead extender may be enough to prevent worsening of infection.[5]

In many cases, especially if the lesion develops slowly without evidence of infection, other surgical measures may be attempted to mitigate the erosion. A reconstructive flap involves grafting a piece of skin over the area of erosion and can be performed by a plastic surgeon.[6] Because of the relatively sparse vasculature of the scalp, these surgeries have a high risk of re-erosion.[7] Cutting the lead itself, to separate the external and intracranial portions, could also prevent intracranial spread without requiring full explantation of the lead.

In a very limited number of cases, in which a small, noninfected lesion can be closely monitored by the physician and caregivers, watchful waiting may be an option. An exposed lead has a high risk for developing an infection, which can quickly spread intracranially and lead to serious illness or death. These risks must be discussed with the patient and weighed against the risks and discomfort of explanting hardware and discontinuing stimulation. In our case, after a flap reconstruction failed and we discussed the risks with the patient, we continued with close monitoring and topical antibiotics. Eventually, a superficial infection did develop, and he needed to have the lead explanted, although watchful waiting allowed for 3 years of stabilization of symptoms before surgery.

PEARLS

- Accurate surgical implantation of the electrode in the chosen target is one of the most important factors affecting successful DBS outcomes. Strategic programming alone is typically insufficient to preclude revision surgery when the lead is not optimally located.
- Delayed skin erosion is a well-recognized long-term complication of DBS surgery. It often occurs around the connector site but can occur in other areas such as the DBS lead cap lock. Skin erosion is a strong risk factor for serious infection, which can quickly spread intracranially, often necessitating urgent antibiotic use and DBS explantation.
- In certain cases of insidious hardware erosion with no evidence of infection, scalp reconstruction with a skin graft to cover and exposed leads may be attempted and is often performed by a plastic surgeon.
- For a limited number of low-risk lesions caused by an eroded lead, long-term management with topical antibiotics may delay explantation of the DBS system. Removal of hardware is warranted if this strategy is unsuccessful in preventing infection. In most cases, it is preferable to explant the system because of the risk for repeated infection that may spread to the brain and other regions. Frequent follow-up and patient education is mandatory because immediate intervention may be needed if the infection occurs.

REFERENCES

1. Doshi PK. Long-term surgical and hardware-related complications of deep brain stimulation. Stereotactic and Functional Neurosurgery 2011;89:89–95.
2. Tolleson C, Stroh J, Ehrenfeld J, Neimat J, Konrad P, Phibbs F. The factors involved in deep brain stimulation infection: a large case series. Stereotactic and Functional Neurosurgery 2014;92:227–233.
3. Hamani C, Lozano AM. Hardware-related complications of deep brain stimulation: a review of the published literature. Stereotactic and Functional Neurosurgery 2006;8:248–251.
4. Hilliard JD, Bona A, Vaziri S, Walz R, Okun MS, Foote KD. Delayed scalp erosion after deep brain stimulation surgery: incidence, treatment, outcomes, and prevention. Neurosurgery 2017;63:156–156.
5. Fily F, Haegelen C, Tattevin P, et al. Deep brain stimulation hardware-related infections: a report of 12 cases and review of the literature. Clinical Infectious Diseases 2011;52:1020–1023.
6. Lanotte M, Verna G, Panciani PP, et al. Management of skin erosion following deep brain stimulation. Neurosurgical Review 2009;32:111–114.
7. Gómez R, Hontanilla B. The reconstructive management of hardware-related scalp erosion in deep brain stimulation for Parkinson disease. Annals of Plastic Surgery 2014;73:291–294.

Case 25

Steroid-Responsive Edema Interfering With Deep Brain Stimulation Programming

PRAVIN KHEMANI AND SHILPA CHITNIS

INDICATION FOR DEEP BRAIN STIMULATION

Parkinson disease (PD) with rest tremor, motor fluctuations, and dyskinesia

CLINICAL HISTORY AND RELEVANT EXAM

A 72-year-old woman with advanced PD underwent bilateral subthalamic nuclei (STN) deep brain stimulation (DBS) implantation to mitigate severe rest tremors, motor fluctuations, and medication-induced dyskinesias. Preoperative evaluation was remarkable for impaired gait and balance primarily due to medication-responsive freezing of gait, and she also had musculoskeletal issues affecting her legs and back. She was aware of the low likelihood of gait and balance improvement following a potential DBS surgery and her preoperative expectations were reasonable. An experienced functional neurosurgery team, which included an electrophysiologist who assisted with microelectrode recording, performed bilateral STN DBS surgery in a single sitting.

COMPLICATIONS

The patient's postoperative course was complicated by a seizure, which was attributed to a small right frontal subdural hematoma. She was treated with antiepileptic medications and discharged home. Other than intermittent gait and balance impairment, her outpatient course remained unremarkable.

She presented for initial electrode screening and monopolar programming in the *off/off* (off PD medications for 12 hours/DBS turned off) state. This programming occurred 5 weeks after DBS lead implantation. She was unable to walk and was wheelchair-bound. Extensive electrode screening in the monopolar state revealed wide stimulation windows at all contacts without side effects but only mild improvement of right-sided tremor and bradykinesia. There was resolution of rigidity at contact 0 of the left STN. Painful dystonic dyskinesias and paresthesias of the left leg were noticed at all contacts of the right STN electrode, at low voltages. Although contact 8 had the largest stimulation window without side effects, the best therapeutic effect was observed with stimulation of contact 9, which was selected because of some improvement in tremor, bradykinesia, and rigidity. She was exhausted after a long monopolar programming session; therefore, bipolar montages were not tested. She had difficulty ambulating independently after programming, but after taking her PD medications, she was able to use a walker. Her overall benefit from programming was suboptimal, although the presence of dyskinesias in the off-medication state when mapping the right STN was considered a favorable outcome.

TROUBLESHOOTING AND MANAGEMENT

Because of poor left STN programming outcome, postoperative brain MRI was ordered to confirm DBS lead location and investigate for a potential intracranial lesion interfering with programming. The brain MRI showed that the electrodes were located in the STN region; however, an abnormal T2 signal hyperintensity was observed surrounding the left STN electrode (Figure 25.1). This finding was not seen in the

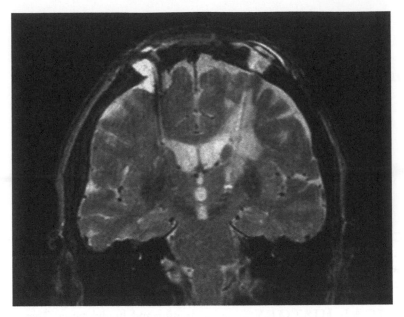

FIGURE 25.1. Magnetic resonance imaging study 4 weeks after deep brain stimulation.

preoperative brain image. The immediate concern was for intracranial infection, and this led to the hospitalization of the patient. The left STN electrode was turned off. Although the patient did not demonstrate typical signs of a brain infection, her gait and balance remained impaired, spinal fluid examination was normal, and a post-contrast computed tomography (CT) scan of the brain did not demonstrate abnormal enhancement. Therefore, antimicrobials were not administered. The suspected diagnosis was a sterile inflammation with edema, and intravenous solumedrol was infused, followed by a short course of oral prednisone. Rehabilitation was also initiated. Her gait and balance improved steadily, and she was discharged home on an oral steroid taper with resumption of her usual PD medication regimen. She was discharged with only unilateral right STN stimulation. The right STN was not reprogrammed because left-sided motor symptoms remained well-controlled.

OUTCOME

Brain MRI performed after steroid treatment showed marked resolution of the abnormal T2 signal around the left STN electrode (Figure 25.2). After completing the oral steroid regimen, monopolar screening of the left STN electrode was repeated and showed wider stimulation thresholds without persistent side effects at all four contacts except contact 3 (contact 3 had close proximity to the internal capsule fibers). The most effective resolution of tremor and bradykinesia was obtained at contact 0 (Table 25.1). That patient continued to require a walker for ambulation, but her motor fluctuations were significantly improved.

DISCUSSION

This case illustrates the phenomenon of sterile steroid-responsive brain edema (SRE) following DBS surgery. SRE is an uncommonly reported and poorly understood sequela of DBS surgery. It can be identified on a postoperative brain MRI as an abnormal T2 signal around one or both electrodes. It can be either clinically silent or cause gait and balance impairment and can be a reason for suboptimal programming outcomes.[1-4] The natural course of SRE is not known, but in our patient, we believe treatment with steroids improved ambulation and facilitated a better clinical course with easier programming. It is also possible that this syndrome would have improved without the use of steroids, and the risks and benefits of this type of therapy need to be considered carefully.

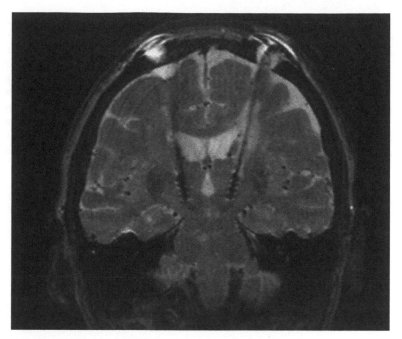

FIGURE 25.2. Brain computed tomography scan after treatment with steroids.

TABLE 25.1. DEEP BRAIN STIMULATION PROGRAMMING PARAMETERS

Initial Settings After Monopolar Mapping

	Electrode Contacts	Amplitude	Pulse Width	Frequency
Left STN	Case + 0 negative	2.3 V	60 μsec	130 Hz
Right STN	Case + 9 negative	2.3 V	60 μsec	130 Hz

Final Settings After Treatment

	Electrode Contacts	Amplitude	Pulse Width	Frequency
Left STN	3+ 1 negative	3.7 V	60 μsec	140 Hz
Right STN	Case + 9 negative	3.5 V	60 μsec	140 Hz

STN = subthalamic nucleus.

PEARLS

- Suboptimal DBS programming outcomes, including narrow therapeutic windows or less than expected improvement of motor symptoms with detailed monopolar programming, or unexplained and rapid deterioration in mobility after DBS surgery should prompt post-surgical brain MRI to verify electrode position and investigate for an intracranial lesion (e.g., edema, hemorrhage, stroke, cysts)
- Knowledge of SRE as a potential sequela of DBS surgery complicating programming is important to prompt rapid imaging, diagnosis, and treatment.
- SRE can be treated with a short course of steroids to improve motor symptoms and programming outcomes, obviating the need for lead revision surgery when the electrodes are well-positioned. It is possible that some cases may resolve without steroids, and practitioners should be careful to exclude infection before administering steroids.

REFERENCES

1. Baizabal Carvallo JF, Mostile G, Almaguer M, Davidson A, Simpson R, Jankovic J. Deep brain stimulation hardware complications in patients with movement disorders: risk factors and clinical correlations. Stereotactic and functional neurosurgery 2012;90:300–306.
2. Deogaonkar M, Nazzaro JM, Machado A, Rezai A. Transient, symptomatic, post-operative, non-infectious hypodensity around the deep brain stimulation (DBS) electrode. Journal of clinical neuroscience: official journal of the Neurosurgical Society of Australasia 2011;18:910–915.
3. Englot DJ, Glastonbury CM, Larson PS. Abnormal T2-weighted MRI signal surrounding leads in a subset of deep brain stimulation patients. Stereotactic and functional neurosurgery 2011;89:311–317.
4. Ryu SI, Romanelli P, Heit G. Asymptomatic transient MRI signal changes after unilateral deep brain stimulation electrode implantation for movement disorder. Stereotactic and functional neurosurgery 2004;82:65–69.

Case 26

The Positive Lesion Effects of Intracranial Hemorrhage on Deep Brain Stimulation Surgery Outcome*

JACQUELINE MEYSTEDT, MALLORY HACKER, AND DAVID CHARLES

INDICATION FOR DEEP BRAIN STIMULATION

Parkinson disease (PD) with rest tremor, bradykinesia, and rigidity

CLINICAL HISTORY AND RELEVANT EXAM

A 55-year-old man with a 5-year history of PD was experiencing progressive worsening of symptoms not adequately controlled by medications. On examination, the symptoms included mild to moderate bilateral resting tremor of the upper extremities, moderate rigidity in the left lower extremity, and bradykinesia that was mild but interfered with activities of daily living. Levodopa treatment had been initiated but resulted in severe motor fluctuations and dyskinesia, and his average duration of good levodopa response had declined to only 60 to 90 minutes. There were no contraindications to deep brain stimulation (DBS) encountered by preoperative testing, and the patient elected to receive DBS therapy. Bilateral subthalamic nucleus (STN) DBS surgery was performed at Vanderbilt University Medical Center (VUMC) under a standardized protocol (Kahn et al., 2011). The VUMC implantation procedure is carried out in three stages, each separated by approximately 1 week: stage I includes target mapping and placement of bone markers; stage II is DBS electrode placement using microelectrode recording (MER) and clinical response; and stage III is internal pulse generator (IPG) implantation.

COMPLICATIONS

Placement of the left STN electrode was well-tolerated, and substantial reductions in tremor, bradykinesia, and rigidity were observed intraoperatively. During STN microelectrode mapping in the right hemisphere, the patient experienced persistent disorientation, confusion, and visual hallucinations, and the remainder of the procedure was aborted without placement of the right electrode.

After surgery, a noncontrast computed tomography (CT) scan revealed a small intracranial hemorrhage (ICH) in the left STN approximately 0.60 cm in diameter around the distal lead (Figure 26.1). The mental status changes noted intraoperatively resolved overnight with observation, and the patient was discharged with a normal mental status following a repeat CT scan showing no change in the ICH. Follow-up evaluation on postoperative day 7 found no adverse effects or neurologic deficits referable to a lesion in the left STN, and a follow-up CT scan revealed resolution of the ICH. However, the patient reported substantial improvements in both tremor and rigidity on the right side even with the stimulator in its off state. These beneficial effects remained until the 12-month follow-up, when the patient reported that the right-sided tremor and rigidity had begun to return.

TROUBLESHOOTING AND MANAGEMENT

The second stage II procedure to implant the electrode in the right STN was delayed until 1 month

* This case report was previously published in the Tennessee Medicine E-Journal, Volume 1, Issue 2 (February 2015).

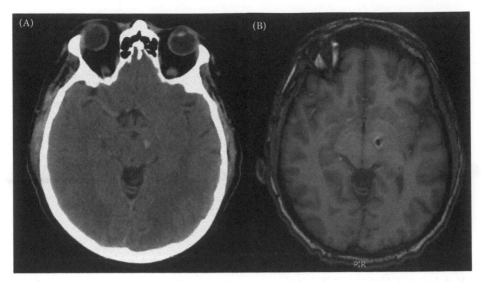

FIGURE 26.1. Computed tomography scan (A) and magnetic resonance imaging (B) performed after intracranial hemorrhage.

after the first procedure in order to allow time for complete resolution of effects from the first electrode placement attempt. Placement of the right STN DBS lead proceeded without complications, and postoperative brain imaging was normal. Implantation of the IPG (stage III) was carried out 1 week later, also without complications. The patient returned for programming and lead interrogation 4 weeks after stage III (>12 hours off medication). He reported substantial reduction of his right-sided tremor with the left STN device remaining in the off state. The right lead was interrogated for efficacy and side effects, and the most distal contact was identified as optimal. Initial programming parameters for the right lead were case positive, contact 0 negative, pulse width of 60 μsec, rate 130 Hz, and amplitude 0.8 V. An optimal contact in the left hemisphere was unable to be located, and that stimulator was not activated.

OUTCOME

The patient returned for follow-up visits at 4, 6, and 10 months, and during this time, he did not exhibit any negative consequences from the ICH. At each follow-up visit, the right brain stimulator was optimized, and the left stimulator remained off because the patient continued to experience a sustained reduction in right-sided symptoms. The patient first noticed a slight reappearance of his right-sided tremor 12 months after implantation. The left STN electrode was interrogated at that time, and an optimal contact was identified.

Initial programming settings of case positive, contact 3 negative, 60 μsec, rate 130 Hz, and amplitude 1.8 V provided a good response and symptomatic relief.

DISCUSSION

This case presents a PD patient who experienced a perioperative focal ICH in the left STN during the DBS lead implantation procedure. Remarkably, the ICH resulted in no observable postoperative adverse effects while conferring substantial reduction of unilateral parkinsonian tremor and rigidity for almost a year.

There are limited reports of PD symptom improvement following a perioperative ICH. Beric and colleagues reported two patients who suffered focal brain hemorrhages intraoperatively followed by improvement in PD symptoms (Beric et al., 2002). The first patient's hemorrhage (about 1 cm in diameter) occurred in the STN and resulted in improved PD symptoms through 26 months of follow-up. This patient, however, also reported an increase in speech dysarthria after surgery. The second patient's ICH occurred in the frontal areas and was fairly large (3 × 4 cm). PD symptom improvement compared with the preoperative condition was observed through 24 months of follow-up, although the patient also experienced confusion and possible seizures (Beric et al., 2002). There has only been one other report of PD symptom improvement following ICH without any long-term adverse effects. In a retrospective review study conducted by Oh and colleagues that examined the potential complications of DBS surgery, one patient was reported to have suffered a small hemorrhage in the thalamic region and thereafter experienced long-term (66 months) arrest of his tremor symptoms without implantation of the pulse generator (Oh, Abosch, Kim, Lang, & Lozano, 2002). No accompanying negative outcomes were reported.

These examples, along with the specific case recounted here, highlight an unusual phenomenon that may occur in DBS for PD. While the exact mechanisms behind the patient's symptom improvement are unknown, the size and location of the ICH are likely important factors in the eventual outcome, and the hemorrhage may have provided benefit in a mechanism similar to that of an intentional lesion surgery.

PEARLS

- While ICH can result in adverse effects, it may not have a negative impact on the patient in all cases. The adverse event may provide some level of improvement in one or more aspects of the patient's condition.
- The improvement that is conferred by an event such as an ICH, regardless of the magnitude of its impact, may only be temporary. It is possible that the patient will need to begin stimulation in the future to treat recurring symptoms. In our case, there was a 12-month delay.
- Conducting postoperative brain imaging is essential after performing DBS lead implantation surgery. Reassessment of the patient will provide the data necessary to decide when and if to commence electrical stimulation.
- Our case revealed a very small hemorrhage without adverse effects, and it is possible that if the hemorrhage were larger there would be a mix of benefits and side effects.

REFERENCES

1. Beric, A., Kelly, P. J., Rezai, A., Sterio, D., Mogilner, A., Zonenshayn, M., & Kopell, B. (2002). Complications of deep brain stimulation surgery. *Stereotactic and Functional Neurosurgery*, 77(1–4), 73–78.
2. Kahn, E., D'Haese, P. F., Dawant, B., Allen, L., Kao, C., Charles, P. D., & Konrad, P. (2011). Deep brain stimulation in early stage Parkinson's disease: operative experience from a prospective randomised clinical trial. *Journal of Neurology, Neurosurgery & Psychiatry*, 83(2), 164.
3. Oh, M. Y., Abosch, A., Kim, S. H., Lang, A. E., & Lozano, A. M. (2002). Long-term hardware-related complications of deep brain stimulation. *Neurosurgery*, 50(6), 1268–1276.

Case 27

Fibrous Scarring and Deep Brain Stimulation Lead Implantation

*VINATA VEDAM-MAI, ANTHONY T. YACHNIS, MICHAEL ULLMAN,
SAMAN P. JAVEDAN, AND MICHAEL S. OKUN*

INDICATION FOR DEEP BRAIN STIMULATION

Tremor-predominant Parkinson disease (PD)

CLINICAL HISTORY AND RELEVANT EXAM

This patient was 74 years old at the time of death. At the time of clinical presentation 6 years prior, he had tremor-predominant PD and underwent deep brain stimulation (DBS) 1 year after diagnosis. His symptoms were progressive, and many of his symptoms did not respond to optimization of medications (carbidopa/levodopa, dopamine agonist patch, and trihexyphenidyl). DBS surgery was set to be bilateral and staged, with subthalamic nucleus (STN) as the target in both hemispheres. The patient underwent DBS implantation on his left side first, with no complications. The electrode was functional for 13 months (monopolar: 2.8 V, 90 μsec pulse width, 185 Hz frequency). Both the patient and clinician perceived benefit in motor symptoms resulting from this DBS lead implantation.

COMPLICATIONS

One and half months later, the second electrode was implanted in the right hemisphere, also with no complications. This electrode was functional for 11 months (bipolar: 2.2 V, 90 μsec pulse width, 195 Hz frequency). However, the patient and clinician perceived only moderate benefit in tremor from this electrode despite multiple adjustments to the settings. One month after the second surgery, the patient was admitted to the emergency department with acute aphasia and mild right hemiparesis resulting from a small stroke in the left hemisphere. The underlying cause of the stroke was diagnosed as atrial fibrillation, and the patient was treated with coumadin after the DBS was deactivated. This management strategy was followed by improvement in both aphasia and hemiparesis symptoms; however, some residual symptoms remained. When the DBS was activated, the patient experienced marginal improvement in tremor on the left side. The patient ultimately died from cardiac arrest. The brain was collected through the University of Florida Brain Tissue Network (UF-BTN) program.

TROUBLESHOOTING AND MANAGEMENT

A review of cases in the UF-BTN program was performed, and of the available 26 cases, one case with a severe collagenous tissue reaction was identified.

Immunohistochemistry

The brain was sectioned for routine neuropathologic diagnosis, and the lead tip blocks were sectioned on a microtome and stained using hematoxylin and eosin for standard diagnosis and Masson's trichrome for confirmation of collagenous deposition [Abcam, Ab150686]. Pathologic diagnosis was confirmed after immunohistochemistry was performed using antibodies to alpha-synuclein (Novocastra), hyperphosphorylated tau (DAKO), and A-beta amyloid (DAKO). Sections were viewed on a standard light microscope (Olympus). Pathology report was prepared by a board certified neuropathologist.

OUTCOME

Gross pathology

Gross examination revealed no significant swelling or atrophy of the brain, which weighed 1,460 g at the time of autopsy. There was significant depigmentation of the substantia nigra and also of the locus coeruleus. DBS defects were observed in both hemispheres, with the right defect located 8 cm from the right frontal pole and 3.5 cm from the vertex and with the left defect located 10.5 cm from the left frontal pole and 3.5 cm from the vertex. Serial sectioning of the DBS tract revealed that the right lead tip was located at the intersection between the STN and substantia nigra, whereas the left lead tip was located at the very ventral part of the STN. There was no evidence of tissue softening or hemorrhage in the vicinity of the DBS lead tracts in either hemisphere. Mild hydrocephalus ex vacuo was detected, and there was clear evidence of cardiovascular disease associated with hypertension and the presence of a fairly large infarct in the left caudate nucleus. Further, there was also a cortical infarct involving the left superior temporal gyrus, which contributed to distinct atrophy of the gyri of the insular cortex and the middle temporal gyrus.

Histopathology

Considerable neuronal loss, along with gliosis, was observed in both the substantia nigra and the locus coeruleus, where there were a few pigmented neurons, and these were positive for the presence of Lewy bodies, with alpha-synuclein. There was no notable change associated with neurodegenerative disease in the cerebral cortex, but there were sparse neuritic plaques present in entorhinal cortex, neocortex, cingulate gyrus. There was evidence of cerebrovascular disease associated with hypertension in the basal ganglia.

The DBS tracts were investigated in detail and showed no evidence of necrosis or hemorrhage. Nevertheless, there was distinct fibrosis at the right DBS lead cavity, and the presence of a fibrocollagenous capsule was detected by trichrome staining (Masson's), Figure 27.1A and B. Minimal hemosiderin deposits were noted around the capsule, and these were composed of mature lymphocytes (Figure 27.1C). Immunohistochemistry for glial fibrillary acidic protein (GFAP) revealed reactive gliosis of the tissue surrounding the capsule (Figure 27.1D); however, healthy neurons were noted adjacent to the capsule. High magnification of lead tip fibrosis with chronic inflammation (Figure 27.1E). The left distal lead tip defect showed only mild gliosis in close proximity to a central cavity. No fibrotic reaction was identified (Figure 27.1F).

DISCUSSION

DBS emerged as a safe and effective alternative to lesion therapy in the late 1990s. It is currently accepted as an effective treatment for movement disorders.[1] DBS involves the stereotactic placement of electrodes into specific brain nuclei. It has proved effective in the treatment not only movement disorders but also of pain, depression, and select neuropsychiatric diseases and has been shown to be safe, with little to no adverse tissue reactions,[2,3] However, its exact mechanism of action still remains unclear. The University of Florida Center for Movement Disorders and Neurorestoration has established a DBS Brain Tissue Network (UF-BTN) to study the electrode–brain interface and changes in tissue as a consequence of DBS.[4] In our cohort, we have observed a single unique case of reactive tissue surrounding the DBS lead, which we present here.

Chronic implantation of stimulation electrodes can result in reactive responses. Several cell types are involved in mounting a "foreign body response" to materials implanted in the central nervous system.[5] Typically, a fibrous tissue layer is observable in the electrode tract on removal[6]; however, the efficacy of DBS has not to date been shown to be negatively affected as a consequence of this pathologic change.[7] The case report presented here details an atypical, exaggerated tissue reaction to a DBS lead placed in the STN of a patient with PD. The usual complications of DBS (infection, hemorrhage) occur during the surgical procedure itself; however, in this case, the pathologic response likely evolved sometime after surgery. Typically, astrocytes become activated on injury and transform themselves into a reactive phenotype, commonly known as reactive gliosis,[8] which describes the changes involved in astrocytes on activation, including upregulation of numbers and an increase in the production of matrix.[9,10] The most common response to long-term electrode implants is an encapsulation layer or glial scar, primarily made up of reactive astrocytes.[11-13] The purpose of the scar formation is still unclear, but it is thought that it helps in maintaining a healthy blood–brain barrier.[9]

The fibrous capsule made up of collagen is, however, a rare occurrence in response to DBS and has not been observed in our DBS Brain Bank, nor has it been reported by any other group.

The advent of upgraded electrode technologies, biocompatible materials, and improved implantation procedures will likely affect the design of electrodes, which will become better suited for minimization of reactive cellular processes.

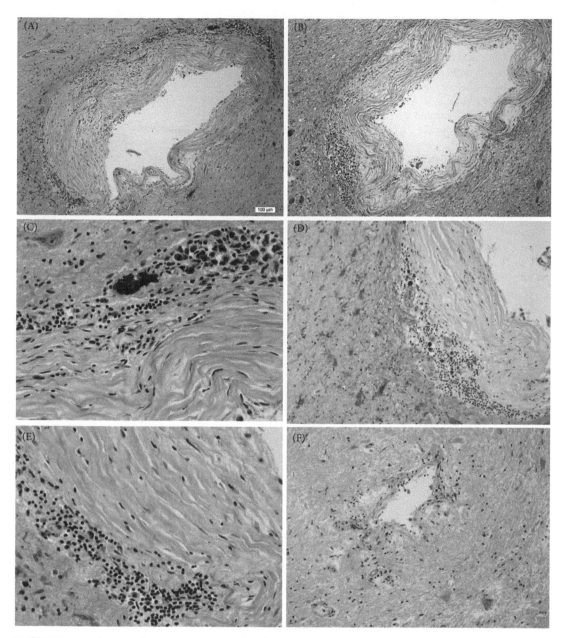

FIGURE 27.1. (A–F) Collagenous reaction to deep brain stimulation placement.

PEARLS

- DBS lead implantation may rarely lead to a severe collagenous fibrous scar.
- It is unknown whether these scars and capsules will affect clinical DBS responses.
- Recent evidence from a large tissue bank[14] suggests that approximately three out of four post-mortem DBS cases exhibited pathologic evidence of at least a mild glial collar or scar present at the ventral DBS lead tip. The amount of gliosis was not significantly associated with duration of DBS. The case presented in this chapter was a severe collagenous change, which seems to be very rare.

REFERENCES

1. Volkmann J. Deep brain stimulation for the treatment of Parkinson's disease. Journal of clinical neurophysiology: official publication of the American Electroencephalographic Society 2004;21:6–17.

2. Haberler C, Alesch F, Mazal PR, et al. No tissue damage by chronic deep brain stimulation in Parkinson's disease. Ann Neurol 2000;48: 372–376.

3. Sun DA, Yu H, Spooner J, et al. Postmortem analysis following 71 months of deep brain stimulation of the subthalamic nucleus for Parkinson disease. J Neurosurg 2008;109:325–329.

4. Vedam-Mai V, Krock N, Ullman M, et al. The national DBS brain tissue network pilot study: need for more tissue and more standardization. Cell Tissue Bank 2011;12(3):219–231.

5. Sahyouni R, Chang DT, Moshtaghi O, Mahmoodi A, Djalilian HR, Lin HW. Functional and histological effects of chronic neural electrode implantation. Laryngoscope investigative otolaryngology 2017;2:80–93.

6. Schultz RL, Willey TJ. The ultrastructure of the sheath around chronically implanted electrodes in brain. Journal of neurocytology 1976;5:621–642.

7. Polikov VS, Tresco PA, Reichert WM. Response of brain tissue to chronically implanted neural electrodes. Journal of neuroscience methods 2005;148:1–18.

8. Giordana MT, Attanasio A, Cavalla P, Migheli A, Vigliani MC, Schiffer D. Reactive cell proliferation and microglia following injury to the rat brain. Neuropathology and applied neurobiology 1994;20:163–174.

9. Landis DM. The early reactions of non-neuronal cells to brain injury. Annual review of neuroscience 1994;17:133–151.

10. Elkabes S, DiCicco-Bloom EM, Black IB. Brain microglia/macrophages express neurotrophins that selectively regulate microglial proliferation and function. J Neurosci 1996;16:2508–2521.

11. Szarowski DH, Andersen MD, Retterer S, et al. Brain responses to micro-machined silicon devices. Brain Res 2003;983:23–35.

12. Biran R, Martin DC, Tresco PA. Neuronal cell loss accompanies the brain tissue response to chronically implanted silicon microelectrode arrays. Exp Neurol 2005;195:115–126.

13. Reier PJ, Perlow MJ, Guth L. Development of embryonic spinal cord transplants in the rat. Brain Res 1983;312:201–219.

14. Vedam-Mai V, Rodgers C, Gureck A, et al. Deep brain stimulation associated gliosis: a post-mortem study. Parkinsonism Relat Disord 2018;54:51–55.

Case 28

Cerebral Venous Infarction After Deep Brain Stimulation Surgery

ANDI NUGRAHA SENDJAJA, TAKASHI MORISHITA, AND TOORU INOUE

INDICATION FOR DEEP BRAIN STIMULATION

Parkinson disease (PD) with motor fluctuations

CLINICAL HISTORY AND RELEVANT EXAM

A 67-year-old woman with a 16-year history of PD underwent staged bilateral subthalamic nucleus (STN) deep brain stimulation (DBS). Her first DBS surgery in the right hemisphere was performed without any complications, and her symptoms improved. A left STN DBS was performed 6 months later. She was discharged on postoperative day 1 without any issues. However, she experienced word-finding difficulties and an altered level of consciousness that same evening after discharge and was brought to the emergency department because the symptoms persisted. On examination, she was diagnosed with incomplete expressive dysfluency and disorientation. A head computed tomography (CT) scan showed cerebral edema and subcortical hemorrhage surrounding the superficial aspect of the DBS lead (Figure 28.1).

COMPLICATIONS

Her neurologic condition deteriorated on postoperative day 1 in a delayed fashion, and the patient had an altered state of consciousness and speech disturbance. The presentation with imaging correlation was typical for venous infarction resulting from DBS lead implantation. A CT scan showed cerebral edema with subcortical hemorrhage along the DBS lead (see Figure 28.1, case 1).

TROUBLESHOOTING AND MANAGEMENT

The patient was conservatively monitored during the clinical course. Management of the condition included optimizing venous return (e.g., elevate the head of the bed 30 degrees), normalizing blood pressure, avoiding dehydration, and initiating early rehabilitation. An emergency craniotomy would have been performed if the hemorrhage were large and life-threatening; however, the hemorrhage was self-limited.

OUTCOME

Dysfluency improved spontaneously within a few days, but confusion persisted for several weeks. While the Unified Parkinson's Disease Rating Scale (UPDRS) motor score in the off-medication state was 38 preoperatively, the patient's PD symptoms improved, leading to a score of 27 on the same scale in the off-medication/on-DBS condition at 4-month follow-up.

DISCUSSION

Diagnosis of venous infarction associated with the DBS surgery can usually be made if neurologic deficits develop in a subacute fashion (on postoperative day 1 or 2) and if cerebral edema is observed around the superficial aspect of the DBS lead and/or subcortical hemorrhage.[1] The incidence of this complication has been reported to be approximately 1%.[1]

Cerebral edema and subcortical hemorrhage are thought to develop as a result of venous hypertension and congestion secondary to obstruction of venous flow. Venous infarction following neurosurgical procedures commonly results from intraoperative injury of cortical veins[1,2] and has been associated with damage of the cortical vein during DBS surgery. The large cortical vein may be injured during dural opening. Therefore, stereotactic planning should be performed carefully to ensure that the blood vessels are not damaged.

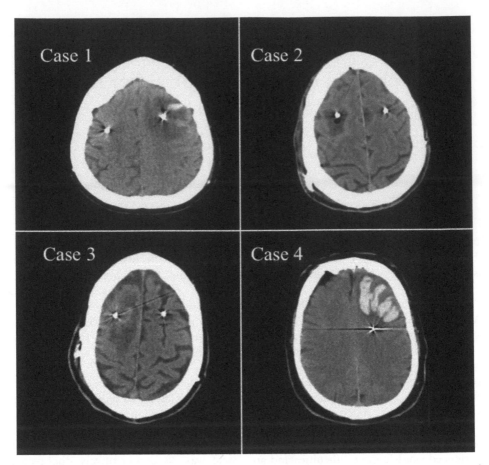

FIGURE 28.1. Computed tomography findings in four cases of post–deep brain stimulation venous infarction. Significant edema around the superficial aspect of the implanted lead is universally present and frequently associated with subcortical hemorrhage. Case 4 shows a classic "flame" hemorrhage commonly seen in venous infarction. (Adapted from Morishita T, Okun MS, Burdick A, Jacobson IV CE, Foote KD. Cerebral venous infarction: a potentially avoidable complication of deep brain stimulation surgery. Neuromodulation: Technology at the Neural Interface 2013:16:407–413, with permission.)

Venous infarction is characterized by a delayed clinical onset with edema and/or hemorrhage along the DBS lead track. During imaging, lesions due to venous infarction are likely to have irregular shapes with poorly differentiated margins, whereas arterial infarctions tend to have sharp, frequently wedge-shaped margins (see Figure 28.1). Head CT may not show an obvious lesion in the immediate postoperative period; therefore, a repeat CT scan may be necessary to confirm diagnosis in cases with neurologic deficits.

An emergency craniotomy may be performed if the hemorrhage is life-threatening. However, conservative therapy with careful observation should be the first-line treatment when this complication is observed. This involves elevating the head of the bed by 30 degrees to optimize venous return, controlling blood pressure to prevent secondary subcortical hemorrhage, avoiding dehydration to optimize blood rheology, administering prophylactic anticonvulsants to diminish the known risk for seizure, and initiating early rehabilitation. Steroids should be avoided because cerebral edema is not a result of inflammation.

The prognosis of cerebral venous infarction is usually good, and full recovery is common. The neurologic conditions of patients can in many cases return to baseline after days to weeks, as presented in this case. The prognostic information is valuable to reassure afflicted patients and their families.

PEARLS

- Venous infarction is a possible complication of DBS surgery. This complication is suspected in patients who complain of neurologic deficits on postoperative day 1 or 2. There may be cerebral edema with or without hemorrhage along the DBS lead.
- Venous infarction is usually an avoidable complication of DBS surgery. Preoperative planning should be supported by optimal visualization of blood vessels using a high-resolution contrasted magnetic resonance imaging or stereotactic CT scan with contrast to avoid injuries to the blood vessels.
- Conservative management is the first-line treatment in the management of venous infarction. The prognosis of cerebral venous infarction is usually good, and full neurologic recovery with optimal treatment is predicted in many, but not all, cases.

REFERENCES

1. Morishita T, Okun MS, Burdick A, Jacobson IV CE, Foote KD. Cerebral venous infraction: a potentially avoidable complication of deep brain stimulation surgery. Neuromodulation: Technology at the Neural Interface 2013;16:407–413.

2. Morishita T, Foote KD, Burdick A, et al. Identification and management of deep brain stimulation intra- and postoperative urgencies and emergencies. Parkinsonism and Related Disorders 2010;16:10.

Case 29

Open Circuits and Loss of Deep Brain Stimulation Benefit in the Setting of Parkinson Disease

ARJUN TARAKAD AND JOOHI JIMENEZ-SHAHED

INDICATION FOR DEEP BRAIN STIMULATION
Parkinson disease (PD) with refractory tremor

CLINICAL HISTORY AND RELEVANT EXAM
The patient is a 67-year-old woman with PD who underwent bilateral subthalamic nucleus (STN) deep brain stimulation (DBS) surgery at age 63 years for tremor that was not responsive to dopaminergic therapy. Preoperative evaluation was significant for the discovery of an intracranial aneurysm, for which she underwent clipping before DBS surgery. The patient had significant improvement of tremor, hand function, and gait following DBS surgery.

COMPLICATIONS
Seven years after the initial surgery, the patient experienced a recurrence of tremor and parkinsonism. Her implantable pulse generator (IPG) was found to have a low voltage and was replaced. During the IPG replacement surgery, the patient was found to have a ruptured breast implant, and treatment with intravenous antibiotics was pursued. Because of this and a fluid collection surrounding the IPG, it was relocated into her abdomen. Return to her previous DBS settings following the surgery did not result in a recapture of the previous improvement in tremor. Interrogation of the DBS system revealed an open circuit at the active anode (contact 0) and high impedance readings at the active cathode (contact 3) of her left STN electrode, which was programmed in a wide bipolar (0– 3+) configuration. Because of the open circuit, a narrower bipolar field (1– 2+) was chosen with some improvement in her tremor, but

no relief of rigidity or bradykinesia, and progressive gait difficulties. She was programmed at these settings for 1½ years with suboptimal benefit. Plain film radiographs did not show any evidence of lead fracture. Electrode revision surgery was being considered, for which the patient was sent for magnetic resonance imaging (MRI) to assess electrode placement, but she was unable to complete this imaging study because of concerns about patient injury related to the open circuit.

TROUBLESHOOTING AND MANAGEMENT
Reassessment of her programming settings revealed a low current delivery (1.84 mA) in the left STN relative to her settings (1– 2+ at 5 V, pulse width of 120 μsec, frequency of 160 Hz) with a therapeutic impedance of 2,700 ohm (normal impedance values per Medtronic reference manual being 250–2,000 ohm). Monopolar programming was attempted at the C+ 1– and C+ 2– configurations. The patient initially developed speech difficulties, which resolved with a reduction in pulse width from 120us to 60us (which is a typical value for initial programming). C+ 2– monopolar configuration provided sustained tremor benefit and improvement of gait and bradykinesia. Despite a reduction in voltage from 5 to 3 V, the current delivery increased from 1.84 to 2 mA.

OUTCOME
The patient has had sustained and durable benefits for 2 years on these DBS settings. Her IPG battery has also continued to function appropriately, without evidence of reduced battery longevity from the open circuit.

DISCUSSION

This case addresses the problem of loss of efficacy of DBS in a PD patient with a previously good response to neuromodulation. While the cause of decline might not always be readily apparent, with reasons ranging from electrode migration to lead fracture,[1] in this case it is reasonable to assume that the open circuit at the active contact was the source of the problem. An open circuit is caused by a disruption in the flow of current between the IPG and the electrode commonly due to a fractured or disconnected wire. It can occur during IPG replacement surgery with inadvertent injury to one of the contacts. It can be identified by high impedance readings seen on diagnostic impedance analysis, which do not fully correct with testing at increasing voltages. In contrast, a short circuit bypasses the flow of current and results in abnormally low impedance readings. Both open circuits and short circuits can result in loss of DBS effectiveness or the development of new side effects.[2-4] While increased battery drain from increase in stimulation amplitude to compensate for loss of efficacy may occur in either case, a short circuit programmed in the constant-voltage mode also has the potential to drain IPG battery independent of changes in stimulation parameters due to shunting of electrical current to a pathway with lower impedance.[5]

DBS electrode revision or removal is not uncommon, with estimates ranging as high as 15 to 34% of surgical cases.[6] Although device malfunction represents only a fraction of revision cases, it can be a potentially costly intervention that confers additional risks associated with brain surgery. While in most cases of acute failure of symptom control due to DBS hardware malfunction, replacement of extension cables or possibly even electrode revision may be necessary, this case demonstrates the possibility that systematic reassessment of DBS programming may recapture sustained clinical benefit without surgical intervention. It is important to note that in this case there was a stable change in current delivery (an open circuit at a specific contact), which was amenable to reprogramming; if loss of efficacy appears to be an active or evolving process, reprogramming alone may not be sufficient.

PEARLS

- When abrupt loss of efficacy in DBS is observed, the cause should be thoroughly evaluated, beginning with DBS interrogation to check for hardware compromise.
  - When a circuit disruption is identified, plain film radiographs may be sufficient to identify a lead fracture.
  - While MRI remains the preferred modality for visualizing brain anatomy, the presence of any circuit abnormality may be a contraindication to MRI (because it could represent a break in the lead, even if not visible on imaging, which can in turn lead to tissue heating). Increased accessibility of software that can merge computed tomography scans to preoperative MRI may be a viable alternative in appropriate cases.
- When a cause for loss of DBS efficacy is found, reprogramming can be tailored around identified problems (e.g., avoidance of the faulty contact; ensuring delivery of sufficient current to the target by checking therapy impedance; or, in the case of a malpositioned electrode, selection of contacts closest to the anatomical target).
- When there is a circuit malfunction, hardware replacement or revision surgery should only be considered if sufficient benefit cannot be achieved with reprogramming in an otherwise stable patient.

REFERENCES

1. Baizabal Carvallo JF, Mostile G, Almaguer M, Davidson A, Simpson R, Jankovic J. Deep brain stimulation hardware complications in patients with movement disorders: risk factors and clinical correlations. Stereotact Funct Neurosurg. 2012;90:300–306.

2. Samura K, Miyagi Y, Okamoto T, et al. Short circuit in deep brain stimulation. J Neurosurg. 2012;117:955–961.

3. Allert N, Reyes Santana M, Karbe H. Short circuit in deep brain stimulation for Parkinson's disease mimicking stroke. Brain Stimul. 2016;9:950–951.

4. Waln O, Jimenez-Shahed J. Rechargeable deep brain stimulation implantable pulse generators in movement disorders: patient satisfaction and conversion parameters. Neuromodulation. 2014;17:425–430.

5. Allert N, Barbe MT, Timmermann L, Coenen VA. Rapid battery depletion and loss of therapy due to a short circuit in bipolar DBS for essential tremor. Acta Neurochir (Wien). 2017;159:795–798.

6. Rolston JD, Englot DJ, Starr PA, Larson PS. An unexpectedly high rate of revisions and removals in deep brain stimulation surgery: analysis of multiple databases. Parkinsonism Relat Disord. 2016;33:72–77.

Case 30

Acute Neuropsychiatric Symptoms and Impulse Control Disorders After Subthalamic Nucleus Deep Brain Stimulation

ADOLFO RAMIREZ-ZAMORA

INDICATION FOR DEEP BRAIN STIMULATION

Progressive and refractory motor fluctuations, tremor, and dyskinesia in the setting of idiopathic Parkinson disease (PD)

CLINICAL HISTORY AND RELEVANT EXAM

A 60-year-old right-handed man with a history of idiopathic PD for 17 years presented with severe motor fluctuations including end-of-dose wearing off, dystonia, freezing of gait, and peak-dose dyskinesia. Medical management included the use of levodopa IR 1,400 mg/day in divided doses, pramipexole 1 mg three times daily, and amantadine 100 mg twice daily. He had no past history of neuropsychiatric disorders or impulse control disorders (ICDs), except for transient history of depression adequately treated with sertraline 100 mg daily for a year (in the remote past). After comprehensive multidisciplinary deep brain stimulation (DBS) assessment, he had uncomplicated, simultaneous bilateral subthalamic nucleus (STN) DBS placement (Medtronic Activa PC DBS implanted with 3,389 leads) using standard trajectory angles and stereotactic approach.[1] The perioperative course was unremarkable. He presented for initial electrode screening and monopolar review 1 month after surgery. His baseline total Unified Parkinson's Disease Rating Scale (UPDRS) Part III score was 41. During initial monopolar review (pulse width [PW] of 60 μsec and frequency of 140 Hz), he noticed a sudden onset of "feeling hyper and euphoria" best defined as a sense of "energy" when activating contact 0 in the right STN at 1.5 to 2 V. A similar feeling was noted with contact 1 around the same voltage.

Additional programming revealed corticobulbar side effects with more dorsal leads at 3 to 4 V. There was improvement in parkinsonism with resolution of resting tremor and marked benefit in bradykinesia and rigidity with all contacts, more notable with contacts 0 and 1. The contralateral, left STN lead revealed a threshold for side effects starting at 2.5 V with ventral contacts and 3 to 4 V with dorsal contacts. Corticospinal side effects, dizziness, and sweatiness were noted with contact 0 and paresthesia with contact 1. Corticospinal side effects were encountered when programing dorsal electrodes as well. The rest of his monopolar review was unremarkable, with improvement in parkinsonism with most contacts but clear reduction in rigidity with contacts 2 and 3 and mild dyskinesia at 2.5 V with contact 2. The initial programming settings in the right STN were unipolar mode with case positive, contact 1 negative, amplitude 2 V, PW 60 μsec, and frequency 140 Hz; and in the left STN, unipolar mode with case positive, contact 2 negative, amplitude 2.5 V, PW 60 μsec, and frequency 140 Hz was used.

COMPLICATIONS

The patient's family contacted our clinic a couple of weeks after the initial programming visit because the patient exhibited a variety of unusual behaviors. His family described the patient as being "hyper or caffeinated," with enlightened mood, distractibility, tachypsychia, and impulsivity. He had increased energy leading to constant running around his house with falls. His family reported insomnia and increased sexual preoccupations along with inability to resist playing scratch-offs at his local convenience store. He noted clear benefit in motor symptoms and fluctuations with unchanged dyskinesia. Reports by family members indicated conflicts resulting from the patient's aberrant behavior and lack of proper judgment. As the patient displayed symptoms of hypomania and ICDs with improvement in motor symptoms, medications were initially adjusted with discontinuation initially of his dopamine agonist followed by amantadine. Despite partial recurrence of motor symptoms including tremors, mild end-of-dose wearing off, and resolution of dyskinesia, impulsive and unusual behaviors persisted. Additional DBS programming was performed using similar contact configuration based on initial adequate motor response reducing amplitude and then switching to bipolar mode (right STN, contact 0+ 1–, 2.3 V, PW 60 μsec, frequency 140 Hz; and left STN contact 2– case +, 2 V, PW 60 μsec, frequency 140 Hz), slowly increasing the amplitude to control rigidity and tremor. He tolerated changes well in clinic with marked improvement in parkinsonism (UPDRS Part III off medications total score of 14). Unfortunately, despite medications and programming changes, the patient reported persistent difficulties controlling impetuous behaviors, increased mood, and intrusive sexual thoughts. There was no evidence of psychosis, dopamine dysregulation syndrome, hallucinations, or depression.

TROUBLESHOOTING AND MANAGEMENT

The patient was diagnosed with an impulse control disorder and hypomania according to the *Diagnostic and Statistical Manual of Mental Disorders,* fourth edition (DSM-IV) criteria using the Mini-International Neuropsychiatric Interview for affective disorders.[2] As previously noted, initial management included medication adjustments as he noted clear improvement in motor control, and STN DBS commonly facilitated medication reduction in the 30 to 50% range. This was followed by levodopa dose reduction to the lowest effective dose to manage motor fluctuations and reduction in STN stimulation, with only partial response in his symptoms. When turning his stimulators off, patient and his family noted improved distractibility and motor and cognitive impulsivity, but this was poorly tolerated by the patient because of worsening parkinsonism and tremors. Multiple reports suggest that stimulation of the substantia nigra reticulata (SNr) and limbic (medioventral) STN territories might induce ICDs and hypomania in patients

with PD. DBS management included reduction in amplitude and using bipolar stimulation with only partial benefit. In his right STN, we then decided to activate the most dorsal contact in unipolar mode, determining amplitude based on motor response (contact 3–, case positive). The patient reported improvement in neuropsychiatric symptoms but noted that increasing parkinsonism and higher voltages induced reproducible corticospinal/corticobulbar side effects associated with stimulation of the internal capsule. We then decided to activate a similar configuration in bipolar mode using first a single and then double contacts to maximize dorsal STN stimulation while reducing lateral-induced side effects. His left STN programming was switched to narrow bipolar (contact 2–, contact 3 positive), and amplitude was adjusted with excellent control of parkinsonism in the right body. A postoperative brain magnetic resonance imaging (MRI) study was reviewed to confirm DBS lead location. The brain MRI showed that the electrodes were located in the STN region bilaterally, but the position of both electrodes, particularly on the right STN, was decisively more medial and deeper than initially planned (Figure 30.1).

OUTCOME

After an initial programming session using more dorsal contacts, the patient noted rapid reduction in impulsive behaviors with a stable response over the following weeks after additional programming sessions adjusting for voltage (using similar settings). Levodopa dose was adjusted accordingly based on response to neurostimulation. His total UPDRS Part III score at 6 months in the off-medication state was 17. Programming using the most ventral contact at 6 months (likely stimulating limbic networks in the STN) consistently reproduced a euphoric and impulsive response in the patient.

DISCUSSION

This case illustrates the complexities of managing de novo neuropsychiatric symptoms after STN DBS and highlights the common overlap among multiple psychiatric symptoms. Unlike striatal territories, there is overlap and convergence between the functional motor, associative, and limbic territories at the level of the STN.[3] STN stimulation mimics both the motor and behavioral effects of dopaminergic drugs, which explains the effects resembling the hyperdopaminergic side effects of dopaminergic drugs

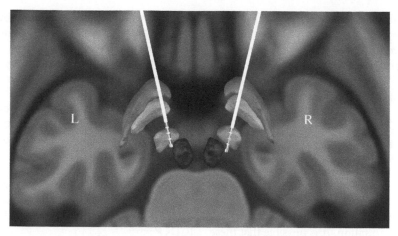

FIGURE 30.1. Schematic representation of normalized, bilateral subthalamic nucleus (STN) deep brain stimulation (DBS) electrode localization. Patient's postoperative imaging indicated a more medial and ventral lead location within the right STN along with a more medial position of DBS contacts in the left STN.

after surgery.[4] This condition in most cases is unrecognized by patients and their relatives, and it spontaneously resolves within a few weeks in most patients.[5] However, prompt identification of reproducible, acute, and consistent psychiatric side effects after STN DBS is critical to initiate correct management. If present, consideration should be given to the possibility of stimulation within the limbic STN territories, SNr, or surrounding fibers, particularly when using high levels of stimulation. In two case reports, voltage higher than 3 V and monopolar stimulation mode were associated with STN DBS–induced mania in ventral contacts. Monopolar stimulation produces a current that runs in multiple parallel paths and may influence a larger volume of tissue, especially when the current density is relatively high.[6,7] In view of the medial, anterior, and ventral location of the limbic territory of the STN, typical double oblique stereotactic trajectories will place the lower contacts more medially, posteriorly, and caudally, thus being closer to the limbic STN. DBS programming can be challenging because other side effects can be encountered, as in this patient, potentially limiting the DBS benefit effect. There are reports of similar motor benefit between ventral and dorsal contacts in STN along with reports of continued used of ventral stimulation in conjunction with pharmacologic therapies despite recurrence of hypomania symptoms because of maximal motor benefit with these contacts.[8] Although rare, the specific treatment approach needs to be individualized based on particular lead and contact locations

and the patient's symptoms. Programming strategies should aim to reduce electrical charge, like reduction of stimulation amplitude or PW or use of bipolar stimulation. Despite imaging and functional limitations when assessing postoperative lead location, stimulation of the SNr has been reported to induce hypomania and behavioral changes mediated by dysfunction of the limbic system, particularly the anterior cingulate cortex and the medial prefrontal cortex.[9] In other studies based on diffusion tensor imaging (DTI), STN DBS–induced reversible acute hypomania might be elicited by inadvertent and unilateral coactivation of putative limbic STN tributaries to the medial forebrain bundle, a recently identified pathway connecting the medial STN to reward circuitry.[6] Even though the risk factors for psychiatric adverse effects of STN DBS are not well established, long-term studies assessing the occurrence of transient hypomania in the perioperative period have identified potential risk factors to develop these side effects, including male gender, relatively early onset of PD, younger age, shorter disease duration, and deeper lead locations in SN.[9,10] The exact prevalence and incidence of hypomania and impulsivity after STN is not known, but where reported, manic symptoms appeared to resolve in most patients after switching from ventromedial to dorsolateral STN stimulation.[11]

The relationship between DBS and ICDs is complex, with conflicting results. This case also illustrates the complex management of ICDs and impulsivity after STN DBS. Dopaminergic drugs (particularly agonists) are a significant risk factor for the development of ICDs, and with medication reduction after STN DBS, this can indirectly improve symptoms. Small retrospective studies of STN DBS have shown conflicting results ranging from noticeable benefit[12-14] to worsening,[15,16] appearance of de novo,[17,18] or no change[15] in ICDs, with most reports published suggesting long-term benefit in selected patients. Mechanisms accounting for ICD improvement in STN DBS beyond dopaminergic medication reduction are under investigation and remain of great interest because they can provide further insight into functional networks involved in reward and inhibition. It is possible that these differing results can be explained by stimulation causing local inhibition of STN neurons while also activating axons of passage or causing antidromic neuronal networks to relieve the symptoms of PD. It is likely that different outcomes in ICDs following DBS depend on multifactorial circumstances ranging from disease duration and severity to premorbid psychiatric conditions and traits, postoperative lead location, medication use, and programming. Finally, although some reports suggest that ICDs are more common with medial STN stimulation, other studies have found no significant correlation between the location of the electrodes and the de novo ICDs.[19,20]

PEARLS

- Acute neuropsychiatric symptoms including hypomania and impulsivity can occur after STN DBS.
- Early identification of consistent, reproducible stimulation-induced behavioral symptoms after STN DBS versus the transient hyperdopaminergic state is critical to initiate appropriate management.
- Impulsivity and hypomania have been reported after STN DBS possibly due to stimulation within the limbic (ventromedial) STN territories, SNr, or surrounding fibers.
- Programming considerations to manage behavioral symptoms include strategies that reduce electrical charge, and another strategy is activation of more dorsal DBS contacts.

REFERENCES

1. Starr PA. Placement of deep brain stimulators into the subthalamic nucleus or Globus pallidus internus: technical approach. Stereotact Funct Neurosurg 2002;79:118–145.
2. Sheehan DV, Lecrubier Y, Sheehan KH, et al. The Mini-International Neuropsychiatric Interview (M.I.N.I.): the development and validation of a structured diagnostic psychiatric interview for DSM-IV and ICD-10. J Clin Psychiatry 1998;59(Suppl 20):22–33; quiz 34–57.
3. Haynes WI, Haber SN. The organization of prefrontal-subthalamic inputs in primates provides an anatomical substrate for both functional specificity and integration: implications for basal ganglia models and deep brain stimulation. J Neurosci 2013;33:4804–4814.
4. Funkiewiez A, Ardouin C, Krack P, et al. Acute psychotropic effects of bilateral subthalamic nucleus stimulation and levodopa in Parkinson's disease. Mov Disord 2003;18:524–530.
5. Antosik-Wojcinska A, Swiecicki L, Dominiak M, Soltan E, Bienkowski P, Mandat T. Impact of STN-DBS on mood, drive, anhedonia and risk of psychiatric side-effects in the population of PD patients. J Neurol Sci 2017;375:342–347.
6. Coenen VA, Honey CR, Hurwitz T, et al. Medial forebrain bundle stimulation as a pathophysiological mechanism for hypomania in subthalamic nucleus deep brain stimulation for Parkinson's disease. Neurosurgery 2009;64:1106–1114; discussion 1114–1105.
7. Tsai ST, Lin SH, Lin SZ, Chen JY, Lee CW, Chen SY. Neuropsychological effects after chronic subthalamic stimulation and the topography of the nucleus in Parkinson's disease. Neurosurgery 2007;61:E1024–1029; discussion E1029–1030.
8. Schilbach L, Weiss PH, Kuhn J, Timmermann L, Klosterkotter J, Huff W. Pharmacological treatment of deep brain stimulation-induced hypomania leads to clinical remission while preserving motor benefits. Neurocase 2012;18:152–159.

9. Ulla M, Thobois S, Llorca PM, et al. Contact dependent reproducible hypomania induced by deep brain stimulation in Parkinson's disease: clinical, anatomical and functional imaging study. J Neurol Neurosurg Psychiatry 2011;82:607–614.

10. Welter ML, Schupbach M, Czernecki V, et al. Optimal target localization for subthalamic stimulation in patients with Parkinson disease. Neurology 2014;82:1352–1361.

11. Chopra A, Tye SJ, Lee KH, et al. Underlying neurobiology and clinical correlates of mania status after subthalamic nucleus deep brain stimulation in Parkinson's disease: a review of the literature. J Neuropsychiatry Clin Neurosci 2012;24:102–110.

12. Lhommee E, Klinger H, Thobois S, et al. Subthalamic stimulation in Parkinson's disease: restoring the balance of motivated behaviours. Brain 2012;135:1463–1477.

13. Amami P, Dekker I, Piacentini S, et al. Impulse control behaviours in patients with Parkinson's disease after subthalamic deep brain stimulation: de novo cases and 3-year follow-up. J Neurol Neurosurg Psychiatry 2015;86:562–564.

14. Gee L, Smith H, De La Cruz P, et al. The influence of bilateral subthalamic nucleus deep brain stimulation on impulsivity and prepulse inhibition in Parkinson's disease patients. Stereotact Funct Neurosurg 2015;93:265–270.

15. Moum SJ, Price CC, Limotai N, et al. Effects of STN and GPi deep brain stimulation on impulse control disorders and dopamine dysregulation syndrome. PLoS One 2012;7:e29768.

16. Lim SY, O'Sullivan SS, Kotschet K, et al. Dopamine dysregulation syndrome, impulse control disorders and punding after deep brain stimulation surgery for Parkinson's disease. J Clin Neurosci 2009;16:1148–1152.

17. Smeding HM, Goudriaan AE, Foncke EM, Schuurman PR, Speelman JD, Schmand B. Pathological gambling after bilateral subthalamic nucleus stimulation in Parkinson disease. J Neurol Neurosurg Psychiatry 2007;78:517–519.

18. Morgan JC, diDonato CJ, Iyer SS, Jenkins PD, Smith JR, Sethi KD. Self-stimulatory behavior associated with deep brain stimulation in Parkinson's disease. Mov Disord 2006;21:283–285.

19. Merola A, Romagnolo A, Rizzi L, et al. Impulse control behaviors and subthalamic deep brain stimulation in Parkinson disease. J Neurol 2017;264:40–48.

20. Kim A, Kim YE, Kim HJ, et al. A 7-year observation of the effect of subthalamic deep brain stimulation on impulse control disorder in patients with Parkinson's disease. Parkinsonism Relat Disord 2018;56:3–8.

Case 31

Improved Outcome on Interleaved Deep Brain Stimulation Settings

SVJETLANA MIOCINOVIC, PRAVIN KHEMANI, REBECCA WHIDDON, AND SHILPA CHITNIS

INDICATION FOR DEEP BRAIN STIMULATION

Parkinson disease (PD) with dyskinesia and motor fluctuations

CLINICAL HISTORY AND RELEVANT EXAM

A 61-year-old man with tremor-predominant PD for 11 years suffered from motor fluctuations and dyskinesias. The off periods were characterized by tremor, marked deterioration of speech, and slowing of gait.

COMPLICATIONS

Bilateral subthalamic nucleus (STN) deep brain stimulation (DBS) was performed after careful evaluation and review of candidate selection criteria but resulted in suboptimal tremor control despite multiple programming sessions. On the postoperative magnetic resonance imaging (MRI) study, the left electrode was found to be medial to the STN (contact 2 was 7 mm lateral, 1 mm posterior, and 1 mm ventral to the mid-commisural point [MCP]). The left STN single monopolar setting only partially improved the tremor. Double monopolar setting at the amplitude and pulse width necessary to control tremor could not be tolerated because of diplopia (Table 31.1).

TROUBLESHOOTING AND MANAGEMENT

The patient underwent standard clinical programming but achieved suboptimal results with conventional techniques and was subsequently managed by interleaving. He maintained stable clinical benefits for at least 3 months on the interleaved settings. He was examined in a clinical programming session to compare therapeutic benefit on interleaved and conventional settings. The interleaved programs were designated as STN1: case positive, contact A negative, voltage V_A, pulse width PW_A, and STN 2: case positive, contact B negative, voltage V_B, pulse width PW_B. Frequency was defaulted to 125 Hz (the maximum allowable by the device). Stimulation settings for the other hemisphere were held constant.

Unified Parkinson's Disease Rating Scale (UPDRS) examination (off medications) was performed for the following stimulation conditions (see Table 31.1): (1) off stimulation (OFF); (2) case positive, contact A negative, voltage V_A, pulse width PW_A (Single Monopolar I); (3) case positive, contact B negative, voltage V_B, pulse width PW_B (Single Monopolar II); (4) case positive, contact A negative, contact B negative, voltage V_A, pulse width PW_A (Double Monopolar I); (5) case positive, contact A negative, contact B negative, voltage V_B, pulse width PW_B (Double Monopolar II); (6) contact B positive, contact A negative, voltage V_A, pulse width PW_A (Bipolar I); (7) contact A positive, contact B negative, voltage V_B, pulse width PW_B (Bipolar II); (8) STN1: case positive, contact A negative, voltage V_A; STN 2: case positive, contact B negative, voltage V_B, pulse width PW_B (Interleaved).

OUTCOME

Interleaving allowed the dorsal contact to be set to a higher amplitude and pulse width, while the contact below was set to a tolerable lower amplitude and pulse width. Together, the two contacts provided complete tremor resolution without side effects. The off-medication UPDRS Part III score was 12 on interleaved setting, while the best conventional setting resulted in a score of 20.

TABLE 31.1. ELECTRODE LOCATIONS AND CLINICAL SCORES ON CONVENTIONAL AND INTERLEAVED SETTINGS

Electrode Location	DBS OFF	Single Monopolar I	Single Monopolar II	Double Monopolar I	Double Monopolar II	Bipolar I	Bipolar II	Interleaved
		C+2−/3.2/90	C+3−/4.2/120	C+2−3−/3.2/90	C+2−3−/4.2/120	3+2−/3.2/90	2+3−/4.2/120	C+2−/3.2/90 C+3−/4.2/120
	UPDRS: 34	UPDRS: 20	UPDRS: 21	UPDRS: 23	UPDRS: 21	UPDRS: 21	UPDRS: 26	UPDRS: 12
	T 3	T 1	T 1	T 1	T 0	T 1	T 2	T 0
	R 2	R 0	R 0	R 0	R 0	R 0	R 0	R 0
	B 2/2/3	B 1/1/2	B 1/2/2	B 1/2/3	B 1/1/3	B 1/1/2	B 1/1/3	B 0/0/1
	S 1	S 1	S 2	S 2	S 2	S 2	S 2	S 1
				Confusion	Diplopia			

On postoperative imaging, the *white arrow* indicates electrode artifact, *gray dotted line* indicates the red nucleus, and *dashed black line* indicates the STN/SNr region (image is axial slice at the level of red nucleus, 4 mm below the MCP). Total UPDRS Part III scores and selected items reported for contralateral side to the interleaved lead using various stimulation settings. T = arm tremor, R = arm rigidity, B = finger taps/hand opening-closing/wrist turning, S = speech. Stimulation frequency was 125 Hz for all settings.

DBS = deep brain stimulation; MCP = mid-commissural point.

UPDRS = Unified Parkinson's Disease Rating Scale.

Reprinted from Miocinovic S, Khemani P, Whiddon R, Zeilman P, Martinez-Ramirez D, Okun MS, Chitnis S. Outcomes, management, and potential mechanisms of interleaving deep brain stimulation settings. Parkinsonism Relat Disord. 2014;20(12):1434–1437, with permission from Elsevier.

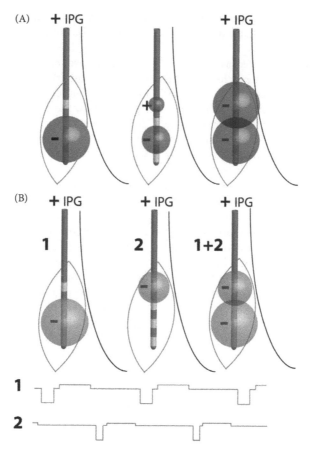

FIGURE 31.1. Graphical representation of the hypothesized mechanisms of interleaving. Spheres represent estimated volume of tissue activated during various deep brain stimulation (DBS) programming settings.[8] In this example, the *dark gray outline* represents subthalamic nucleus (STN), and the *black curve* is the corticospinal tract. Top section (A) demonstrates conventional settings: monopolar stimulation at contact 1 (*left*) does not stimulate a sufficiently large area of the nucleus and does not provide complete resolution of symptoms. Changing to bipolar setting (*middle*) provides some additional activation around contact 3, but it is overall insufficient because bipolar stimulation results in a narrower field. Double monopolar (*right*) provides sufficient coverage of the nucleus but also stimulates corticospinal tract, causing side effects. Bottom section (B) illustrates interleaved programming: user specifies two programs, which are applied interchangeably. Bottom tracings show shape and timing of the stimulation pulses applied to each contact (large negative pulse activates neurons, while small positive afterpulse recovers charge). For each program, user defines specific contacts, amplitude, and pulse width, although frequency is limited up to 125 Hz by the device. This allows greater freedom in selecting different stimulation settings for the two contacts while still benefiting from monopolar field. In this example, interleaving provides sufficient stimulation of the nucleus while avoiding the corticospinal tract. The small overlap area experiences stimulation at twice the frequency because it is seeing pulses from both programs, but the clinical utility of this phenomenon is unknown.[2] IPG = implantable pulse generator.

DISCUSSION

Although DBS technology has not changed fundamentally since its inception, the latest neurostimulator upgrades of Activa PC, Activa RC, and Activa SC (Medtronic Inc., Minneapolis, MN) offer increased programming functionality with an interleaving feature. Interleaving refers to activating two stimulation programs that rapidly alternate from pulse to pulse between each other (Figure 31.1). Each of the two interleaving programs can specify the active electrode contacts, pulse width, and pulse amplitude. The frequency for each program must be the same, and it is limited by the device up to 125 Hz. One or both electrodes can be interleaved, but no more than two programs can be used for each electrode.

Interleaving can be used with both constant voltage (traditional method) and constant current modes.[1]

Interleaving has been suggested as a strategy when conventional programming techniques fail to achieve desired results. Undesirable results may or may not be due to factors such as suboptimal positioning of the lead. When clinicians struggle to program a DBS device, they often employ various additional techniques, including bipolar settings, double monopolar or tripolar settings, and alternative pulse widths and frequencies. The goal of each of these techniques is to shape the electric field in order to maximize therapeutic response while minimizing side effects. If there is a suboptimally positioned lead, interleaving may help to avoid a repeat surgical procedure. Interleaving provides an alternative method to alter the shape of the electrical fields and possibly maximize benefits.

Mechanism of action

The most important feature of interleaving is that it enables the use of multiple negative (cathodal) contacts, but at different amplitudes (see Figure 31.1B). The standard double monopolar setting (two negative contacts with the IPG set as case positive or anodal) forces both contacts on the DBS lead to be set at the same amplitude (and pulse width), which can result in adverse reactions because frequently both contacts cannot be programmed at high settings (see Figure 31.1A, right). One may also set a double monopolar amplitude below the side effect thresholds for both contacts, or a programmer may alternatively choose a single monopolar or bipolar setting. These approaches, however, may not in all cases provide sufficient spread of current for an optimal therapeutic response (see Figure 31.1A, left and middle). Even though pulses from the two programs are offset from each other, they are likely creating an effective electrical field that is a result of the combination of the two individual fields.[2]

Several published reports on interleaving have employed the technique as a means of using different amplitudes at two negative contacts. Wojtecki and colleagues published a case report of a PD patient whose rigidity and bradykinesia responded to STN stimulation at contact 1 at 3.9 V; however, the tremor responded best to stimulation at contact 3 at 1.5 V.[3] Double monopolar stimulation at 3 V or higher resulted in unacceptable dysarthria, so an interleaving strategy was employed. Kovacs and colleagues similarly reported a case series of four patients with dystonia in whom interleaving was more beneficial than monopolar (either single or double) stimulation.[4] In this series, the authors argued that the use of different voltages at each contact maximized the amount of current necessary to control dystonia. Weiss and colleagues used interleaving in a study of gait and balance in PD patients with STN DBS, and the strategy employed was to simultaneously stimulate STN and SNr.[5] Interleaving was used so that both nuclei could be stimulated together; however, higher current was delivered to the contact in the STN, and lower voltages were programmed for the SNr. Another use of interleaving was demonstrated by Barbe and colleagues, who compared dysarthria in ventral intermediate (Vim) nucleus DBS patients set to interleaving using the same amplitude at each active contact (referred to as "non-current-shaped interleaving") versus those set to interleaving with unequal amplitudes ("current-shaped interleaving").[6] Barbe and colleagues demonstrated that current-shaped interleaving, using the same contacts and the same total amount of current, could improve dysarthria in select cases. This strategy suppressed tremor while at the same time directing more current to the dorsal contact in an attempt to lessen dysarthria.

It is unknown whether interleaving provides any additional advantage over simply allowing use of different amplitudes at different contacts. Interleaved settings with identical amplitudes and pulse widths at two different contacts would be similar to double monopolar settings; however, pulses at each contact would be offset by 4 msec (125 Hz equals 8 msec interpulse interval). We do not know whether the effect of the two programs in an interleave is simply the sum of the effects of the individual fields, or if the phase delay may provide an enhanced, synergistic outcome.[2] Baumann and colleagues used interleaving in one patient with essential tremor (ET) and PD to stimulate STN and Vim.[7] Interestingly, the authors reported that single monopolar stimulation was effective for relieving ET when the active contact was the most dorsal, in the Vim. Single monopolar stimulation was effective against PD when the active contact was the most ventral, in the STN. In this case, double monopolar settings using both contacts did not alleviate either symptom, but also did not evoke side effects. The authors proposed that "the importance of pulse timing (simultaneous vs interleaving) may be related to temporal integration in the receiving brain areas." Because single monopolar DBS was therapeutic for each individual symptom, this would imply that the double monopolar setting was causing some sort of undesirable interference. This presumed interference would likely be at downstream targets because the volumes of stimulation from two distal contacts could not overlap except at higher voltages (even with the narrow-spacing 3389 electrode). As a result, interleaving potentially could be argued to have synergistic effects that may be either clinically beneficial or deleterious.

The potential synergistic effect of interleaving (either positive or negative) may in part be due to the area of overlap between the two electric fields that is intentionally created by the interleaved programs. If active contacts are sufficiently close together, and amplitudes sufficiently large, there will be a volume of tissue that will be exposed to pulses from both programs, and effectively will be stimulated at double the interleaved frequency. The device manufacturer has set the maximum interleaving frequency to 125 Hz, so the maximum frequency that neuronal elements in the overlapped area can be stimulated would be 250 Hz. Although such frequencies are unlikely to be harmful to neurons, there is a potential concern that additive charge density at high frequencies and high pulse widths may exceed safety limits.[2] Limiting the frequency to 125 Hz may affect clinical symptoms, particularly tremor, which may require higher stimulation frequencies. Another shortcoming is that the use of interleaving restricts the frequency at which the other hemisphere can be stimulated (unless the patient has two independent IPGs).

In clinical practice, interleaving is most likely to be useful in two scenarios: (1) different contacts are beneficial for specific symptoms, but each is beneficial at different stimulation amplitude, and one contact may have side effects at higher amplitude; or (2) symptoms are resolved incompletely, and further voltage increase is limited by side effects. There are also potential drawbacks to interleaving; in some cases, it may drain the neurostimulator battery faster than the conventional settings, and it limits frequency to 125 Hz, which may be suboptimal for tremor control. Interleaving may be most beneficial in cases in which there is a suboptimal lead placement; however, long-term interleaving settings may not always hold benefit. Interleaving should be thought of as one more tool that may augment outcomes and possibly obviate the need for surgical revisions.

In addition to the Medtronic system, two additional companies (Abbott and Boston Scientific) now provide commercially available DBS systems for the US market. They do not have an interleaving option, but both provide other methods to sculpt the electric field and minimize side effects. The Boston Scientific system has multiple independent current control (MICC) so that each contact can be set to its own stimulation amplitude. The Abbott system has segmented contacts so that one or more select segments can be activated rather than the entire circular contact.

PEARLS

- Interleaving is a programming technique available in Medtronic DBS neurostimulators that allows two sets of stimulation parameters to be applied interchangeably (on a millisecond level).
- Interleaving can in select cases provide differential improvement in motor benefits with the possibility of limiting side effects.
- Interleaving may be most beneficial in cases in which there is a suboptimal lead placement and possibly obviate the need for surgical revision.

REFERENCES

1. Medtronic. Activa® SC, Activa® PC and Activa® RC Online Learning. http://professional.medtronic.com/activatraining. Accessed on Mar 16, 2014.
2. Montgomery EB. Deep Brain Stimulation Programming: Principles and Practice. Oxford, UK: Oxford University Press, 2010.
3. Wojtecki L, Vesper J, Schnitzler A. Interleaving programming of subthalamic deep brain stimulation to reduce side effects with good motor outcome in a patient with Parkinson's disease. Parkinsonism Relat Disord. 2011;17(4):293–294.
4. Kovács N, Janszky J, Nagy F, Balás I. Changing to interleaving stimulation might improve dystonia in cases not responding to pallidal stimulation. Mov Disord. 2012;27(1):163–165.
5. Weiss D, Walach M, Meisner C, Fritz M, Scholten M, Breit S, et al. Nigral stimulation for resistant axial motor impairment in Parkinson's disease? A randomized controlled trial. Brain. 2013;136(Pt 7):2098–2108.
6. Barbe MT, Dembek TA, Becker J, Raethjen J, Hartinger M, Meister IG, et al. Individualized current-shaping reduces DBS-induced dysarthria in patients with essential tremor. Neurology. 2014;82(7):614–619.
7. Baumann CR, Imbach LL, Baumann-Vogel H, Uhl M, Sarnthein J, Sürücü O. Interleaving deep brain stimulation for a patient with both Parkinson's disease and essential tremor. Mov Disord. 2012;27(13):1700–1701.
8. McIntyre CC, Mori S, Sherman DL, Thakor NV, Vitek JL. Electric field and stimulating influence generated by deep brain stimulation of the subthalamic nucleus. Clin Neurophysiol. 2004;115(3):589–595.

Case 32

Deep Brain Stimulation Targeting the Ventral Intermediate Nucleus of the Thalamus for Parkinsonian Tremor and Later Adding the Globus Pallidus Interna for Parkinson Disease Features

QIANG ZHANG AND TERI R. THOMSEN

INDICATIONS FOR DEEP BRAIN STIMULATION

Severe tremor uncontrolled with medication; parkinsonian motor fluctuations

CLINICAL HISTORY AND RELEVANT EXAM

A 69-year-old right-handed gentleman with history of tremor presented to the University of Iowa Movement Disorders Clinic for consideration for deep brain stimulation (DBS) surgery. His tremor began 8 years ago in his right hand and gradually progressed to involve his left hand. He first noticed these symptoms when he was working as a locksmith, and the tremor interfered with the performance of fine motor tasks. He retired 3 years ago because of severe tremor. The tremor is worse with action but also present at rest. Of note, carbidopa/levodopa was helpful with his tremor control initially, although the effect wore off, and the medication was discontinued because of side effects emerging at higher dosage. He also tried propranolol, primidone, benzodiazepines, ropinirole, and amantadine; however, all these medications were ineffective, and he discontinued all medications 5 years ago. At the time of initial presentation to us, he had trouble with handwriting, eating, and fastening buttons. On exam, he had severe resting, postural, and kinetic tremors in both hands, but worse on the right. He also had bradykinesia and cogwheeling rigidity, worse on the right. He had a shuffling gait with stooped posture and decreased arm swing bilaterally, particularly on the right. He carried the diagnosis of essential tremor (ET), but we revised his diagnosis to right-dominant, tremor-predominant idiopathic Parkinson disease (PD) at first visit. We restarted carbidopa/levodopa and had an extensive discussion about surgical options targeting tremor (ventral intermediate [Vim] nucleus of thalamus) versus parkinsonism (subthalamic nucleus [STN] or globus pallidus internus [GPi]). Eventually, we decided to proceed with bilateral Vim DBS placement because the patient was not bothered by other features of parkinsonism, and a levodopa *off/on* test showed less than 40% improvement in Unified Parkinson's Disease Rating Scale (UPDRS) score (59 > 52). After Vim DBS placement, his tremor was adequately controlled (Figures 32.1 and 32.2). However, after 2 years, his parkinsonian symptoms progressed, and he developed dyskinesia and motor fluctuations requiring a higher dosage of levodopa/carbidopa. He also required higher DBS settings for tremor control, which caused significant dysarthria. Therefore, we decided to proceed with bilateral GPi DBS placement, in the hope of alleviating parkinsonian motor fluctuations and achieving better tremor control without stimulation-related side effects (Figure 32.3).

COMPLICATION

Dysarthria

TROUBLESHOOTING AND MANAGEMENT

For the patient's initial programming of bilateral Vim DBS, we used monopolar settings on both sides, and he had adequate tremor control (Table 32.1). His tremor gradually worsened by the time he came back for a second programming. We

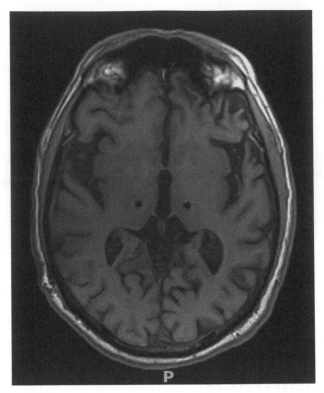

FIGURE 32.1. Magnetic resonance imaging after ventral intermediate nucleus of the thalamus deep brain stimulation placement surgery.

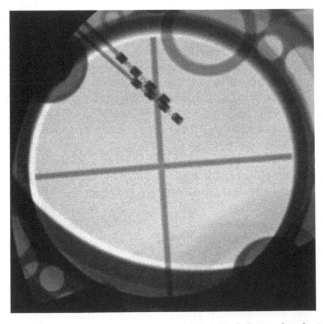

FIGURE 32.2. Fluoroscopy during ventral intermediate nucleus of the thalamus deep brain stimulation placement surgery.

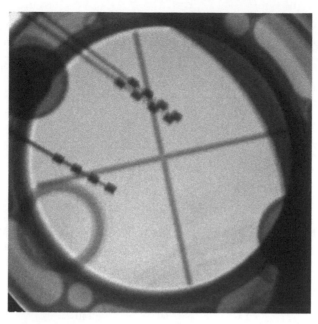

FIGURE 32.3. Fluoroscopy during globus pallidus interna deep brain stimulation placement surgery.

changed left Vim DBS settings to double monopolar and changed the right Vim DBS contact from 11 to 10 (more ventral contact), and this achieved adequate tremor control (Table 32.2). We gradually increased the amplitude over time, with adequate tremor control (Table 32.3); however, 2 years later, the same settings that provided good tremor control also caused worsening dysarthria (Table 32.4). The patient's parkinsonian symptoms also continued to worsen. He developed dyskinesia and motor fluctuations and required an increasing dosage of levodopa/carbidopa. Therefore, we performed a second DBS surgery targeting the bilateral GPi. For the first DBS programming of GPi DBS, we used double monopolar settings with pulse width of 90 μsec and frequency of 180 Hz (Table 32.5B). We were also able to decrease the settings on his Vim DBS, and dysarthria improved significantly (Table 32.5A). For the second DBS programming of GPi DBS, his parkinsonian symptoms worsened as microlesion benefits subsided; therefore, we further adjusted the settings of his GPi DBS (Table 32.6B). This also facilitated a decrease in the Vim DBS settings without affecting tremor control and with further improvement in dysarthria (Table 32.6A).

OUTCOME

This case presents a possible option for consideration of Vim DBS in a PD patient with severe tremor, followed by rescue bilateral GPi DBS for other motor symptoms of PD. The patient continues to follow up in our clinic. With a combination of Vim and GPi DBS therapy, he has good control of his motor symptoms, including resting tremor, kinetic tremor, rigidity, and bradykinesia. He has good balance with very rare falls, and he does not need a cane or a walker for ambulation. His tremor control has allowed him to resume some work as a locksmith at the age of 73 years. The speech issues he experienced previously have also resolved because we were able to decrease the Vim DBS settings after GPi DBS placement and adjustment. In our last clinic visit, 12 years after the onset of his tremors, his UPDRS Part III score was 29.

DISCUSSION

Although the majority of ET patients do not develop parkinsonism over time, a subset of ET patients may develop PD.[1] Epidemiologic studies reported 3% to 19% of ET patients eventually developing PD.[2-4] On the other hand, although PD patients usually have a resting tremor, kinetic tremor is also a frequent feature in PD. One study showed that only 1.3% of 870 PD patients did not have kinetic tremor as evaluated by a spiral drawing task. Interestingly, the study also showed that among 29 PD patients without postural or resting tremor, eight had moderate and four had severe kinetic tremor on spiral drawing.[5] Our patient initially carried the diagnosis of essential tremor;

TABLE 32.1. VENTRAL INTERMEDIATE NUCLEUS OF THE THALAMUS DEEP BRAIN
STIMULATION PARAMETERS AFTER INITIAL PROGRAMMING (9/2015)

	Electrode Configuration	Voltage (V)	Pulse Width (μsec)	Frequency (Hz)	Therapeutic Effects
Left Vim	2–	2.5	60	130	Adequate tremor control
Right Vim	11–	1.4	60	130	

Vim = ventral intermediate nucleus of the thalamus.

TABLE 32.2. VENTRAL INTERMEDIATE NUCLEUS OF THE THALAMUS DEEP BRAIN
STIMULATION PARAMETERS AFTER SECOND PROGRAMMING (10/2015)

	Electrode Configuration	Voltage (V)	Pulse Width (μsec)	Frequency (Hz)	Therapeutic Effects
Left Vim	2–, 3–	2.8	60	140	Improved tremor control
Right Vim	10–	1.7	60	140	

Vim = ventral intermediate nucleus of the thalamus.

TABLE 32.3. VENTRAL INTERMEDIATE NUCLEUS OF THE THALAMUS DEEP BRAIN
STIMULATION PARAMETERS AFTER THIRD PROGRAMMING (12/2015)

	Electrode Configuration	Voltage (V)	Pulse Width (μsec)	Frequency (Hz)	Therapeutic Effects
Left Vim	2–, 3–	3.3	60	140	Improved tremor control
Right Vim	10–	2.0	60	140	

Vim = ventral intermediate nucleus of the thalamus.

TABLE 32.4. VENTRAL INTERMEDIATE NUCLEUS OF THE THALAMUS DEEP BRAIN
STIMULATION PARAMETERS BEFORE BILATERAL GLOBUS PALLIDUS INTERNA DEEP
BRAIN STIMULATION SURGERY (5/2017)

	Electrode Configuration	Voltage (V)	Pulse Width (μsec)	Frequency (Hz)	Therapeutic Effects
Left Vim	2–, 3–	4.15	60	140	Adequate tremor control, moderate dysarthria
Right Vim	10–	2.0	60	140	

Vim = ventral intermediate nucleus of the thalamus.

TABLE 32.5A. VENTRAL INTERMEDIATE NUCLEUS OF THE THALAMUS DEEP BRAIN STIMULATION PARAMETERS AFTER BILATERAL GLOBUS PALLIDUS INTERNA DEEP BRAIN STIMULATION SURGERY (9/2017)

	Electrode Configuration	Voltage (V)	Pulse Width (μsec)	Frequency (Hz)	Therapeutic Effects
Left Vim	2–, 3–	2.8	60	140	Adequate tremor control, improved dysarthria
Right Vim	10–	2.5	60	140	

Vim = ventral intermediate nucleus of the thalamus.

TABLE 32.5B. GLOBUS PALLIDUS INTERNA DEEP BRAIN STIMULATION PARAMETERS AFTER FIRST PROGRAMMING (9/2017)

	Electrode Configuration	Voltage (V)	Pulse Width (μsec)	Frequency (Hz)	Therapeutic Effects
Left GPi	2–	2.7	90	180	Improved tremor, bradykinesia, and rigidity
Right GPi	10–	1.5	90	180	

GPi = globus pallidus interna.

TABLE 32.6A. VENTRAL INTERMEDIATE NUCLEUS OF THE THALAMUS DEEP BRAIN STIMULATION PARAMETERS DURING THE SECOND GLOBUS PALLIDUS INTERNA DEEP BRAIN STIMULATION PROGRAMMING (1/2018)

	Electrode Configuration	Voltage (V)	Pulse Width (μsec)	Frequency (Hz)	Therapeutic Effects
Left Vim	2–, 3–	2.6	60	140	Adequate tremor control, improved dysarthria
Right Vim	10–	2.3	60	140	

Vim = ventral intermediate nucleus of the thalamus.

TABLE 32.6B. GLOBUS PALLIDUS INTERNA DEEP BRAIN STIMULATION PARAMETERS DURING THE SECOND PROGRAMMING (1/2018)

	Electrode Configuration	Voltage (V)	Pulse Width (μsec)	Frequency (Hz)	Therapeutic Effects
Left GPi	2–	3.5	90	180	Improved tremor, bradykinesia, and rigidity
Right GPi	10–	2.65	90	180	

GPi = globus pallidus interna.

however, given the age of onset (61 years) and appearance of his clinical features, this tremor was most likely of parkinsonian etiology.

Vim DBS is a well-established therapy for medication-refractory ET, while PD patients may also benefit from Vim (tremor only) or from DBS targeting either the STN or GPi.[6,7] Concurrent GPi and Vim DBS has also been reported in patients with dystonic tremor.[8]

Previous work has shown that GPi DBS is effective for parkinsonian motor symptoms including tremor, while Vim DBS is effective for tremor control in PD, but not as effective with the other aspects of parkinsonian motor symptoms, including bradykinesia, rigidity, and postural instability.[6,7] However, it is unclear whether GPi and Vim DBS can work synergistically in tremor control. In our case, we clearly see a synergistic effect not only with improved tremor control but also with reduced settings on the Vim DBS programming, which led to significant improvement in the DBS-induced dysarthria.

GPi DBS and STN DBS have equivalent efficacy in treating parkinsonian motor symptoms.[7] However, because of the concerns of cognitive issues associated with STN DBS, we chose GPi DBS as the target. Partly owing to the larger volume, GPi DBS usually tends to drain battery faster. To that point, our patient had his implantable pulse generator (IPG) for GPi DBS replaced 2 years after surgery. In the meanwhile, the IPG

for his Vim DBS is still functional 4 years after surgery.

Tremor in PD usually responds to dopaminergic medication and DBS targeting GPi or STN. For severe tremors, medications used in ET, including propranolol, primidone, topiramate, gabapentin, and benzodiazepines, may also provide additional benefit.[9] For DBS programming, usually higher frequency stimulation correlates with better tremor control, but unfortunately, it is also associated with higher incidence of balance issues as well as dysarthria. Here we report a PD case with very severe, medication-refractory tremor in which Vim DBS was initially effective for tremor control but 2 years later resulted in severe dysarthria due to increased settings for tremor control. We introduced a second DBS surgery targeting GPi, and GPi DBS worked synergistically with Vim DBS to provide improved tremor control with lower Vim DBS settings and improved dysarthria.

In summary, Vim DBS and GPi DBS can be safely implanted simultaneously, and they may work synergistically to improve tremor control. While Vim DBS may be considered for refractory tremor in PD, a second rescue DBS surgery is possible that targets GPi or STN to address other PD-related motor symptoms. It is unclear in our case why the Vim DBS could not be weaned off, but it could be either because the lead of the GPi DBS was suboptimal or the postural-action tremor was severe enough to necessitate a Vim target.

PEARLS

- For PD patients with severe, medication-refractory tremor and relatively mild bradykinesia and rigidity, Vim DBS implantation may be considered.
- For patients with Vim DBS implantation for tremor control who later develop parkinsonian symptoms, a second rescue surgery targeting GPi or STN may be considered.
- GPi DBS and Vim DBS may work synergistically on tremor control and achieve good overall symptomatic therapeutic outcome with significant improvement of stimulation-related side effects. In many cases, only one target is required if leads are optimally placed.
- If a patient has a grade 2 or more postural-action tremor Vim DBS may be necessary because STN and GPi DBS are more effective in resting tremor.

REFERENCES

1. Shahed J, Jankovic J. Exploring the relationship between essential tremor and Parkinson's disease. Parkinsonism Relat Disord 2007;13:67–76.

2. Geraghty JJ, Jankovic J, Zetusky WJ. Association between essential tremor and Parkinson's disease. Ann Neurol 1985;17:329–333.

3. Koller WC, Busenbark K, Miner K. The relationship of essential tremor to other movement disorders: report on 678 patients. Essential Tremor Study Group. Ann Neurol 1994;35:717–723.

4. Cleeves L, Findley LJ, Koller W. Lack of association between essential tremor and Parkinson's disease. Ann Neurol 1988;24:23–26.

5. Kraus PH, Lemke MR, Reichmann H. Kinetic tremor in Parkinson's disease: an underrated symptom. J Neural Transm (Vienna) 2006;113:845–853.

6. Benabid AL, Pollak P, Gao D, et al. Chronic electrical stimulation of the ventralis intermedius nucleus of the thalamus as a treatment of movement disorders. J Neurosurg 1996;84:203–214.

7. Williams NR, Foote KD, Okun MS. STN vs. GPi deep brain stimulation: translating the rematch into clinical practice. Mov Disord Clin Pract 2014;1:24–35.

8. Schadt CR, Charles PD, Davis TL, Konrad PE. Thalamotomy, DBS-Vim, and DBS-GPi for generalized dystonia: a case report. Tenn Med 2007;100:38–39.

9. Louis ED. Diagnosis and management of tremor. Continuum (Minneap Minn) 2016;22:1143–1158.

Case 33

Expected Improvement in Sleep Quality and Unexpected Improvement in Severe Nightmares After Deep Brain Stimulation in Parkinson Disease

LAURICE YANG

INDICATION FOR DEEP BRAIN STIMULATION

Motor fluctuations in Parkinson disease (PD)

CLINICAL HISTORY AND RELEVANT EXAM

A 68-year-old man with a history of PD, hypertension, and hyperlipidemia presented for evaluation for deep brain stimulation (DBS) surgery. His parkinsonian symptoms started 12 years prior with left-sided bradykinesia, rigidity, and rest tremor. Over the course of his disease, he developed a shuffling gait, and his rest tremor progressed to his right hand. The patient described that for most of his life, he had issues with severe nightmares about his childhood past. These dreams would occur several times a week and would increase in frequency when he was more stressed at work or at home.

Preoperative evaluation was remarkable for levodopa-responsive bradykinesia, rigidity, and rest tremor. He had no exclusion criteria and was approved to move forward with surgery. We discussed with him that it was unclear whether he would have improvement in nonmotor symptoms, such as mood or nightmares. He understood and underwent bilateral subthalamic nucleus (STN) DBS with the Medtronic DBS system.

COMPLICATIONS

No complications occurred from this surgery.

TROUBLESHOOTING AND MANAGEMENT

At the time of the initial programming, the patient experienced a *microlesion effect* whereby he had improvement in his tremors and bradykinesia but also noted a decrease in the frequency of his nightmares. Additionally, he felt generally happier and less stressed after the surgery. We started with monopolar settings: C+ 1– on the right and C+ 9– on the left, with a pulse width of 60 μsec, frequency of 130 Hz, and voltage of 1 V. At the second programming session, his bradykinesia and rest tremor had improved, and interestingly, his sleep quality and nightmares had improved as well; he experienced only two nightmares in the last 2 months since his initial programming session. Although he was very grateful that his motor symptoms had improved, he was tearfully overjoyed that his nightmares had mostly resolved with DBS surgery, which had been refractory to medications in the past.

OUTCOME

He was seen for about one year after the DBS was placed, but was lost to follow up after that. Over the course of the year, the voltage was increased slowly up to 2.7 V on the left electrode and 2.2 V on the right electrode with good motor response; his nightmares had largely disappeared.

DISCUSSION

The effects of DBS on nonmotor symptoms has been a topic of great discussion. Although there is limited evidence on whether nonmotor symptoms respond to deep brain stimulation, it has been suggested that nonmotor symptoms like fatigue, pain, and anxiety improve with STN stimulation[1,3–5] and that the benefit of nonmotor symptoms is greater in those that have a larger symptomatic motor improvement after stimulation.[1] In this case, the patient's motor symptoms were very responsive to DBS. Although there is limited literature on the effects of DBS stimulation on nightmares, stimulation could improve sleep quality in patients who have either bilateral[6] or unilateral[4,7] STN stimulation. One study showed that patients in their cohort with more left-sided symptoms had worse sleep quality at baseline and received the best sleep outcome after unilateral STN DBS surgery.[4] Interestingly, this patient did have symptoms that were worse on the left side. Although there is still more research needed to be done in this field, it is thought-provoking that the laterality of motor symptoms could be associated with more sleep symptoms. Furthermore, it is also possible to adjust DBS programming to mitigate nonmotor symptoms, such as mood where using the active site in the ventral contracts in STN DBS stimulation could improve mood and sleep symptoms.[8,9]

There are theories on why sleep quality would improve with stimulation. Improvement in sleep can be due to several factors which include changes in mood, mobility, anti-parkinsonian medications and sleep patterns.[4] One article suggests that DBS could affect the limbic STN, which regulates emotional pathways.[5] This could increase pain tolerance[5] and consequently, enhance sleep quality.[10,11] Improvement in sleep could also be simply related to feeling more comfortable and relaxed after the decrease of motor symptoms with DBS.[12] In either case, future studies are required to better understand how DBS can affect sleep physiology and how this could influence future treatment strategies.

PEARLS

- There is a large array of nonmotor symptoms in patients with PD that significantly affect quality of life, and among them is sleep quality.
- Nonmotor PD symptoms, such as mood and, as our case illustrates, sleep quality could potentially improve with STN DBS stimulation.
- Further studies are needed to explore the effect of STN and globus pallidus interna implantation on sleep and other nonmotor symptoms in PD.
- The mechanism of improvement in the lifelong nightmares in our patient is unknown at this time.

REFERENCES

1. Fabbri M, Coelho M, Guedes L, Rosa M, Abreu D, Goncalves N, et al. Acute response of non motor symptoms to subthalamic deep brain stimulation in Parkinson's disease. Parkinsonism Relat Disord 2017;41:113–117.
2. Kim H, Jeon B, Paek S. Non motor symptoms and subthalamic deep brain stimulation in Parkinson's disease. J Mov Disord 2015;8(2):83–91.
3. Wolz M, Hauschild J, Fauser M, Klingelhofer L, Schacker G, Reichmann H, et al. Immediate effects of deep brain stimulation of the subthalamic nucleus on nonmotor symptoms in Parkinson's disease. Parkinsonism Relat Disord 2012;18(8):994–997.
4. Amara A, Standaert D, Futhrie S, Cutter G, Watts R, Walker H. Unilateral subthalamic nucleus deep brain stimulation improves sleep quality in Parkinson's disease. Parkinsonism Relat Disord 2012;18:63–68.
5. Marques A, Chassin O, Morand D, Pereira B, Derost P, Ulla M, et al. Central pain modulation after subthalamic nucleus stimulation. Neurology 2013;81(7):633–640.
6. Hjort N, Ostergaard K, Dupont E. Improvement of sleep quality in patients with advanced Parkinson's disease treated with deep brain stimulation of the subthalamic nucleus. Mov Disord 2004;19(2):196–199.
7. Chahine L, Ahmed A, Sun Z. Effects of STN DBS for Parkinson's disease on restless leg syndrome

and other sleep related measures. Parkinsonism Relat Disord 2011;17(3):208–211.

8. Dafsari H, Petry-Schmelzer J, Ray-Chaudhri K, Ashkan K, Weis L, Dembek, M., et al. Non-motor outcomes of subthalamic stimulation in Parkinson's disease depend on location of active contacts. Brain Stim 2018;11:904–912.

9. York M, Wilde E, Simpson R, Jankovic J. Relationship between neuropsychological outcome and DBS surgical trajectory and electrode location. J Neurol Sci 2009;287(1–2):159–171.

10. Keskindag B, Karaaziz M. The association between pain and sleep in fibromyalgia. Saudi Med J 2017;38(5):465–475.

11. Gerhard J, Burns J, Post K, Smith D, Porter L, Burgess H, et al. Relationships between sleep quality and pain-related factors for people with chronic low back pain: tests of reciprocal and time of day effects. Ann Behav Med 2017;51(3):365–375.

12. Eugster L, Bargiotas P, Bassetti C, Schuepbach W. Deep brain stimulation and sleep-wake functions in Parkinson's disease: A systematic review. Parkinsonism Relat Disord 2016;32:12–19.

13. Witt K, Daniels C, Reiff J, Krack P, Volkmann J, Pinsker M, et al. Neuropsychological and psychiatric changes after deep brain stimulation for Parkinson's disease: a randomized multicentre study. Lancet Neurol 2008;7:605–614.

14. Castelli L, Perozzo P, Zibetti M, Crivelli B, Vorabito U, Lanotte M, et al. Chronic deep brain stimulation of the subthalamic nucleus for Parkinson's disease: effects on cognition, mood, anxiety, and personality traits. Eur Neurol 2006;55:136–144.

SECTION 4

Dystonia

Case 34

Patient Selection Criteria for Deep Brain Stimulation for Dystonia

LAURA S. SURILLO DAHDAH, RASHEDA EL-NAZER,
RICHARD B. DEWEY, JR., PADRAIG O'SUILLEABHAIN,
AND SHILPA CHITNIS

CANDIDATE SCREENING AND SELECTION

Dystonia is defined as a movement disorder characterized by sustained or intermittent muscle co-contractions causing abnormal, often repetitive, movements, postures, or both. Dystonic movements are typically patterned, twisted, and frequently tremulous. Dystonia can be precipitated or worsened by voluntary action and is associated with overflow activation of distant muscle groups.[1] A recent revision of the dystonia diagnostic criteria now classifies dystonia into two axes: (1) clinical characteristics (age at onset, temporal pattern, body distribution—whether focal, segmental, or generalized; as well as associated features) and (2) etiology, whether idiopathic/genetic or secondary to other neurologic/medical diseases.[1] Pharmacologic treatments for dystonia remain generally unsatisfactory and consist of various combinations of levodopa, anticholinergics, muscle-relaxants, benzodiazepines, and botulinum toxin injections (particularly for focal and segmental dystonia). The outcomes of medical treatment are frequently suboptimal as a result of limited effectiveness and the potential for significant side effects, such as sedation and cognitive impairment. A humanitarian-device exemption through the US Food and Drug Administration was approved for the treatment of medically refractory symptoms of generalized dystonia with deep brain stimulation (DBS). Bilateral globus pallidus interna (GPi) DBS surgery has been shown in many small studies to be effective for both generalized and focal dystonia, which includes cervical dystonia and tardive dystonia.[2,3] The effects of using DBS in tardive dystonia may

be more immediate in contrast to other forms of dystonia, where the positive effects could be delayed by many weeks or even months. DBS may in select cases be an appropriate treatment for the disabling symptoms of generalized, cervical, tardive, and other dystonias with suboptimal responses to pharmacotherapy or botulinum toxin injections (when applicable). The presence of fixed contractures may limit DBS effectiveness, but symptoms such as pain may have the potential for improvement.[4,5] Rigorous patient selection and careful management of comorbidities are essential for favorable outcomes when using DBS to treat dystonia.

In general, patients with primary (idiopathic) dystonia tend to respond better to DBS than patients with secondary forms, with the exception of tardive dystonia. This observation uses for its basis the old terminology for primary and secondary dystonia. It should also be noted that some genetic forms of dystonia may have a good response to DBS (e.g., DYT1 dystonia).[6] Multidisciplinary teams can be used to clarify the diagnosis preoperatively using aspects of the history along with brain magnetic resonance imaging (MRI), diagnostic drug trials (such as with levodopa in the correct clinical setting), and in select cases, even genetic testing.

The examination before dystonia surgery should confirm, exclude, or clarify the reducibility of potential joint contractures. This examination in rare cases requires anesthesia. Contractures that fail to reduce by physical manipulation usually do not have a robust response to DBS surgery.[4]

Patients considering DBS generally experience functional impairment and disability from their dystonia. This functional impairment may include compromised movements, pain, and social isolation. It is suggested that examining clinicians use quantitation of baseline severity of dystonia with validated scales such as the Burke–Fahn–Marsden Dystonia Rating Scale (BFMDRS), the Unified Dystonia Rating Scale, and the Toronto Western Spasmodic Torticollis Rating Scale (TWSTRS).[7] The applicable scales should also be performed at specific intervals postoperatively to assess DBS response and to facilitate quality improvement. Currently, there is no consensus regarding threshold scores for disability, dystonia, and pain severity, and therefore each case should be carefully selected by using a multidisciplinary approach. A quality of life (QoL) scale may also be helpful to quantitate baseline and clinical responses to DBS.

DBS surgery should only be considered after appropriate drug trials and botulinum toxin injections (when applicable) have failed to provide a level of improvement to address the disability.[7] Drug classes often used in dystonia include anticholinergics, benzodiazepines, antiepileptics, and antispasmodic agents.[7] The typical dystonia patient selected for surgical intervention should have failed trials of levodopa, anticholinergics, baclofen, benzodiazepines, and tetrabenazine, although many centers with expertise in specific movement disorders do not feel that all classes of medications need to be trialed in every patient.[8] There are no consensus criteria regarding which drugs or what doses are needed before considering DBS surgery. The clinician should use the multidisciplinary team and clinical judgment to decide what therapies will offer a favorable risk-to-benefit ratio to justify a therapeutic trial. In cases of generalized dystonia particularly in children, it is advisable not to wait too long to consider DBS because fixed skeletal deformities can develop if the dystonia is left untreated. Overall, selection criteria for GPi DBS in dystonia remain ambiguous.[4,9]

Candidate evaluation for DBS should ideally include a multidisciplinary team (neuropsychology, neurosurgery, psychiatry, and rehabilitation) as well as neuroimaging assessment.[10,11] Additionally, a videotaped clinical evaluation using a standardized dystonia rating scale can be useful.[7] Centers with access to social workers and financial counselors would contribute greatly to the multidisciplinary team. Nutritionists are useful especially for patients whose body weight falls below 100 lb.

DIAGNOSIS AND ETIOLOGY OF DYSTONIA

In evaluating a dystonic patient for DBS, the history and examination should focus on the identification of possible secondary causes of dystonia. Secondary dystonia, with the exception of tardive dystonia, is in general less responsive to DBS. The physician should question the patient about birth, early development, medication use, toxin exposure (e.g., manganese and carbon monoxide), family history, and trauma.[12–15] Metabolic disorders such as Wilson disease, glutaric aciduria, propionic acidemia, and methylmalonic aciduria should be excluded (but may also be partially responsive to DBS in select patients, or DBS may offer relief from opisthotonus). Patients should be tested for the *DYT1* gene (testing for this is commercially available) if the dystonia is generalized and onset was documented to occur before age 26 years.[16] Many centers also now test for *DYT6*. Imaging may be required to exclude secondary causes of dystonia.[15,17,18] The optimal brain target for secondary dystonia is unknown. In select cases such as cerebral palsy and iron deposition diseases, DBS may provide a palliative option.[16]

Identifying which patients will respond to DBS is challenging because there have been few controlled studies examining predictors of outcome. Nevertheless, it is known that some forms of dystonia respond better than others (primary generalized, cervical/segmental, and tardive show greater response than secondary dystonia). Because patients with secondary dystonia are less likely to benefit from DBS, it is important to classify the type and cause of dystonia before referring a patient for a DBS evaluation.[7,19]

SYMPTOMS THAT RESPOND TO DEEP BRAIN STIMULATION

Idiopathic dystonia

Currently, there is level I evidence supporting the benefit of DBS in inherited/idiopathic generalized/segmental dystonia. This level of evidence was reached in one class I study and one class II study showing 40 to 50% motor improvement after 3 months in sham- controlled, double-blinded evaluations.[4,20] In 2005, Vidailhet and colleagues reported 22 patients with idiopathic generalized dystonia who had a significant improvement in dystonia severity with GPi DBS. This result was derived from a double-blind evaluation with and without stimulation at 3 months of follow-up in a multicenter, prospective, controlled study.[20] A year later, Kupsch and colleagues published a multicenter, randomized, sham-controlled study that showed a significant improvement in the severity of dystonia in 20 patients who had generalized/segmental idiopathic dystonia at 3-month follow-up after bilateral GPi DBS.[21] In 2012, Volkmann and colleagues showed that 3 years and 5 years after surgery, pallidal stimulation continued to be an effective and relatively safe treatment option for patients with severe idiopathic dystonia, with a 50 to 60% motor improvement.[22] In these published cohorts, the accumulated experience suggested that younger age and less severe dystonia were correlated with better motor improvement, but not with function at outcome.

Many papers currently support the efficacy of bilateral GPi DBS for dystonia. In a double-blind, sham-controlled trial evaluating 22 patients with idiopathic or inherited, isolated, generalized dystonia who underwent bilateral GPi DBS, the motor and disability scores of the BFMDRS improved by 47 and 34% in the neurostimulation group compared with 25 and 24% in the sham-stimulation group, respectively, at 3 months after surgery. The face, speech, and swallowing scores did not change in the cohort, and the *DYT1* status did not influence the therapy outcome.[20] An open-label, long-term follow-up study of the same cohort observed that the motor improvement was maintained at 3 years, with a mean improvement in the BFMDRS of 58%.[23] Another double-blind, sham-controlled multicenter study led by a German group analyzed 40 patients with idiopathic or inherited, isolated, segmental, or generalized dystonia. The motor and disability scores of the BFMDRS improved by 39.3 and 37.5% in the neurostimulation group compared with 4.9 and 8.3% in the sham-stimulation group, respectively, at 3 months after surgery. The patients were switched to the on-stimulation phase, and after 6 months the dystonic symptoms were reduced by 48%. No clinical characteristic, including the *DYT1* mutation, predicted the motor outcome.[9] To evaluate the long-term GPi DBS effect, a prospective study evaluated 38 patients for 5 years after surgery. The motor and disability scores of the BFMDRS improved by 57.8 and 47%, respectively. All motor symptoms, except for speech and swallowing, improved. All QoL measures improved after DBS, except for the social and emotional functioning.[21]

Several other studies also evaluated the long-term effects of GPi DBS in idiopathic, DYT1, and DYT6 generalized dystonia and found an improvement in the motor BFMDRS scores ranging from 42 to 80% and in the disability scores ranging from 23 to 70%.[24-31] A recent study was reported that had the longest available follow-up, with patients followed up to 19 years after surgery.[29] The motor and disability scores on the BFMDRS improved by 57 and 23.3% at the last follow-up, respectively. There was no difference between DYT1 and isolated idiopathic dystonia in outcome. A recent meta-analysis of GPi DBS efficacy in isolated dystonia (including cervical dystonia) reported a mean absolute improvement in motor BFMDRS of 23.8 points at 6 months to 26.6 points at the last follow-up (mean, 32.5 months; range, 6–72 months).[32]

In cervical dystonia, a single class I, randomized, sham-controlled trial by Volkmann and colleagues in 2012 showed that after 3 months of bilateral GPi DBS, cervical dystonia severity and related disability were reduced by 26%.[22]

In 2007, a well-designed, blinded-rater study reported outcomes in 10 patients at 12 months after surgery, showing 44%, 64%, and 65% mean improvements in TWSTRS severity, disability, and pain subscores, respectively.[33] Hung and colleagues[34] reported long-term sustained benefit in a series of 10 cervical dystonia patients up to 3 years after surgery. Although most reports suggested overall improvement, there were several reports suggesting only minor improvements in head and neck position but significant improvement in associated neck pain.

In 2002, a prospective single-blind study showed an initial improvement in the TWSTRS severity score by 38% in five patients after 3 months of GPi DBS, with subsequent amelioration of 63% after 20 months. The disability score also improved by 69%.[35] There was one prospective, randomized, sham-controlled trial in which 62 patients with cervical dystonia were evaluated before and 3 months after surgery. The TWSTRS severity and disability scores improved by 26 and 41% in the neurostimulation group compared with 6 and 11% in the sham-stimulation group.[36] Four studies have confirmed the long-term benefit of GPi DBS in cervical dystonia, with a mean improvement ranging from 47.6 to 70% (follow-up 2.5–10 years after surgery).[24,37-39] QoL has also been shown by several studies to improve in the long term.

Rarely, the GPi target in dystonia DBS has been associated with parkinsonism. Additionally, new targets have been emerging for dystonia DBS (generalized and cervical), including the STN. STN DBS in cervical dystonia may lead to reversible dyskinesia (corrected by decreasing the current density or the location of stimulation). It is likely that we will see an expansion in targets for specific disorders.

Other types of isolated focal dystonia, including dystonic camptocormia,[40] focal hand dystonia,[41,42] and Meige syndrome.[43] Overall, these disorders have been associated with favorable outcomes after GPi DBS. The benefit of orofacial dystonia, including speech and swallowing problems, after GPi DBS is inferior to that of limb and neck dystonia, and in many cases there is no response or even worsening.[20,21] Nevertheless, several reports have described favorable short-term results of patients with refractory Meige syndrome.[44–47] Even in the long term, as retrospectively analyzed in 12 patients with Meige syndrome, the motor BFMDRS improved by 53% after 6.5 years. The subscores for eyes were improved by 47%, for mouth by 56%, and for speech/swallowing by 64%.[43] Moreover, another recent long-term analysis in patients with Meige syndrome showed a 58.9% improvement in the BFMDRS scores after a mean follow-up of 66 months.[48]

Secondary dystonia

In general, there is less evidence for the effectiveness of DBS in secondary and neurodegenerative dystonias than in idiopathic focal generalized/segmental forms. The reduced benefit observed in these disorders is likely related to progression of the underlying disease. Individuals with neurodegenerative dystonia are also thought to be at greater risk for side effects from DBS. There are no clear guidelines defining suitable patients for DBS in the secondary dystonia groups of disorders.

Tardive dystonia can cause significant disability in some individuals, and surgical treatment has been performed with promising results. In 2007, Damier and colleagues published a class III study demonstrating the effectiveness of bilateral GPi DBS in tardive dystonia. The results were confirmed by a double-blind evaluation of 10 patients showing a mean decrease of 50% in the Extrapyramidal Symptoms Rating Scale score when stimulation was applied compared with the absence of stimulation at 6 months postoperatively.[49] Collectively, several studies have been done to confirm the efficacy and safety of this treatment for tardive dystonia,[50] including one from Pouclet-Courtemanche and colleagues, published in 2016.[51] Tardive dystonia has been known to respond to both pallidotomy and DBS. The clinical experience and studies have shown that the improvement may be immediate compared with the long delays in other dystonic disorders treated with DBS.

In cerebral palsy (CP), there is some evidence for mild improvement with the application of DBS. One study prospectively analyzed the effect of bilateral GPi DBS in 13 patients with CP and showed 24% improvement in the motor BFMDRS 12 months after surgery. The subscore analysis revealed that axial (neck and trunk) and limb function improved, while face, speech, and swallowing did not. Functional disability, pain, and mental health–related QoL were also significantly improved. It is important to highlight that these patients did not experience any worsening of cognition or mood after DBS.[52] A meta-analysis of 20 studies involving 68 patients with CP treated with GPi DBS found improvements in the BFMDRS motor scale of 23.6% after a mean follow-up of 12 months. The improvement in the disability component of the same scale was less impressive but still significant at 9.2%. The authors observed a significant negative correlation between severity of dystonia and clinical outcome.[53] Experts have commented that the improvements following DBS in cerebral palsy may be beneficial to individual patients and families even if not captured by conventional rating scales.

Secondary dystonia DBS has had one class III study in eight patients with different etiologies (CP, after encephalitis, after anoxic damage, sepsis, neuroleptics, stroke, and radiation treatment). Results were overall positive, showing improvement in six subjects on the Unified Dystonia Rating Scale (reduction from preoperative score of 40 to 26.4 after surgery), but results also confirmed the clinical experience that secondary/neurodegenerative dystonias are generally less responsive to DBS than idiopathic dystonia again, with the exception of tardive dystonia.[54]

Myoclonus-dystonia syndrome may be associated with a genetic mutation, particularly in the epsilon sarcoglycan gene, or can manifest with another underlying disorder (e.g., mitochondrial). In general, treatment with either GPi or thalamic ventral intermediate (Vim) DBS has been effective regardless of the etiology. With respect to fewer adverse, stimulation-induced events of GPi DBS in comparison with Vim DBS, GPi DBS seems to be preferable. Combined GPi DBS and Vim DBS can be useful in cases of incapacitating myoclonus, refractory to GPi DBS alone.[55]

RISKS OF DEEP BRAIN STIMULATION SURGERY AND PATIENT AND FAMILY EXPECTATIONS

Risks

The most common serious complications with DBS include stroke, infection, and lead fracture. Most of the rates quoted for these complications are derived from mixed populations of patients and not specifically for dystonia. For all patients considering DBS surgery, the common quote is a 1 to 2% risk for symptomatic hemorrhagic stroke per brain hemisphere, a 5 to 10% risk for device-related infection at times severe enough to require further surgery for hardware removal, and a 1 to 2% per year risk for lead fracture.[56]

These numbers are general estimates derived collectively from many studies and assume that most DBS centers have reasonable quality controls.

The previously described studies conclude that GPi DBS is a generally well-tolerated procedure. However, speech difficulties deserve attention, especially in patients with previous speech disturbances, because dysarthria has been observed in most of the reported series. Permanent speech problems were reported in four patients in a retrospective series, and the number increased to seven of 60 patients in the prospective study by Volkmann and colleagues.[22] Other complications included transient lethargy, somnolence, stupor, involuntary movement disorders, hemiparesis, cervical pain, electrode dislocation and misplacement, and a depressive episode requiring psychiatric treatment.[22,57]

One strategy to reduce complications has been to stage the procedure. Performing one hemisphere and waiting a few weeks or longer to implant the second hemisphere may be better tolerated and reduce DBS-related side-effect issues.

Expectations

The response to DBS in dystonia can be variable and might depend on several clinical,[32] genetic,[58] and electrophysiologic[59] factors. The current evidence ranges from class I evidence for isolated generalized dystonia to class IV evidence for some acquired combined dystonia. Thus, considering a patient with dystonia for DBS sometimes may not be straightforward because reliable predictive factors remain murky. Overall, patients with idiopathic or inherited, isolated, focal, segmental, or generalized dystonia, tardive dystonia, and myoclonus dystonia seem to respond well to DBS, while acquired dystonia and other combined dystonias secondary to brain injuries and to neurodegenerative disorders are typically less responsive, if at all. Even among the "good" DBS candidates, other factors, including skeletal deformities or secondary disabilities (e.g., myelopathy), disease duration, age, genetic subtype, baseline motor impairment, and the connectivity between the stimulation site and other brain regions, may influence the outcomes. These factors should be considered before surgery.[32,35,60,61]

In most cases, patients should undergo surgery before the onset of fixed skeletal deformities, which are expected to limit functional improvement even when dystonia symptoms are ameliorated.[62]

Patients need to be taught that, unlike PD and ET, dystonia symptoms often show delayed improvements and require repeated programming sessions. These sessions may need to persist 6 to 12 months or even longer. Patients should be aware that there is no clear symptom a clinician can use in the office to gauge programming, so it may take longer to assess outcome and optimize programming settings.

MEDICAL COMORBIDITIES AND DEEP BRAIN STIMULATION

Please refer to Case 7 on candidate selection for deep brain stimulation in patients with Parkinson disease and essential tremor. In general, all medical comorbidities should be assessed by a multidisciplinary team. Heart, lung, diabetes, and diseases that contribute to immunocompromise may all affect risk.

PSYCHIATRIC ILLNESS AND COGNITIVE IMPAIRMENT AND DEEP BRAIN STIMULATION

Neuropsychological testing and psychiatric assessment are critical components of the evaluation process.[63] Psychiatric assessment is considered a necessity because mood disorders such as depression and anxiety can worsen following surgery. In patients with psychiatric comorbidities, suicide has been rarely reported after GPi DBS.[9,64] Patients with severe, unresolved psychotic symptoms should be excluded at least until optimized.[7] Neuropsychological evaluation can also screen for mood disorders and impulse control issues that may not be obvious during clinical evaluations. Also, these screenings may pick up on histories of recreational drug use and prior hospitalizations for psychiatric reasons. In general, neuropsychological testing is important because preexisting psychiatric illness and cognitive impairment may worsen after surgery and result in a diminished motor benefit, lead to poor cooperation during awake surgical procedures, and affect postsurgical programming.

Nonetheless, even though few studies have addressed specifically the effects of DBS on nonmotor symptoms in dystonia, two small series reported marked improvement in the pain score[61,62] and in depression after GPi DBS in cervical dystonia.[65] Another study with 12 patients that had isolated focal or segmental dystonia demonstrated improvements in working memory, executive function, anxiety, and depression.[66] Other studies have shown significant decline in verbal fluency in one patient and in verbal memory in another,[64] or reported no change in cognitive function.[67] A neuropsychological assessment conducted in a prospective multicenter trial reported reduction in word fluency 12 months after surgery for cervical dystonia.[68] The other domains were not affected.

A long-term neuropsychiatric study using psychiatric interviews and *Diagnostic and Statistical Manual of Mental Disorders,* fourth edition (DSM-IV) diagnostic criteria in 57 patients with inherited or acquired, isolated or combined dystonia reported no significant changes after surgery (mean follow-up, 24.4 ± 19.6 months).[69] These results in general support the psychiatric stability of dystonic patients treated with GPi DBS.

Overall, the available data suggests that GPi DBS is safe from a cognitive and psychiatric perspective but only if screening and optimization are adequately performed. From the class IV studies available, the incidence of suicide after DBS was very low; however, postoperative monitoring of neuropsychiatric symptoms and frequent follow-up visits may contribute to this low rate.[9]

PREOPERATIVE MAGNETIC RESONANCE IMAGING

The presence of minor structural abnormalities in the basal ganglia in idiopathic dystonia is not in most cases a contraindication for DBS. Brain imaging is considered mandatory in the preoperative selection process for subjects with dystonia who are considering DBS in order to support the diagnosis of primary or secondary dystonia and to examine the presence or absence of viable surgical targets.[9] In cervical dystonia, recurrent involuntary neck movements may contribute to osteoarthritic cervical spondylosis, which is an independent risk factor for neck pain. Thus, cervical spine plain films and MRI may be helpful preoperatively to assess the degree of arthritic spinal disease. In addition, skeletal imaging might be useful to quantify spinal deformities in children with primary dystonia.[70–75]

PEARLS

- GPi DBS is now well-established for the treatment of generalized or segmental idiopathic dystonia, especially after failure of medical treatments.
- New brain targets for primary and secondary dystonia are emerging (e.g., STN, thalamus, globus pallidus externa).
- A multidisciplinary approach to screening and management should always be employed.
- It is important to address patient expectations and to have a discussion of the likely delay in clinical benefit requiring multiple programming visits over many months.
- Patients with idiopathic/inherited dystonias are likely to have the best outcome from DBS surgery. This is especially true in the younger patients with less severe dystonia at baseline.
- DYT1 dystonia in some cases may be associated with a positive outcome.
- In focal cervical dystonia after failure of botulinum toxin injections, DBS can be considered a good option with both GPi and STN DBS emerging as options.
- STN DBS seems to be associated with cervical dyskinesia. GPi DBS may rarely be associated with parkinsonism.
- For patients with secondary dystonias, the surgical alternative should be carefully considered by a multidisciplinary team.
- The DBS approach is generally less effective, although tardive dystonia responds robustly and immediately in most GPi DBS cases.
- Myoclonus dystonia also seems to respond briskly to both GPi and Vim thalamic DBS.
- Patients and families should weigh the expected outcomes and be counseled to have reasonable expectations.
- Symptom improvement in dystonia cases frequently will span weeks to months, unless it is tardive dystonia or dystonia myoclonus.
- Ideal dystonia DBS candidates have few medical comorbidities, no dementia, no active psychiatric disease, and no fixed contractures.

REFERENCES

1. Albanese, A., Bhatia, K., Bressman, S. B., DeLong, M. R., Fahn, S., Fung, V. S., . . . Lang, A. E. (2013). Phenomenology and classification of dystonia: a consensus update. Movement disorders, 28(7), 863–873.
2. Loher, T. J., Capelle, H. H., Kaelin-Lang, A., Weber, S., Weigel, R., Burgunder, J. M., & Krauss, J. K. (2008). Deep brain stimulation for dystonia: outcome at long-term follow-up. Journal of neurology, 255(6), 881–884.
3. Trottenberg, T., Volkmann, J., Deuschl, G., Kühn, A. A., Schneider, G. H., Müller, J., . . . Kupsch, A. (2005). Treatment of severe tardive dystonia with pallidal deep brain stimulation. Neurology, 64(2), 344–346.
4. Coubes, P., Cif, L., El Fertit, H., Hemm, S., Vayssiere, N., Serrat, S., . . . Frerebeau, P. (2004). Electrical stimulation of the globus pallidus internus in patients with primary generalized dystonia: long-term results. Journal of neurosurgery, 101(2), 189–194.
5. Cif, L., Valente, E. M., Hemm, S., Coubes, C., Vayssiere, N., Serrat, S., . . . Coubes, P. (2004). Deep brain stimulation in myoclonus–dystonia syndrome. Movement disorders: official journal of the Movement Disorder Society, 19(6), 724–727.
6. Rodriguez, R. L., Fernandez, H. H., Haq, I., & Okun, M. S. (2007). Pearls in patient selection for deep brain stimulation. The neurologist, 13(5), 253–260.
7. Marks Jr., W. J. (Ed.). (2015). Deep brain stimulation management. Cambridge, UK: Cambridge University Press.
8. Albanese, A., Barnes, M. P., Bhatia, K. P., Fernandez-Alvarez, E., Filippini, G., Gasser, T., . . . Valls-Solè, J. (2006). A systematic review on the diagnosis and treatment of primary (idiopathic) dystonia and dystonia plus syndromes: report of an EFNS/MDS-ES Task Force. European journal of neurology, 13(5), 433–444.
9. Bronte-Stewart, H., Taira, T., Valldeoriola, F., Merello, M., Marks Jr., W. J., Albanese, A., . . . Moro, A. E. (2011). Inclusion and exclusion

criteria for DBS in dystonia. Movement disorders, 26(S1), S5–S16.

10. Tagliati, M., Shils, J., Sun, C., & Alterman, R. (2004). Deep brain stimulation for dystonia. Expert review of medical devices, 1(1), 33–41.

11. Volkmann, J., & Benecke, R. (2002). Deep brain stimulation for dystonia: patient selection and evaluation. Movement disorders: official journal of the Movement Disorder Society, 17(S3), S112–S115.

12. Kostić, V. S., Svetel, M., Kabakci, K., Ristić, A., Petrović, I., Schüle, B., . . . Klein, C. (2006). Intrafamilial phenotypic and genetic heterogeneity of dystonia. Journal of the neurological sciences, 250(1-2), 92–96.

13. Pierro, M. M., Bollea, L., Di Rosa, G., Gisondi, A., Cassarino, P., Giannarelli, P., . . . Stortini, M. (2005). Anoxic brain injury following near-drowning in children. Rehabilitation outcome: three case reports. Brain injury, 19(13), 1147–1155.

14. O'Riordan, S., & Hutchinson, M. (2004). Cervical dystonia following peripheral trauma. Journal of neurology, 251(2), 150–155.

15. Tan, M. H., & Lim, E. (2004). Post-encephalitic segmental dystonia with apraxia of eyelid opening. Parkinsonism & related disorders, 10(3), 173–175.

16. Bressman, S. B., Fahn, S., Ozelius, L. J., Kramer, P. L., & Risch, N. J. (2001). The DYT1 mutation and nonfamilial primary torsion dystonia. Archives of neurology, 58(4), 681–682.

17. Crompton, D. E., Chinnery, P. F., Bates, D., Walls, T. J., Jackson, M. J., Curtis, A. J., & Burn, J. (2005). Spectrum of movement disorders in neuroferritinopathy. Movement disorders: official journal of the Movement Disorder Society, 20(1), 95–99.

18. Meunier, S., Lehéricy, S., Garnero, L., & Vidailhet, M. (2003). Dystonia: lessons from brain mapping. Neuroscientist, 9(1), 76–81.

19. Fox, M. D., & Alterman, R. L. (2015). Brain stimulation for torsion dystonia. JAMA neurology, 72(6), 713–719.

20. Vidailhet, M., Vercueil, L., Houeto, J. L., Krystkowiak, P., Benabid, A. L., Cornu, P., . . . Blond, S. (2005). Bilateral deep-brain stimulation of the globus pallidus in primary generalized dystonia. New England Journal of Medicine, 352(5), 459–467.

21. Kupsch, A., Benecke, R., Müller, J., Trottenberg, T., Schneider, G. H., Poewe, W., . . . Pinsker, M. O. (2006). Pallidal deep-brain stimulation in primary generalized or segmental dystonia. New England Journal of Medicine, 355(19), 1978–1990.

22. Volkmann, J., Wolters, A., Kupsch, A., Müller, J., Kühn, A. A., Schneider, G. H., . . . Deuschl, G. (2012). Pallidal deep brain stimulation in patients with primary generalised or segmental dystonia:

5-year follow-up of a randomised trial. Lancet Neurology, 11(12), 1029–1038.

23. Vidailhet, M., Vercueil, L., Houeto, J. L., Krystkowiak, P., Lagrange, C., Yelnik, J., . . . Grand, S. (2007). Bilateral, pallidal, deep-brain stimulation in primary generalised dystonia: a prospective 3 year follow-up study. Lancet Neurology, 6(3), 223–229.

24. Mehrkens, J. H., Bötzel, K., Steude, U., Zeitler, K., Schnitzler, A., Sturm, V., & Voges, J. (2009). Long-term efficacy and safety of chronic globus pallidus internus stimulation in different types of primary dystonia. Stereotactic and functional neurosurgery, 87(1), 8–17.

25. Cif, L., Vasques, X., Gonzalez, V., Ravel, P., Biolsi, B., Collod-Beroud, G., . . . Coubes, P. (2010). Long-term follow-up of DYT1 dystonia patients treated by deep brain stimulation: an open-label study. Movement disorders, 25(3), 289–299.

26. Panov, F., Gologorsky, Y., Connors, G., Tagliati, M., Miravite, J., & Alterman, R. L. (2013). Deep brain stimulation in DYT1 dystonia: a 10-year experience. Neurosurgery, 73(1), 86–93.

27. FitzGerald, J. J., Rosendal, F., De Pennington, N., Joint, C., Forrow, B., Fletcher, C., . . . Aziz, T. Z. (2014). Long-term outcome of deep brain stimulation in generalised dystonia: a series of 60 cases. Journal of Neurology, Neurosurgery, and Psychiatry, 85(12), 1371–1376.

28. Brüggemann, N., Kühn, A., Schneider, S. A., Kamm, C., Wolters, A., Krause, P., . . . Lozano, A. M. (2015). Short-and long-term outcome of chronic pallidal neurostimulation in monogenic isolated dystonia. Neurology, 84(9), 895–903.

29. Meoni, S., Fraix, V., Castrioto, A., Benabid, A. L., Seigneuret, E., Vercueil, L., . . . Moro, E. (2017). Pallidal deep brain stimulation for dystonia: a long term study. Journal of Neurology, Neurosurgery, and Psychiatry, 88(11), 960–967.

30. Valldeoriola, F., Regidor, I., Mínguez-Castellanos, A., Lezcano, E., García-Ruiz, P., Rojo, A., . . . Martí, M. J. (2010). Efficacy and safety of pallidal stimulation in primary dystonia: results of the Spanish multicentric study. Journal of Neurology, Neurosurgery, and Psychiatry, 81(1), 65–69.

31. Lettieri, C., Rinaldo, S., Devigili, G., Pisa, F., Mucchiut, M., Belgrado, E., . . . Eleopra, R. (2015). Clinical outcome of deep brain stimulation for dystonia: constant-current or constant-voltage stimulation? A non-randomized study. European journal of neurology, 22(6), 919–926.

32. Moro, E., LeReun, C., Krauss, J. K., Albanese, A., Lin, J. P., Walleser Autiero, S., . . . Vidailhet, M. (2017). Efficacy of pallidal stimulation in isolated dystonia: a systematic review and meta-analysis. European journal of neurology, 24(4), 552–560.

33. Kiss, Z. H., Doig-Beyaert, K., Eliasziw, M., Tsui, J., Haffenden, A., & Suchowersky, O. (2007). The Canadian multicentre study of deep brain stimulation for cervical dystonia. Brain, *130*(11), 2879–2886.

34. Hung, S. W., Hamani, C., Lozano, A. M., Poon, Y. W., Piboolnurak, P., Miyasaki, J. M., . . . Moro, E. (2007). Long-term outcome of bilateral pallidal deep brain stimulation for primary cervical dystonia. Neurology, *68*(6), 457–459.

35. Krauss, J. K., Loher, T. J., Pohle, T., Weber, S., Taub, E., Bärlocher, C. B., & Burgunder, J. M. (2002). Pallidal deep brain stimulation in patients with cervical dystonia and severe cervical dyskinesias with cervical myelopathy. Journal of Neurology, Neurosurgery, and Psychiatry, *72*(2), 249–256.

36. Volkmann, J., Mueller, J., Deuschl, G., Kühn, A. A., Krauss, J. K., Poewe, W., . . . Schneider, G. H. (2014). Pallidal neurostimulation in patients with medication-refractory cervical dystonia: a randomised, sham-controlled trial. Lancet Neurology, *13*(9), 875–884.

37. Loher, T. J., Capelle, H. H., Kaelin-Lang, A., Weber, S., Weigel, R., Burgunder, J. M., & Krauss, J. K. (2008). Deep brain stimulation for dystonia: outcome at long-term follow-up. Journal of neurology, *255*(6), 881–884.

38. Skogseid, I. M., Ramm-Pettersen, J., Volkmann, J., Kerty, E., Dietrichs, E., & Røste, G. K. (2012). Good long-term efficacy of pallidal stimulation in cervical dystonia: a prospective, observer-blinded study. European journal of neurology, *19*(4), 610–615.

39. Walsh, R. A., Sidiropoulos, C., Lozano, A. M., Hodaie, M., Poon, Y. Y., Fallis, M., & Moro, E. (2013). Bilateral pallidal stimulation in cervical dystonia: blinded evidence of benefit beyond 5 years. Brain, *136*(3), 761–769.

40. Reese, R., Knudsen, K., Falk, D., Mehdorn, H. M., Deuschl, G., & Volkmann, J. (2014). Motor outcome of dystonic camptocormia treated with pallidal neurostimulation. Parkinsonism & related disorders, *20*(2), 176–179.

41. Goto, S., Shimazu, H., Matsuzaki, K., Tamura, T., Murase, N., Nagahiro, S., & Kaji, R. (2008). Thalamic Vo-complex vs pallidal deep brain stimulation for focal hand dystonia. Neurology, *70*(16 Pt 2), 1500–1501.

42. Doshi, P. K., Ramdasi, R. V., Karkera, B., & Kadlas, D. B. (2017). Surgical interventions for task-specific dystonia (writer's dystonia). Annals of Indian Academy of Neurology, *20*(3), 324.

43. Reese, R., Gruber, D., Schoenecker, T., Bäzner, H., Blahak, C., Capelle, H. H., . . . Schrader, C. (2011). Long-term clinical outcome in Meige syndrome treated with internal pallidum deep brain stimulation. Movement disorders, *26*(4), 691–698.

44. Bereznai, B., Steude, U., Seelos, K., & Bötzel, K. (2002). Chronic high-frequency globus pallidus internus stimulation in different types of dystonia: a clinical, video, and MRI report of six patients presenting with segmental, cervical, and generalized dystonia. Movement disorders, *17*(1), 138–144.

45. Capelle, H. H., Weigel, R., & Krauss, J. K. (2003). Bilateral pallidal stimulation for blepharospasm-oromandibular dystonia (Meige syndrome). Neurology, *60*(12), 2017–2018.

46. Ostrem, J. L., Marks Jr., W. J., Volz, M. M., Heath, S. L., & Starr, P. A. (2007). Pallidal deep brain stimulation in patients with cranial–cervical dystonia (Meige syndrome). Movement disorders, *22*(13), 1885–1891.

47. Limotai, N., Go, C., Oyama, G., Hwynn, N., Zesiewicz, T., Foote, K., . . . Okun, M. S. (2011). Mixed results for GPi-DBS in the treatment of cranio-facial and cranio-cervical dystonia symptoms. Journal of neurology, *258*(11), 2069–2074.

48. Horisawa, S., Ochiai, T., Goto, S., Nakajima, T., Takeda, N., Kawamata, T., & Taira, T. (2018). Long-term outcome of pallidal stimulation for Meige syndrome. Journal of neurosurgery, *130*(1), 84–89.

49. Damier, P., Thobois, S., Witjas, T., Cuny, E., Derost, P., Raoul, S., . . . Nguyen, J. M. (2007). Bilateral deep brain stimulation of the globus pallidus to treat tardive dyskinesia. Archives of general psychiatry, *64*(2), 170–176.

50. Spindler, M. A., Galifianakis, N. B., Wilkinson, J. R., & Duda, J. E. (2013). Globus pallidus interna deep brain stimulation for tardive dyskinesia: case report and review of the literature. Parkinsonism & related disorders, *19*(2), 141–147.

51. Pouclet-Courtemanche, H., Rouaud, T., Thobois, S., Nguyen, J. M., Brefel-Courbon, C., Chereau, I., . . . Laurencin, C. (2016). Long-term efficacy and tolerability of bilateral pallidal stimulation to treat tardive dyskinesia. Neurology, *86*(7), 651–659.

52. Vidailhet, M., Yelnik, J., Lagrange, C., Fraix, V., Grabli, D., Thobois, S., . . . Ardouin, C. (2009). Bilateral pallidal deep brain stimulation for the treatment of patients with dystonia-choreoathetosis cerebral palsy: a prospective pilot study. Lancet Neurology, *8*(8), 709–717.

53. Koy, A., Hellmich, M., Pauls, K. A. M., Marks, W., Lin, J. P., Fricke, O., & Timmermann, L. (2013). Effects of deep brain stimulation in dyskinetic cerebral palsy: a meta-analysis. Movement Disorders, *28*(5), 647–654.

54. Katsakiori, P. F., Kefalopoulou, Z., Markaki, E., Paschali, A., Ellul, J., Kagadis, G. C., . . . Constantoyannis, C. (2009). Deep brain

stimulation for secondary dystonia: results in 8 patients. Acta neurochirurgica, *151*(5), 473.

55. Gruber, D., Kühn, A. A., Schoenecker, T., Kivi, A., Trottenberg, T., Hoffmann, K. T., . . . Asmus, F. (2010). Pallidal and thalamic deep brain stimulation in myoclonus-dystonia. Movement disorders, *25*(11), 1733–1743.

56. Ostrem, J. L., & Starr, P. A. (2008). Treatment of dystonia with deep brain stimulation. Neurotherapeutics, *5*(2), 320–330.

57. Munhoz, R. P., Picillo, M., Fox, S. H., Bruno, V., Panisset, M., Honey, C. R., & Fasano, A. (2016). Eligibility criteria for deep brain stimulation in Parkinson's disease, tremor, and dystonia. Canadian Journal of Neurological Sciences, *43*(4), 462–471.

58. Aravamuthan, B. R., Waugh, J. L., & Stone, S. S. (2017). Deep brain stimulation for monogenic dystonia. Current opinion in pediatrics, *29*(6), 691–696.

59. Neumann, W. J., Horn, A., Ewert, S., Huebl, J., Brücke, C., Slentz, C., . . . Kühn, A. A. (2017). A localized pallidal physiomarker in cervical dystonia. Annals of neurology, *82*(6), 912–924.

60. Andrews, C., Aviles-Olmos, I., Hariz, M., & Foltynie, T. (2010). Which patients with dystonia benefit from deep brain stimulation? A metaregression of individual patient outcomes. Journal of Neurology, Neurosurgery, and Psychiatry, *81*(12), 1383–1389.

61. Horn, A., Reich, M., Vorwerk, J., Li, N., Wenzel, G., Fang, Q., . . . Kühn, A. A. (2017). Connectivity predicts deep brain stimulation outcome in Parkinson disease. Annals of neurology, *82*(1), 67–78.

62. Isaias, I. U., Alterman, R. L., & Tagliati, M. (2008). Outcome predictors of pallidal stimulation in patients with primary dystonia: the role of disease duration. Brain, *131*(7), 1895–1902.

63. Zhang, L., Sperry, L., & Shahlaie, K. (2012). Deep brain stimulation: a minimally invasive surgical option for movement disorders. Journal of Nurse Life Care Planning, *12*(2).

64. Foncke, E. M., Schuurman, P. R., & Speelman, J. D. (2006). Suicide after deep brain stimulation of the internal globus pallidus for dystonia. Neurology, *66*(1), 142–143.

65. Kiss, Z. H., Doig-Beyaert, K., Eliasziw, M., Tsui, J., Haffenden, A., & Suchowersky, O. (2007). The Canadian multicentre study of deep brain

stimulation for cervical dystonia. Brain, *130*(11), 2879–2886.

66. de Gusmao, C. M., Pollak, L. E., & Sharma, N. (2017). Neuropsychological and psychiatric outcome of GPi-deep brain stimulation in dystonia. Brain stimulation, *10*(5), 994–996.

67. Hung, S. W., Hamani, C., Lozano, A. M., Poon, Y. W., Piboolnurak, P., Miyasaki, J. M., . . . Moro, E. (2007). Long-term outcome of bilateral pallidal deep brain stimulation for primary cervical dystonia. Neurology, *68*(6), 457–459.

68. Dinkelbach, L., Mueller, J., Poewe, W., Delazer, M., Elben, S., Wolters, A., . . . Volkmann, J. (2015). Cognitive outcome of pallidal deep brain stimulation for primary cervical dystonia: one year follow up results of a prospective multicenter trial. Parkinsonism & related disorders, *21*(8), 976–980.

69. Meoni, S., Zurowski, M., Lozano, A. M., Hodaie, M., Poon, Y. Y., Fallis, M., . . . Moro, E. (2015). Long-term neuropsychiatric outcomes after pallidal stimulation in primary and secondary dystonia. Neurology, *85*(5), 433–440.

70. Konrad, C., Vollmer-Haase, J., Anneken, K., & Knecht, S. (2004). Orthopedic and neurological complications of cervical dystonia–review of the literature. Acta neurologica scandinavica, *109*(6), 369–373.

71. Hirose, G., & Kadoya, S. (1984). Cervical spondylotic radiculo-myelopathy in patients with athetoid-dystonic cerebral palsy: clinical evaluation and surgical treatment. Journal of Neurology, Neurosurgery, and Psychiatry, *47*(8), 775–780.

72. Waterston, J. A., Swash, M., & Watkins, E. S. (1989). Idiopathic dystonia and cervical spondylotic myelopathy. Journal of Neurology, Neurosurgery, and Psychiatry, *52*(12), 1424–1426.

73. Polk, J. L., Maragos, V. A., & Nicholas, J. J. (1992). Cervical spondylotic myeloradiculopathy in dystonia. Archives of physical medicine and rehabilitation, *73*(4), 389–392.

74. Hagenah, J. M., Vieregge, A., & Vieregge, P. (2001). Radiculopathy and myelopathy in patients with primary cervical dystonia. European neurology, *45*(4), 236–240.

75. Lumsden, D. E., Gimeno, H., Elze, M., Tustin, K., Kaminska, M., & Lin, J. P. (2016). Progression to musculoskeletal deformity in childhood dystonia. European journal of paediatric neurology, *20*(3), 339–345.

Case 35

Deep Brain Stimulation for Dystonia

Basic Programming Pearls

MITESH LOTIA

INTRODUCTION

Dystonia is a movement disorder characterized by sustained or intermittent muscle co-contractions causing abnormal, often repetitive movements, postures, or both. Dystonic movements are typically patterned, twisting, and tremulous. Dystonia is often initiated or worsened by voluntary action and associated with overflow muscle activation.[1] This updated definition attempts to differentiate dystonia clinically from tremors or chorea and to offer precise treatment options. Although levodopa for dopamine-responsive dystonia or high-dose trihexyphenidyl in generalized dystonia has been helpful, failure of medical therapies is commonly reported due to poor tolerability or lack of consistent benefits.[2] Botulinum toxin is the first-line therapy for focal or segmental dystonia.[3,4] However, for a refractory or generalized primary dystonia, deep brain stimulation (DBS) is approved by the US Food and Drug Administration (FDA) for humanitarian use (humanitarian device exemption [HDE]). For a successful outcome, patient selection, appropriate stimulation techniques, and precise targeting are critical components, especially because the clinical effects can often be delayed by weeks to months.

SELECTION CRITERIA AND INDICATIONS FOR DEEP BRAIN STIMULATION IN DYSTONIA

Various surgical techniques, including pallidotomy, thalamotomy, and DBS, have been proved to be useful for the treatment of dystonia. However, DBS of the global pallidus interna (GPi) has emerged as the treatment of choice for patients with idiopathic progressive dystonia.[5] There are many classifications of dystonia, and appropriate patient selection is critical to a successful outcome. The selection depends not only on the etiology (primary vs. secondary) but also on the age, presence of other clinical features (dystonia plus), and other comorbidities (neuropsychiatric, musculoskeletal).[6]

Most patients with primary dystonia respond better to DBS compared with secondary dystonia.[5] DYT1 patients have had earlier and more significant improvement along with long-term benefits.[7,8] The responses in other isolated genetic dystonia syndromes have been variable. There is a less predictable response in patients with DYT6[9] and no response in patients with DTY24 dystonic tremor, whereas patients with DYT11[10] and DYT28[11] have been reported to improve significantly. Furthermore, DYT12 dystonia patients consistently demonstrate a lack of efficacy.[12] Therefore, it is important, when possible, to establish a preoperative genetic diagnosis for accurate prediction of surgical outcomes.[13] Currently, there is no cutoff score for the severity of symptoms, but DBS is often recommended for patients with functional limitations due to motor impairment, pain, or disability. Patients of all ages may benefit from the procedure, even though there are few reports of the surgery for the patients younger than 7 years. For childhood dystonia, patients with primary dystonia of shorter duration seem to respond better with GPi DBS, although this is questionable given the paucity of data.[14] DBS in children with cerebral palsy has mixed outcomes, possibly owing to lack of quantifiable data, which challenges the judgment of outcome.[15] The neuropsychiatric comorbidities (depression and suicide) should be aggressively treated preoperatively[6] because these are likely to influence long-term outcomes.

GPi DBS should be considered for primary cervical dystonia associated with pain and for severe neck deformity despite adequate botulinum toxin trial. A recent meta-analysis of 115 patients with craniofacial dystonia with pallidal/ subthalamic stimulation showed significant improvement on the Burke–Fahn–Marsden Dystonia Rating Scale—Movement (BFMDRS-M) (21.5 ± 11.0 vs. 8.6 ± 6.9, $p < 0.001$) and disability scores compared with the baseline scores.[16] Patients with focal dystonia referred for "botulinum injection resistance" should be carefully evaluated for potential benefits from different muscle selection, a modified dosing plan, or even a different toxin (type B vs. type A). While DBS can be beneficial in patients with acquired causes (tardive dystonia,[17,18] pantothenate kinase-associated neurodegeneration [PKAN][19]), patients with secondary dystonia from structural lesions[20] and those with fixed skeletal deformities[21] may not have as robust a response.

PRESURGICAL PLANNING

The importance of detailed presurgical planning cannot be overemphasized. Besides considering the factors mentioned earlier, a careful clinical examination should include using standardized rating scales such as the BFMDRS-M and Toronto Western Spasmodic Torticollis Scale (TWSTRS).[22] Detailed video documentation outlining task-specific limitations such as writing, using utensils, speech, and other fine motor movements is beneficial for long-term follow-up. The exam should also include documentation of tremors, myoclonus, and bradykinesia, along with any speech impairment. This type of documentation not only helps document the findings but also facilitates an opportunity for appropriate presurgical counseling. Presurgical magnetic resonance imaging (MRI) for stereotactic target localization with coronal and axial sections through the basal ganglia is helpful. Further details of stereotactic localization are beyond the scope of this chapter.

A detailed neuropsychological evaluation will help to identify cognitive impairment across different domains and also aid in recognizing underlying mood/thought disorder. Treatment of neuropsychiatric symptoms is essential because it may affect the postsurgical experience.

I highly recommend discussing and carefully documenting the expectations from the surgery with patients and families because the outcomes can be variable based on the many factors described previously. The overall goals should be to (1) minimize the abnormal posturing, thus improving quality of life and reducing disability; (2) reduce the pain related to abnormal posturing; (3) provide effective stimulation with minimal side effects; and (4) deliver efficient use of the stimulation (i.e., prolong battery life).

TARGET SELECTION

While subthalamic nucleus (STN) and ventral intermediate (Vim) nucleus of the thalamus have been useful for dystonia treatment, pallidal DBS has been the most frequently used target for the treatment of dystonia. With increasing experience, different regions within the pallidum have been described. A wide variety of stimulation parameters and various algorithms, along with computer-assisted brain mapping, have been employed.[23,24] The posteroventral region is thought to represent the sensorimotor territory[25,26] and is most frequently targeted in dystonia.[27] Some of the recent trials with effects of subthalamic stimulation on dystonia are summarized in Table 35.1.

INITIAL PROGRAMMING

Several factors render DBS programming for dystonia more unique than in tremor or parkinsonism (Table 35.2). The microlesion is often less evident in patients with dystonia, except in a small subset of patients in which eight out of nine patients with dystonia reported transient improvement in their symptoms after the surgery and continual benefits at 6 months.[28] While there are no controlled trials, reimbursement patterns and logistical health strategies usually dictate the use of immediate inpatient versus outpatient postoperative programming. However, to allow postoperative recovery and to minimize the potential microlesion effect, it is advisable to wait for 2 to 4 weeks before initiating the initial programming. Unlike in patients with tremor or Parkinson disease (PD), there is usually no reason to hold any dystonia medications before the programming.

It is always a good practice to examine the scalp and implantable pulse generator (IPG) site incisions for their integrity and to verify appropriate healing. It is useful to measure and to document the electrode impedance, which is an indicator of the proper functioning of the device. Excessively high impedance may point toward an open circuit from a lead fracture or a persistent

TABLE 35.1. SUBTHALAMIC NUCLEUS DEEP BRAIN STIMULATION FOR DYSTONIA

Study	Design	Dystonia Type	N	Amplitude (V)	Pulse Width (μsec)	Frequency (Hz)	Scales	Results	Comments
Cao et al. (2013)[59]	Retrospective, blinded raters 3- to 10-year follow-up	Primary dystonia	27	2–3.6	90–120	135–195 (1 pt at 60)	BFMDRS. SF-36	Improvement in BFMDRS: 55% at 1 month, 70% at 1 year, 79% at 3–10 years Sustained improvement in SF-36	- Side effects - 22.2% (lead fracture, malpositioning, transient depression and dyskinesia) - Improved battery life compared to GPi
Ostrem et al. (2017)[60]	Prospective, blinded rater, 3-year follow=up	Isolated (cranial, cervical, segmental)	20	2.5 (±1.2)	65.5 (±13.4)	129.3 (±30.1) (1 pt at 60)	BFMDRS, TWSTRS, SF-36, CGI	At 36 months, Improvement in BFMDRS: 70.4% Improvement in TWSTRS: 66.6% Improved SF-36 and CGI	- No infection or bradykinesia - dyskinesias in all patients
Zhan et al. (2018)[61]	Retrospective, blinded rater	Meige syndrome	15	1.95–3.75	60–120	135–185	BFMDRS SF-36	Improvement in BFMDRS: 74% Improved SF-36	
Deng et al. (2018)[62]	Retrospective, 10-year follow-up	Primary dystonias	14	2.4 (±0.4)	73.6–80.7 (±16.9)	141.4–142.5 (±18.2)	BFMDRS SF-36	Improvement in BFMDRS: 50% at 1 month, 79.1% at 1 year, 86.5% at 5 years, 88.5% at last follow-up Sustained improvement in SF-36	8/14 developed side effects—infection, displacements, transient depression,

BFMDRS = Burke-Fahn-Marsden Rating Scale; SF-36 = Short Form 36 questions for quality of life; CGI = Clinical Global Impression; TWSTRS = Toronto Western Spasmodic Torticollis Rating Scale.

TABLE 35.2. DIFFERENCE BETWEEN DEEP BRAIN STIMULATION PROGRAMMING IN
DYSTONIA AND TREMOR/PARKINSONISM

	Dystonia	Tremor/Parkinsonism
Microlesion effect	Minimal to none	Mostly present for 2–4 weeks
Withhold medications before programming	Generally not recommended	Stop antitremor and dopaminergic medications for at least 12 hours before the programming (some are long-acting, and this is not as big an issue as in Parkinson disease)
Onset of benefits	Usually delayed by hours to weeks to months	Usually immediate (seconds to minutes) improvement in tremor, rigidity, and bradykinesia
Medication changes	Relatively slow tapering	Antitremor/anti-dyskinetic medications can be weaned after initial programming Dopaminergic medications can be slowly lowered over time based on the lead location

pneumocephalus,[29] whereas a low impedance may indicate a short circuit.

Evidence-based recommendations for initial programming in dystonia are lacking, mainly because of the lack of controlled studies and paucity of cases. However, several approaches have been proposed, such as monopolar stimulation,[18] monopolar stimulation of two adjacent contacts,[30] short bursts of increasing amplitudes with high-frequency stimulation,[31] or prolonged test periods of monopolar stimulation review at low frequency.[32] Moro and colleagues studied the acute effects of various stimulation parameters in patients with bilateral GPi DBS for cervical dystonia patients in a double-blinded fashion.[33] After attempting 10 different stimulation settings, the amplitude and the frequency changes were observed to provide the most significant antidystonic benefits. A progressive increase in the amplitude and frequency was associated with better outcomes in this study of eight cervical dystonia patients.

The initial DBS contacts can be chosen with the help of intraoperative microelectrode recordings and postoperative imaging data (Figure 35.1). A systematic unipolar review with a slower amplitude increment at ventral contacts while keeping the pulse width and frequency constant at 90 to 120 μsed and 60 to 130 Hz, respectively, is a reasonable approach.[34] Often, tonic side effects may become apparent during programming, and these can guide the electrode selection by moving dorsally, during the first programming. Many experts use variations of the previous approach.

If no side effects emerge, patients can be discharged on reasonable settings of 1.5 to 2.5 V, 90 to 150 μsec, and 130 Hz. Many patients may require higher pulse widths. Many experts also offer a few weeks on low-frequency settings (<100 Hz).[35,36] On return in 2 to 4 weeks, further adjustments can be made depending on the effects.

SUBSEQUENT PROGRAMMING

The follow-up programming can be planned every 2 to 4 weeks for a minimum of 3 months, but in most dystonia cases programming may need to occur from implant to 6 to 12 months, given the frequent delay in benefits. One other advantage to frequent programming sessions is the opportunity to monitor for neuropsychiatric side effects. If there are benefits from the first programming session, further amplitude increments can be made. The amplitude increment usually increases the volume of tissue activation. The pulse width defines the duration of each electrical pulse within a specified field of tissue activation. Therefore, pulse width increment is presumed to increase the neuronal recruitment within the volume activated by the amplitude. If the amplitude is already approximately 2.5 to 3 V, many experts consider increasing the pulse width (with monopolar stimulation). If no benefits emerge, double monopolar stimulation can be useful for recruiting additional nuclei. Alternatively, one may consider low-frequency (50–90 Hz) stimulation because previous trials have also shown benefits

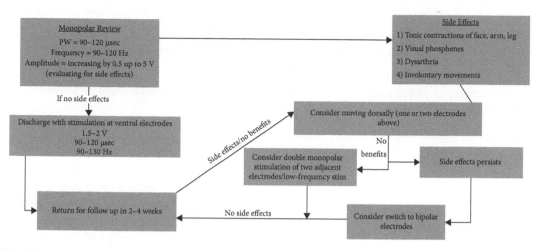

FIGURE 35.1. Approach to initial programming. PW = pulse width.

at lower (60 Hz) frequencies, with benefits lasting at least up to 1 year.[32] Finally, the use of interleaving or multiple monopolar independent contacts has also been recently used.

A recent systematic review of pallidal DBS summarized mean voltage, pulse width, and frequencies parameters for primary generalized and secondary dystonia.[37] While amplitude (3.3 ± 0.6 V) and frequencies (131 ± 5 Hz) were standard for most patients, there was a wide variation in the range of pulse width (112 ± 31, 203 ± 22, 446 ±8 μsec) across multiple studies. The longer pulse widths were more common among generalized dystonia, whereas shorter pulse widths were more frequent in focal and acquired dystonia. Occasionally, very long pulse widths of 450 μsec can be effective. Approaches to programming in dystonia vary between experts, and there is no one right pathway. It is most important to be slow and deliberate and to inform families of the time required for improvements to potentially emerge.

POSTPROGRAMMING MEDICATION MANAGEMENT

Successful DBS surgeries for dystonia are, in many cases, associated with a reduction in medications.[38,39] Most often, the medications are minimally effective in dystonia, and in children, the anticholinergics may affect school function.[2] After the abnormal postures and the related pain improve, one should consider reducing the medications. Typically, muscle relaxants, opioids, and benzodiazepines can be minimized or slowly tapered. Trihexyphenidyl and dopaminergic medications should be carefully titrated down to avoid withdrawal symptoms. Botulinum toxin injections may be considered for focal dystonia (hand or cervical dystonia) in patients with generalized dystonia if they fail to improve despite optimal DBS programming. One common scenario is a patient with improvement from DBS who may still require botulinum toxin for foot dystonia.

TROUBLESHOOTING

The most common causes for suboptimal clinical response in carefully selected patients include suboptimal lead placement followed by improper programming.[40] However, a careful evaluation of the lead location and systematic approach to programming can often help improve success. Okun and colleagues described the experience of two movement disorder centers where nearly half of patients (51%) with "failed" DBS procedures had improved outcomes with appropriate intervention, whereas nearly one-third (34%) of them did not improve despite maximal intervention.[41] DBS complications can be divided into hardware-related complications and stimulation-related side effects, as summarized in Table 35.3. Failure to benefit in dystonia is a complex determination given the possibility that benefits may emerge months after programming.

If there is a presence of persistent side effects at lower current densities across all DBS contacts, imaging should be considered to evaluate for poor electrode placement (Figure 35.3).[42] If there are mild side effects, the use of dorsal contacts or a bipolar configuration can be considered. If there

TABLE 35.3. STIMULATION-RELATED SIDE EFFECTS AND THEIR MANAGEMENT

Side Effect	Structure Stimulated	Likely DBS Lead Location	Management Strategy
Visual phosphenes (flashing lights)	Optic tract	Too inferior	Stimulate dorsal electrodes
Tonic muscle contractions at lower stimulation	Corticospinal tracts	Too posteromedial	Reduce the amplitude, move dorsally or change to bipolar electrode
Dysarthria	Corticobulbar tracts	Too posterior	Consider reducing the amplitude or bipolar configuration
Dyskinesia	Dorsal GPi/GPe		Stimulation of ventral contacts if no capsular effects or consider bipolar configuration
Bradykinesia	Ventral GPi		Stimulate dorsal leads
Gait disorder	Too anterior Ventral GPi		Stimulate dorsal leads

DBS = deep brain stimulation; GPe = globus pallidus externa; GPi = globus pallidus interna.

are no benefits at all contacts after 3 to 6 months of programming with adequate charge density, one should consider reimaging to evaluate for suboptimal lead placement or for lead migration. One should carefully review the details from each programming session. Additionally, leads may dorsally migrate during battery changes or from growth in children. A benefit that fades days after programming and cannot be recaptured may be a clue to a suboptimally placed lead.

Sudden loss of benefits after initial improvement often points toward a hardware failure. Check the electrode and therapy impedance. If the impedance is significantly higher, it could be from a lead fracture/migration, infection, or a failed IPG. Postoperative lead migration is higher in dystonia patients presumably because of severe head movements,[43] and this issue may adversely affect the outcomes in dystonia.[44] The risk for wound infections has been variable, ranging from 1 to 15% across multiple studies.[45-47] Careful surgical techniques, appropriate use of perioperative antibiotics, routine incisional precautions, and avoidance of heavy weight-lifting/heavy physical activity for a few weeks can help minimize some of these complications. End of life of the IPG battery can often lead to severe acute exacerbation of dystonia or status dystonicus.[48] Therefore, routine evaluation of a dual-channel battery should be performed at least every 6 months. In younger patients, the use of rechargeable batteries should be considered for longevity because these have been shown to be cost-effective (in Europe).[49]

STIMULATION-INDUCED ADVERSE EFFECTS

Figure 35.2 summarizes various side effects related to the stimulation of GPi and STN, along with surrounding structures,[50] and Table 35.2 outlines management strategies to minimize each of these side effects. While visual phosphenes are often present with the ventral contacts, they are useful to identify in the first programming session.[42] Chronic stimulation of posteroventral lateral GPi has been postulated to cause general alteration of neuronal activity in striato-pallido-thalamo-cortical motor pathways.[51] Bradykinesia and impaired postural stability with chronic GPi stimulation have been reported.[52,53] These changes should be carefully evaluated and may warrant further adjustment by moving the active electrodes dorsally or by employing other strategies.[54] In GPi DBS, stimulation-induced bradykinesia is rare; however, in STN DBS for dystonia, stimulation-induced dyskinesia is common. The dyskinesia can be addressed by decreasing the current density.

Furthermore, dyskinesia induction has been reported with stimulation of the dorsal GPi/globus pallidus externa (GPe).[55] Amplitude reduction, bipolar configuration and widening the pulse width, or moving the stimulating electrodes ventrally all may be helpful. Posteriorly and sometimes medially activated electrodes have been found to alter motor aspects of speech.[56] However, speech fluency, intelligibility,

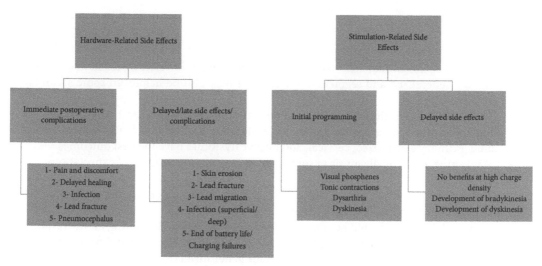

FIGURE 35.2. Side effects of globus pallidus interna stimulation.

and critical aspects of hyperkinetic and hypoki-netic dysarthria showed dualistic effects of GPi DBS in a study by Rusz and colleagues.[57] These authors suggested that lower stimulation param-eters (i.e., current densities) and more lateral electrical stimulation would likely minimize the side effects of hypokinetic dysarthria and dysflu-ency. Awareness of these side effects can help to identify and possibly avoid them. There is a scar-city of systematized data on dystonia program-ming and its potential side effects. The biggest challenge is the lack of an acute clinical marker during programming that might indicate the best contact or stimulation setting. This scenario is where physiology with local field potentials may be useful in the future.[58]

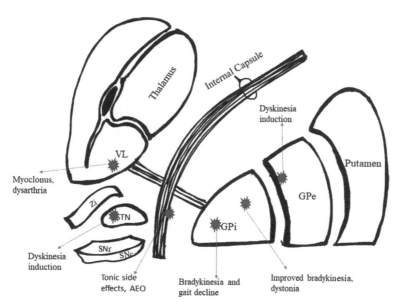

FIGURE 35.3. Stimulation-related effects by anatomic location. AEO = Apraxia of eyelid opening; GPe = globus pallidus externa; GPi = globus pallidus interna; SNc = Substantia Nigra pars compacta; SNr = Substantia Nigra pars reticulata; STN = subthalamic nucleus; VL = Ventral Lateral Nucleus; Zi = Zona inserta. (Adapted from Baizabal-Carvallo JF, Jankovic J. Movement disorders induced by deep brain stimulation. *Parkinsonism & Related Disorders.* 2016;25:1–9.)

PEARLS

- DBS is a well-established, effective, and safe for treatment of select medication-refractory primary generalized and segmental dystonias. It may also be helpful in some secondary dystonias.
- Careful patient selection is the most important predictive factor for a successful clinical outcome. Contractures, speech, facial, and swallowing features may have a less robust outcome. Primary generalized, cervical, and tardive dystonias have the best outcomes.
- Establishing a genetic diagnosis in some cases can inform discussion of expectations.
- A monopolar review with increasing the amplitude, while keeping the pulse width and frequency constant, in a ventral electrode is suggested for initial programming, although there is no standard accepted approach.
- Further adjustments should be considered every 2 to 4 weeks, depending on the response. Some experts suggest using a shorter pulse width for focal or acquired dystonia, whereas longer pulse widths may be more beneficial for generalized dystonia. There is a paucity of cases to guide management, and often an empirical open-minded trial-and-error approach over many months is required.
- Stimulation-induced side effects such as bradykinesia, hypokinetic dysarthria, and gait changes are possible, especially with more ventral GPi stimulation, whereas dyskinesia induction is likely from more dorsal GPi stimulation. STN DBS in dystonia is commonly associated with dyskinesia.
- Standardized scales should be performed before and after surgery to assess the outcomes.
- Patients and families should be counseled that there frequently are delayed benefits and side effects, and a long-term trial-and-error approach is the best course. Patients and families should also understand that the field lacks an immediate clinical marker during programming in most cases (e.g., atremor in essential tremor or PD).

REFERENCES

1. Albanese A, Bhatia K, Bressman SB, et al. Phenomenology and classification of dystonia: a consensus update. *Movement Disorders.* 2013;28(7):863–873.
2. Jankovic J. Medical treatment of dystonia. *Movement Disorders.* 2013;28(7):1001–1012.
3. Hallett M, Albanese A, Dressler D, et al. Evidence-based review and assessment of botulinum neurotoxin for the treatment of movement disorders. *Toxicon.* 2013;67:94–114.
4. Albanese A, Asmus F, Bhatia KP, et al. EFNS guidelines on diagnosis and treatment of primary dystonias. *European Journal of Neurology.* 2011;18(1):5–18.
5. Albanese A, Di Giovanni M, Lalli S. Dystonia: diagnosis and management. *European Journal of Neurology.* 2019;26(1):5–17.
6. Bronte-Stewart H, Taira T, Valldeoriola F, et al. Inclusion and exclusion criteria for DBS in dystonia. *Movement Disorders.* 2011;26(S1):S5–S16.
7. Vidailhet M, Jutras M-F, Grabli D, Roze E. Deep brain stimulation for dystonia. *Journal of Neurology, Neurosurgery, and Psychiatry.* 2013;84(9):1029–1042.
8. Panov F, Gologorsky Y, Connors G, Tagliati M, Miravite J, Alterman RL. Deep brain stimulation in DYT1 dystonia: a 10-year experience. *Neurosurgery.* 2013;73(1):86–93; discussion 93.
9. Bruggemann N, Kuhn A, Schneider SA, et al. Short- and long-term outcome of chronic pallidal neurostimulation in monogenic isolated dystonia. *Neurology.* 2015;84(9):895–903.
10. Roze E, Vidailhet M, Hubsch C, Navarro S, Grabli D. Pallidal stimulation for myoclonus-dystonia: ten years' outcome in two patients. *Movement Disorders.* 2015;30(6):871–872.
11. Zech M, Jech R, Havránková P, et al. KMT2B rare missense variants in generalized dystonia. *Movement Disorders.* 2017;32(7):1087–1091.
12. Albanese A, Di Giovanni M, Amami P, Lalli S. Failure of pallidal deep brain stimulation in DYT12-ATP1A3 dystonia. *Parkinsonism & Related Disorders.* 2017;45:99–100.
13. Jinnah HA, Alterman R, Klein C, et al. Deep brain stimulation for dystonia: a novel perspective on

the value of genetic testing. *Journal of Neural Transmission (Vienna)*. 2017;124(4):417–430.

14. Badhiwala JH, Karmur B, Elkaim LM, et al. Clinical phenotypes associated with outcomes following deep brain stimulation for childhood dystonia. *Journal of Neurosurgery Pediatrics*. 2019;1–9.

15. Sanger TD. Deep brain stimulation for cerebral palsy: where are we now? *Developmental Medicine and Child Neurology*. 2020;62(1):28–33.

16. Wang X, Zhang Z, Mao Z, Yu X. Deep brain stimulation for Meige syndrome: a meta-analysis with individual patient data. *Journal of Neurology*. 2019;266(11):2646–2656.

17. Gruber D, Sudmeyer M, Deuschl G, et al. Neurostimulation in tardive dystonia/dyskinesia: a delayed start, sham stimulation-controlled randomized trial. *Brain Stimulation*. 2018;11(6):1368–1377.

18. Gruber D, Trottenberg T, Kivi A, et al. Long-term effects of pallidal deep brain stimulation in tardive dystonia. *Neurology*. 2009;73(1):53–58.

19. Svetel M, Tomic A, Dragasevic N, et al. Clinical course of patients with pantothenate kinase-associated neurodegeneration (PKAN) before and after DBS surgery. *Journal of Neurology*. 2019;266(12):2962–2969.

20. Mohammad SS, Paget SP, Dale RC. Current therapies and therapeutic decision making for childhood-onset movement disorders. *Movement Disorders*. 2019;34(5):637–656.

21. Isaias IU, Alterman RL, Tagliati M. Outcome predictors of pallidal stimulation in patients with primary dystonia: the role of disease duration. *Brain*. 2008;131(7):1895–1902.

22. Comella CL, Fox SH, Bhatia KP, et al. Development of the comprehensive cervical dystonia rating scale: methodology. *Movement Disorders Clinical Practice*. 2015;2(2):135–141.

23. Reich MM, Horn A, Lange F, et al. Probabilistic mapping of the antidystonic effect of pallidal neurostimulation: a multicentre imaging study. *Brain*. 2019;142(5):1386–1398.

24. Cheung T, Noecker AM, Alterman RL, McIntyre CC, Tagliati M. Defining a therapeutic target for pallidal deep brain stimulation for dystonia. *Annals of Neurology*. 2014;76(1):22–30.

25. Cacciola A, Milardi D, Bertino S, et al. Structural connectivity-based topography of the human globus pallidus: Implications for therapeutic targeting in movement disorders. *Movement Disorders*. 2019;34(7):987–996.

26. Starr PA, Turner RS, Rau G, et al. Microelectrode-guided implantation of deep brain stimulators into the globus pallidus internus for dystonia: techniques, electrode locations, and outcomes. *Journal of Neurosurgery*. 2006;104(4):488–501.

27. Vidailhet M, Vercueil L, Houeto J-L, et al. Bilateral deep-brain stimulation of the globus pallidus in primary generalized dystonia. *New England Journal of Medicine*. 2005;352(5):459–467.

28. Cersosimo MG, Raina GB, Benarroch EE, Piedimonte F, Aleman GG, Micheli FE. Micro lesion effect of the globus pallidus internus and outcome with deep brain stimulation in patients with Parkinson disease and dystonia. *Movement Disorders*. 2009;24(10):1488–1493.

29. Lyons MK, Neal MT, Patel NP. Intraoperative high impedance levels during placement of deep brain stimulating electrode. *Operative Neurosurgery (Hagerstown)*. 2019;17(6):E264–E266.

30. Krauss JK, Pohle T, Weber S, Ozdoba C, Burgunder J-M. Bilateral stimulation of globus pallidus internus for treatment of cervical dystonia. *Lancet*. 1999;354(9181):837–838.

31. Kupsch A, Benecke R, Müller J, et al. Pallidal deep-brain stimulation in primary generalized or segmental dystonia. *New England Journal of Medicine*. 2006;355(19):1978–1990.

32. Alterman RL, Miravite J, Weisz D, Shils JL, Bressman SB, Tagliati M. Sixty hertz pallidal deep brain stimulation for primary torsion dystonia. *Neurology*. 2007;69(7):681–688.

33. Moro E, Piboolnurak P, Arenovich T, Hung SW, Poon Y-Y, Lozano AM. Pallidal stimulation in cervical dystonia: clinical implications of acute changes in stimulation parameters. *European Journal of Neurology*. 2009;16(4):506–512.

34. Marks Jr WJ. *Deep brain stimulation management*. Cambridge, UK: Cambridge University Press; 2015.

35. Baizabal-Carvallo JF, Alonso-Juarez M. Low-frequency deep brain stimulation for movement disorders. *Parkinsonism & Related Disorders*. 2016;31:14–22.

36. Ostrem JL, Markun LC, Glass GA, et al. Effect of frequency on subthalamic nucleus deep brain stimulation in primary dystonia. *Parkinsonism & Related Disorders*. 2014;20(4):432–438.

37. Magown P, Andrade RA, Soroceanu A, Kiss ZHT. Deep brain stimulation parameters for dystonia: a systematic review. *Parkinsonism & Related Disorders*. 2018;54:9–16.

38. Volkmann J, Wolters A, Kupsch A, et al. Pallidal deep brain stimulation in patients with primary generalised or segmental dystonia: 5-year follow-up of a randomised trial. *Lancet Neurology*. 2012;11(12):1029–1038.

39. Moro E, Gross RE, Krauss JK. What's new in surgical treatment for dystonia? *Movement Disorders*. 2013;28(7):1013–1020.

40. Pauls KAM, Krauss JK, Kampfer CE, et al. Causes of failure of pallidal deep brain stimulation in cases

with pre-operative diagnosis of isolated dystonia. *Parkinsonism & Related Disorders.* 2017;43:38–48.

41. Okun MS, Tagliati M, Pourfar M, et al. Management of referred deep brain stimulation failures: a retrospective analysis from 2 movement disorders centers. *Archives of Neurology.* 2005;62(8):1250–1255.

42. Kupsch A, Tagliati M, Vidailhet M, et al. Early postoperative management of DBS in dystonia: programming, response to stimulation, adverse events, medication changes, evaluations, and troubleshooting. *Movement Disorders.* 2011;26(Suppl 1):S37–S53.

43. Yianni J, Nandi D, Shad A, Bain P, Gregory R, Aziz T. Increased risk of lead fracture and migration in dystonia compared with other movement disorders following deep brain stimulation. *Journal of Clinical Neuroscience.* 2004;11(3):243–245.

44. Morishita T, Hilliard JD, Okun MS, et al. Postoperative lead migration in deep brain stimulation surgery: Incidence, risk factors, and clinical impact. *PLoS One.* 2017;12(9):e0183711–e0183711.

45. Fenoy AJ, Simpson RK. Risks of common complications in deep brain stimulation surgery: management and avoidance. *Journal of Neurosurgery.* 2014;120(1):132.

46. Crosley KM. Perioperative care during deep brain stimulation surgery. *AORN Journal.* 2018;108(2):148–153.

47. Sillay K, Larson P, Starr P. Deep brain stimulator hardware-related infections: incidence and management in a large series. *Neurosurgery.* 2008;62:360–367.

48. Hyam JA, de Pennington N, Joint C, et al. Maintained deep brain stimulation for severe dystonia despite infection by using externalized electrodes and an extracorporeal pulse generator. *Journal of Neurosurgery.* 2010;113(3):630–633.

49. Perez J, Gonzalez V, Cif L, Cyprien F, Chan-Seng E, Coubes P. Rechargeable or nonrechargeable deep brain stimulation in dystonia: a cost analysis. *Neuromodulation: Technology at the Neural Interface.* 2017;20(3):243–247.

50. Baizabal-Carvallo JF, Jankovic J. Movement disorders induced by deep brain stimulation. *Parkinsonism & Related Disorders.* 2016;25:1–9.

51. Wolf ME, Capelle HH, Bazner H, Hennerici MG, Krauss JK, Blahak C. Hypokinetic gait changes induced by bilateral pallidal deep brain stimulation for segmental dystonia. *Gait & Posture.* 2016;49:358–363.

52. Huebl J, Brucke C, Schneider GH, Blahak C, Krauss JK, Kuhn AA. Bradykinesia induced by frequency-specific pallidal stimulation in patients with cervical and segmental dystonia. *Parkinsonism & Related Disorders.* 2015;21(7):800–803.

53. Berman BD, Starr PA, Marks WJ Jr., Ostrem JL. Induction of bradykinesia with pallidal deep brain stimulation in patients with cranial-cervical dystonia. *Stereotactic and Functional Neurosurgery.* 2009;87(1):37–44.

54. Schrader C, Capelle HH, Kinfe TM, et al. GPi-DBS may induce a hypokinetic gait disorder with freezing of gait in patients with dystonia. *Neurology.* 2011;77(5):483–488.

55. Elkouzi A, Tsuboi T, Burns MR, Eisinger RS, Patel A, Deeb W. Dorsal GPi/GPe stimulation induced dyskinesia in a patient with Parkinson's disease. *Tremor and Other Hyperkinetic Movements (NY).* 2019;9:10.7916/tohm.v7910.7685.

56. Pauls KAM, Brockelmann PJ, Hammesfahr S, et al. Dysarthria in pallidal deep brain stimulation in dystonia depends on the posterior location of active electrode contacts: a pilot study. *Parkinsonism & Related Disorders.* 2018;47:71–75.

57. Rusz J, Tykalova T, Fecikova A, Stastna D, Urgosik D, Jech R. Dualistic effect of pallidal deep brain stimulation on motor speech disorders in dystonia. *Brain Stimulation.* 2018;11(4):896–903.

58. Thompson JA, Lanctin D, Ince NF, Abosch A. Clinical implications of local field potentials for understanding and treating movement disorders. *Stereotactic and Functional Neurosurgery.* 2014;92(4):251–263.

59. Cao C, Pan Y, Li D, Zhan S, Zhang J, Sun B. Subthalamus deep brain stimulation for primary dystonia patients: a long-term follow-up study. *Movement Disorders.* 2013;28(13):1877–1882.

60. Ostrem JL, San Luciano M, Dodenhoff KA, et al. Subthalamic nucleus deep brain stimulation in isolated dystonia: a 3-year follow-up study. *Neurology.* 2017;88(1):25–35.

61. Zhan S, Sun F, Pan Y, et al. Bilateral deep brain stimulation of the subthalamic nucleus in primary Meige syndrome. *Journal of Neurosurgery.* 2018;128(3):897–902.

62. Deng Z, Pan Y, Zhang C, et al. Subthalamic deep brain stimulation in patients with primary dystonia: a ten-year follow-up study. *Parkinsonism & Related Disorders.* 2018;55:103–110.

Case 36

Choosing a Target for Deep Brain Stimulation in Dystonia-Associated Tremor

MUSTAFA S. SIDDIQUI AND STEPHEN B. TATTER

INDICATIONS FOR DEEP BRAIN STIMULATION

Dystonia-associated tremor and cervical dystonia

CLINICAL HISTORY AND RELEVANT EXAM

A 67-year-old right-handed white male was referred with a 20-year history of primary generalized dystonia. His symptoms of cervical dystonia and bilateral arm tremors were disabling and significantly affected his quality of life. His most bothersome symptom was severe neck pain. Tremors of his arms prevented him from holding a cup of water or eating without spilling. Writing was impossible, and he could barely put a pen on the paper because of the tremor. He required help with most chores. He also had bilateral leg tremors but felt that these tremors were not disabling. He tried baclofen up to 45 mg per day and trihexyphenidyl 15 mg per day without any meaningful benefit. A trial of levodopa 300 mg per day and clonazepam 1 mg twice daily did not make a meaningful difference.

His past medical history was remarkable for anterior cervical discectomy with fusion at C4-5, C5-6, and C6-7, along with diabetes and hypertension. He reported some weakness in the right hand. He also reported a popping and cracking sensation in his neck. Magnetic resonance imaging (MRI) of the cervical spine showed C3-4 disk degeneration without any cord compression. He had moderate cervical stenosis. A radiograph of the cervical spine following anterior fusion of C4-7 showed no pathologic motion in flexion/extension films. He denied any radicular pain. He did not have any bowel or bladder symptoms.

On examination, he had a 25-degree chin deviation to the left, moderate left shoulder elevation, a 20-degree head tilt to the left, and slight anterocollis. He assessed his neck pain as varying between 5 and 10, with 10 being the most intense. The pain was located in the left occipital region and along the left trapezius ridge. He had lateral neck shift to the right. On the Toronto Western Spasmodic Torticollis Scale (TWSTRS), he had a Torticollis Severity Score of 22.

He had grade 4 rest, action, and postural tremors in the right arm and grade 3 rest, action, and postural tremors in the left arm. Tremors were dystonic in nature; they were intermittent and more pronounced in action and specific postures. On maintaining certain postures, his tremors decreased. He had grade 3 rest tremor in the right leg and grade 1 in left leg. He scored 63 points on the Fahn–Tolosa–Marin Tremor Rating Scale (TRS).

Based on these findings, we diagnosed the patient with medication-refractory primary generalized dystonia and offered deep brain stimulation (DBS) to target his cervical dystonia and limb tremors. He had no behavioral or cognitive contraindications to DBS. The patient was very reluctant to undergo brain surgery, and instead opted for botulinum toxin injections to address the symptoms of cervical dystonia. He tested negative for Wilson disease. Genetic testing for the *DYT1* gene mutation was offered, but he declined because of cost.

For 5 years, he continued to obtain satisfactory relief of cervical dystonia symptoms with regular botulinum toxin therapy. However, the patient finally opted for DBS because the bilateral arm tremors severely limited his ability to perform activities of daily living.

We explained to the patient the strategies of targeting the globus pallidus interna (GPi) versus the ventral intermediate (Vim) nucleus: namely, that the former was likely to improve his cervical dystonia but might not improve his arm tremors; whereas the latter strategy was likely to improve the arm tremors but not the cervical dystonia. To address both conditions, we discussed the option of multiple leads. After the patient passed the preoperative interdisciplinary evaluation (including neuropsychological evaluation), we offered him DBS surgery.

COMPLICATIONS
There were no complications.

TROUBLESHOOTING AND MANAGEMENT
Preoperatively, the neurologist (who was also the intraoperative neurophysiologist) and the surgeon planned to first target the right GPi and then to place a second lead in the right Vim if the tremor did not improve. Our surgical team decided not to place a lead in the left hemisphere until his postoperative response from the right hemispheric leads could be evaluated. The team also was hesitant to implant three leads and thus increase the patient's risk for postoperative confusion.

The patient's head was placed in a CRW stereotactic frame, and a volumetric computed tomography (CT) scan was obtained. The CT scan and MRI sets were then fused. These were in turn fused with the Cranial Vault Atlas using a nonrigid co-registration algorithm and to the Schaltenbrand-Wahren human stereotactic brain atlas, with reference to the anterior commissure and to the posterior commissure. The internal segment of the globus pallidus was targeted 20.5 mm lateral, 1 mm anterior, and 3 mm inferior to the mid-commissural point. The Vim nucleus of the thalamus was targeted 14 mm lateral, 5.7 mm posterior, and 0 mm inferior to the mid-commisural point.

Microelectrode recording (MER) was carried out using the FHC Guideline 4000 microtargeting system (FHC Inc.) and the FHC D-Zap mTD microelectrode. MER confirmed a 7.5-mm span of GPi. After MER, the microelectrode was withdrawn by more than 10 mm, and a cannula was advanced with the microelectrode drive by 10 mm to achieve the same depth as the microelectrode (then withdrawn). We used the tip of the microelectrode cannula for stimulation to determine the efficacy and thresholds for side effects. We used a stimulation setting of 150 μsec pulse width at 130-Hz frequency. We increased the electrical current gradually and determined the

tremor efficacy and thresholds for stimulation-related effects. The optic tract was identified after the patient reported visualization of light flashes on stimulation. After satisfactory thresholds for stimulation and verification of the optic tract were achieved, we placed a DBS lead (Model 3389, Medtronic Inc., Minneapolis, MN) within the right GPi based on physiologic mapping. Motor thresholds were low enough to predict programmability. However, no meaningful decreases in tremor occurred after employing both the cannula tip and the DBS lead for stimulation. The lead was secured to the Stimloc cove, as recommended by the manufacturer.

As preplanned, the team moved on intraoperatively to target the right Vim. Physiologic mapping defined a target 2 mm deep and 2 mm medial to the imaging target. We used the cannula tip and DBS lead (Model 3389, Medtronic Inc.) for stimulation as described previously. This completely captured tremor of the left arm with satisfactory stimulation thresholds for side effects. A second DBS lead (Model 3389, Medtronic Inc.) was placed in the new right Vim target based on physiologic mapping. The electrode was secured to the Stimloc cover by removing one of the foot plates from the protective cover. The distal ends of both electrodes were shielded with protective covers, the Vim cut short, and tunneled right laterally beneath the galea.

Following a standard protocol, 3 weeks later, the patient underwent placement of an implantable pulse generator (Model Activa PC, Medtronic Inc.) on the right side of the chest. Electrodes 0 to 3 were connected with the right GPi, and contacts 8 to 11 were connected with the right Vim. Under the scalp, the right Vim electrode/extension set connection was covered with a white opaque protective cover, and the right GPi electrode/extension was covered with a translucent protective cover. We confirmed electrical continuity of the leads, and all contacts had normal impedances.

OUTCOME
The right Vim lead was programmed to target tremor and resulted in immediate and almost complete tremor capture of the left arm and leg (see later discussion for programming parameters).

The right GPi lead was programmed to address cervical dystonia (see programming parameters discussed later). The patient obtained satisfactory improvement; his cervical dystonia was no longer bothersome and no longer required medications or botulinum toxin therapy. His pain level improved from 10 to 0 on a self-reported visual analog scale. No cognitive, behavioral, speech, or gait worsening was observed postoperatively. Subjectively, the patient described less of a feeling of pulling in the neck, which he had described as disabling before surgery.

As part of routine clinical care, surgical outcomes were evaluated 6 months after surgery. Based on TRS ratings, the left arm tremor improved by 91% and the left leg tremor by 100% (contralateral to the side of stimulation).

The patient's cervical dystonia on the TWSTRS Torticollis Severity Scale improved by 22%. Neck pain improved from 10 to 0 on a self-reported visual analog scale. He discontinued all medications and botulinum toxin injections.

Given this encouraging response, the patient then opted for a second DBS procedure targeting the left Vim to address his right arm and leg tremor. He felt that his existing right pallidal lead provided sufficient relief of his cervical dystonia and hence did not feel the need for a left GPi lead.

Seven months after the placement of the right hemispheric GPi and Vim leads, the patient underwent left Vim lead placement (Model 3389, Medtronic Inc.), which was connected 3 weeks later to a single-channel implantable pulse generator (Model Activa SC, Medtronic Inc.) in the left chest. The right arm tremor improved by 75% and the right leg tremor by 100% following the left Vim procedure. No perioperative or postoperative complications were reported.

We have followed this patient regularly for more than 3 years after the second procedure. He continues to obtain very good symptom relief for both cervical dystonia and tremors and has not required botulinum toxin therapy for the cervical dystonia.

The programming parameters at 6 months were as follows:

Right VIM lead (right Activa IPG electrode contacts 8–11): montage: 8+, 9–, amplitude 4 V, pulse width 90 μsec, frequency 180 Hz

Right target GPi (right Activa electrode contacts 0–3): montage: case +, 1–, amplitude 3.1 V, pulse width 60 μsec, frequency 180 Hz

Left Vim (left Activa electrode contacts 0–3): montage: case+, 1 and 2– (double cathodes), amplitude 2.2 V, pulse width 90 μsec, frequency 160 Hz

We localized the active DBS contacts by fusing the postoperative head CT scan with the preoperative brain MRI. The active contact in the right Vim lead was in the Zi region (Figure 36.1B). The active contact in the right GPi lead was in the most ventral portion of that region (Figure 36.1A). The left Vim lead, which was programmed on a double cathode monopolar montage, had one active contact in the Vim region and the other in zona incerta (Zi)/subthalamic nucleus (STN) region (Figure 36.2)

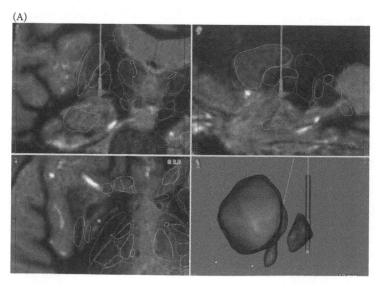

Figure 1(A) Right GPi lead's active contact 1 in ventral GPi

FIGURE 36.1. Multiple right hemispheric leads.

(B)

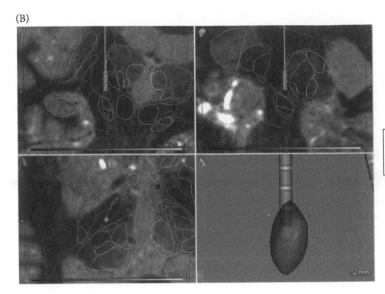

Figure 1(B) Right VIM lead's active contact 1 (8) in the zona incerta region

FIGURE 36.1. Continued

DISCUSSION

GPi is the most frequently used target for primary dystonia. Its effects on dystonic tremor are mixed; some studies show good benefit,[1] and others do not.[2] However, the Vim target has a predictable and robust antitremor effect,[2,3] but does not significantly improve symptoms of dystonia.[2,4] Recent reports describing DBS of the STN show results similar to those for GPi, although effects on dystonic tremor have been less clear.[1,5] Case reports of multiple targets including GPi combined with Ventralis Oralis Posterior (VOP)/Vim nucleus have shown successful treatment of mixed dystonic symptoms.[6,7]

In the case described here, the active contacts (double cathode montage) in the left Vim lead were in the Vim and Zi/STN region (Figure 36.2). The active contact in the right Vim lead was in the Zi region (Figure 36.1B). The caudal Zi, posterior subthalamic area, and STN regions have been reported as efficacious targets for essential tremor.[8] In our case, it appeared that targeting these regions was also efficacious for dystonic tremor. Whether this can be extrapolated to other patients would require larger studies.

The active contact in the right GPi lead was in the most ventral portion of that region (Figure 36.1A). This has been previously reportedly as the most efficacious region for dystonia. In contrast, for Parkinson disease (PD), the most efficacious region has been reported as more dorsal.[9]

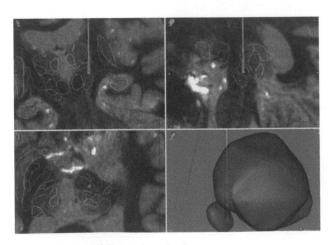

Left VIM Lead Active contact 1 in zona incerta /subthalamic nucleus region. Active Contact 2 in the VIM region.

FIGURE 36.2. Left hemispheric lead.

PEARLS

- Primary generalized dystonia, unlike essential tremor and PD, is not a single disease entity, but rather a heterogeneous clinical syndrome.
- It is important to identify which dystonic symptoms are most disabling for the patient, so these can be specifically targeted.
- In the absence of data for the best DBS target, the best option may be adopting a systematic approach and carefully employing the brain target most likely to address the disabling symptoms.
- There are cases of GPi DBS in which tremor has been shown to be suppressed, so understanding the most disabling symptom and employing a safe and systematic approach to adding DBS leads is a good strategy.

REFERENCES

1. Fasano A, Bove F, Lang AE. The treatment of dystonic tremor: a systematic review. *Journal of Neurology, Neurosurgery, and Psychiatry* 2014;85(7):759–769.
2. Hedera P, Phibbs FT, Dolhun R, et al. Surgical targets for dystonic tremor: considerations between the globus pallidus and ventral intermediate thalamic nucleus. *Parkinsonism & Related Disorders* 2013;19(7):684–686.
3. Pauls KAM, Hammesfahr S, Moro E, et al. Deep brain stimulation in the ventrolateral thalamus/subthalamic area in dystonia with head tremor. *Movement Disorders* 2014;29(7):953–959.
4. Cury RG, Fraix V, Castrioto A, et al. Thalamic deep brain stimulation for tremor in Parkinson disease, essential tremor, and dystonia. *Neurology* 2017;89(13):1416–1423.
5. Mills KA, Starr PA, Ostrem JL. Neuromodulation for dystonia: target and patient selection. *Neurosurgery Clinics of North America* 2014;25(1):59–75.
6. Goulenko V, da Costa PL, Niemeyer P. Unilateral thalamic and pallidal deep brain stimulation for idiopathic hemidystonia: results of individual and combined stimulations. Case report. *Neurosurgical Focus* 2017;43(1):E2.
7. Ramirez-Zamora A, Okun MS. Deep brain stimulation for the treatment of uncommon tremor syndromes. *Expert Review of Neurotherapeutics* 2016;16(8):983–997.
8. Deuschl G, Raethjen J, Hellriegel H, Elble R. Treatment of patients with essential tremor. *Lancet Neurol* 2011;10(2):148–161.
9. Isaias IU, Alterman RL, Tagliati M. Deep brain stimulation for primary generalized dystonia: long-term outcomes. *Arch Neurol* 2009;66(4):465–470.

Case 37

Stimulation-Induced Dyskinesia, Interleaving Settings, and Management of Subthalamic Nucleus Deep Brain Stimulation in DYT1 Dystonia

KYLE T. MITCHELL, KRISTEN A. DODENHOFF, PHILIP A. STARR, AND JILL L. OSTREM

INDICATION FOR DEEP BRAIN STIMULATION

Generalized dystonia secondary to the *DYT1* genetic mutation

CLINICAL HISTORY AND RELEVANT EXAM

A 16-year-old boy with genetically confirmed DYT1 dystonia presented with worsening cervical and right arm dystonia and was referred for evaluation of DBS candidacy. Since early childhood, he held his pencil differently from his peers and had difficulty writing in cursive. At age 13 years, he noticed involuntary extension at the wrist when throwing a ball and poor accuracy when kicking a soccer ball. These symptoms progressed and included right foot inversion when walking and difficulty holding objects. One year later, he developed severe involuntary downward pulling of the neck, which worsened with stress and resulted in difficulty swallowing. A 6-week trial of levodopa provided about a 10% subjective improvement in neck pulling and improvement in right-sided dystonic symptoms. Trihexyphenidyl resulted in similar benefits. Baclofen helped with pain but not the involuntary movements. Botulinum toxin injections into the bilateral sternocleidomastoid muscles did not provide relief of anterocollis. Preoperative evaluation revealed spasmodic adductor dysphonia, severe anterocollis, opisthotonic posture, action-induced dystonia of the right hand when writing, and left foot inversion when walking. Anterocollis worsened with speech and when he played his trombone.

He underwent bilateral subthalamic nucleus (STN) deep brain stimulation (DBS) placement using an interventional magnetic resonance imaging (MRI)-guided technique.[1] Postoperative brain imaging showed accurate electrode placement in bilateral STN (Figure 37.1). The STN target was chosen as opposed to traditional pallidal stimulation given his phenomenology of primarily axial dystonia and as part of a prospective study.[2] This decision was also based on a pilot study of STN DBS for cervical dystonia, which revealed similar efficacy to published pallidal stimulation outcomes. Additionally, early studies showed a potential for reduced stimulation-induced bradykinesia.[3]

COMPLICATIONS

Bilateral Activa single-channel implantable pulse generators (IPGs) were programmed 3 weeks after lead implantation with conservative parameters (bilateral monopolar C+ 1−, amplitude of 1 V, pulse width of 90 μsec, frequency of 130 Hz). On these settings, the patient developed severe generalized dyskinesia, which resolved when the stimulation was deactivated. Stimulation amplitudes higher than 0.5 V resulted in a return of dyskinesia, and he had no meaningful improvement in his dystonia on the low settings.

TROUBLESHOOTING AND MANAGEMENT

Because of a low stimulation-induced threshold to develop dyskinesia, the patient underwent extensive programming at follow-up visits using bipolar configurations, which resulted in some improvement in anterocollis. With a gradual increase of stimulation amplitude to 3 V over the following 2 months, he had near-complete

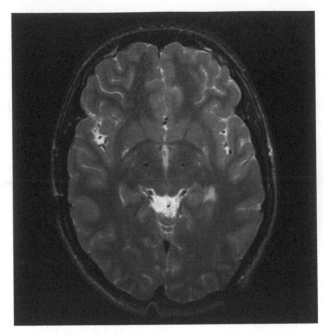

FIGURE 37.1. Postoperative T2-weighted magnetic resonance imaging confirming bilateral subthalamic nucleus lead placement.

resolution in right arm and truncal dystonia but persistent cervical dystonia when speaking or eating. Attempts to further increase the voltage resulted in a return of right arm dyskinesia. Programming the right STN DBS with double monopolar configurations of ventral contacts to relieve anterocollis due to left-sided neck muscle involvement resulted in dysarthria and left arm dyskinesia.

Right-sided dyskinesia was observed as a slow, writhing anterior shifting, and alternating internal and external rotation of the left shoulder was typically delayed by 3 to 5 minutes after reaching an amplitude threshold at which limb and neck dystonia was effectively alleviated. Left-sided dyskinesia was mild and only manifested during walking as irregular, jerky distal movements of the arm in contrast to the shoulder movements.

After a year, cervical dystonia improved with a gradual increase in amplitude in a double monopolar configuration of the right STN (Table 37.1). With these settings, he had near-complete resolution of cervical dystonia and dysarthria; however, improvement of right arm action-induced dystonia gradually diminished over the course of 2 years. Higher amplitude stimulation in left STN led to improvement in dystonia but return of dyskinesia. Lower frequencies were

tried but resulted in dysarthria related to dystonic platysma activation, neck flexion, and lower jaw thrusting. Attempts at using dorsal contacts in double monopolar configurations for potential antidyskinetic effects of zona incerta were not helpful.

He was eventually programmed with interleaved settings (see Table 37.1), with inclusion of the most dorsal contact in left STN, and this resulted in complete resolution of right arm dystonia without dyskinesia.

OUTCOME

At the most recent follow-up visit, 6 years after implantation, the patient had no abnormal exam findings aside from mild intermittent straining of the voice when initiating speech. See Table 37.1 for programming settings and corresponding improvement in Burke–Fahn–Marsden Dystonia Rating Scale (BFMDRS) and Toronto Western Spasmodic Torticollis Rating Scale (TWSTRS) over time.

DISCUSSION

This case is an example of a robust response of primary dystonia to bilateral STN DBS. The patient's young age and diagnosis of DYT1 dystonia, which is known to respond well to pallidal

TABLE 37.1. PROGRAMMING SETTINGS AND DYSTONIA SCALES AT BASELINE AND LONG-TERM FOLLOW-UP

Outcome	Baseline	1 year	6 years
Programming settings	N/A	Left: 0+ 1–, 2.8 V, 60 μsec, 130 Hz Right: C+ 1– 2–, 1.4 V, 60 μsec, 130 Hz	Left STN1: C+ 3–, 3 V, 60 μsec, 125 Hz Left STN2: C+ 1–, 1 V, 60 μsec, 125 Hz Right STN1: C+ 1–, 0.9 V, 60 μsec, 120 Hz Right STN2: C+ 2, 1.1 V, 60 μsec, 120 Hz
BFMDRS	Severity 35*, disability 2	Severity 6.5*, disability 2	Severity 0.5, disability 1
TWSTRS	43*	6.5*	0

*Burke–Fahn–Marsden Dystonia Rating Scale (BFMDRS) and Toronto Western Spasmodic Torticollis Rating Scale (TWSTRS) severity scores were determined by blinded raters of video exams at baseline and 1-year follow-up; higher scores show increased severity of illness.

stimulation,[4–6] suggest that he would have similarly improved with pallidal stimulation. Our large prospective controlled trial on the STN target revealed excellent response in dystonia severity compared with baseline, which persisted at the 3-year follow-up. The two younger patients (mean age, 11 years) with DYT1 dystonia had a larger percentage of clinical improvement than the two older patients (mean age, 29.5 years) with the same diagnosis; however, the sample sizes were small, which limited outcome interpretation.[2]

Interestingly, stimulation-induced dyskinesia occurred in all 20 treated patients in this trial. Programming with a bipolar configuration using contact 3, which was likely dorsal to STN in zona incerta (based on microelectrode recording), and reducing voltage were successful in relieving dyskinesia in a majority of patients.[2] Several patients, including this case, required more advanced programming with interleaved settings in order to avoid dyskinesia and ultimately control the dystonia. This case also demonstrates a variety of possible STN stimulation-induced movements—both patterned, diphasic, writhing right shoulder movements and jerky, irregular left hand movements. Further, a limb unaffected by dystonia preoperatively (left arm in this case) still should be considered possibly susceptible to the development of dyskinesia.

This case illustrates the potential of STN DBS as an alternative target to pallidal stimulation in DYT1 dystonia. Initial stimulation-induced severe dyskinesia may occur but can be overcome with a slow increase of stimulation amplitude and use of bipolar or interleaved configurations involving dorsal contacts. STN stimulation-induced dyskinesia in primary dystonia will likely increase the time and complexity of DBS programming in many cases.

PEARLS

- STN is a possible target for dystonia patients.
- The STN target in dystonia commonly leads to stimulation-induced dyskinesia, even in cases with severe limb dystonia.
- Complex programming may be required to manage these cases, and interleaving settings should be considered.

REFERENCES

1. Starr PA, Markun LC, Larson PS, Volz MM, Martin AJ, Ostrem JL. Interventional MRI-guided deep brain stimulation in pediatric dystonia: first experience with the ClearPoint system. *J Neurosurg Pediatr.* 2014;14(4):400–408.
2. Ostrem JL, San Luciano M, Dodenhoff KA, et al. Subthalamic nucleus deep brain stimulation in isolated dystonia: a 3-year follow-up study. *Neurology.* 2017;88(1):25–35.
3. Ostrem JL, Racine CA, Glass GA, et al. Subthalamic nucleus deep brain stimulation in primary cervical dystonia. *Neurology.* 2011;76(10):870–878.
4. Haridas A, Tagliati M, Osborn I, et al. Pallidal deep brain stimulation for primary dystonia in children. *Neurosurgery.* 2011;68(3):738–743; discussion 743.
5. Coubes P, Roubertie A, Vayssiere N, Hemm S, Echenne B. Treatment of DYT1-generalised dystonia by stimulation of the internal globus pallidus. *Lancet.* 2000;355(9222):2220–2221.
6. Coubes P, Cif L, El Fertit H, et al. Electrical stimulation of the globus pallidus internus in patients with primary generalized dystonia: long-term results. *J Neurosurg.* 2004;101(2):189–194.

Case 38

Deep Brain Stimulation Targeting the Globus Pallidus Interna for Dystonic Tremor in the Setting of Generalized Dystonia

QIANG ZHANG AND TERI R. THOMSEN

INDICATION FOR DEEP BRAIN STIMULATION

Severe dystonic tremor uncontrolled with medication

CLINICAL HISTORY AND RELEVANT EXAM

A 31-year-old right-handed man presented to the University of Iowa Movement Disorders Clinic for evaluation of left arm tremor and pain after left arm injury sustained a year prior. He had a left arm injury after a fall at work, following which he started to experience pain in his left arm, and he later developed a tremor in his left arm. On examination, the patient had tremor and dystonic posturing of the left hand and arm. He also had a mild writer's cramp in his right hand. We diagnosed him with generalized dystonia and a coexistent dystonic tremor and started him on a trial of botulinum toxin injections. However, the patient received minimal benefit from these injections, and his symptoms continued to progress and eventually involved the left leg a year later, which resulted in balance issues and falls. Because of these symptoms, the patient was unable to work. Physical therapy made the pain and cramps worse. He also failed trials of medications, including trihexyphenidyl, carbidopa-levodopa, and tizanidine. Because of severe generalized dystonia and dystonic tremor, we decided to proceed with bilateral globus pallidus interna (GPi) deep brain stimulation (DBS) lead placement. The patient's tremor and dystonia were well controlled, and he was able to go back to work. At his last visit 3 years after DBS placement, he was functioning well and performing adequately at his job at a heavy machine factory.

COMPLICATIONS

Tremor, balance issues, and falls

TROUBLESHOOTING AND MANAGEMENT

For his initial programming of the bilateral GPi DBS, we used a frequency of 130 Hz and monopolar settings on both sides, which achieved adequate tremor control (Table 38.1). The patient also had relief of his dystonia as well as his pain. One month later, we increased the amplitude on both sides of his GPi DBS, and his residual dystonia and tremor symptoms were well controlled (Table 38.2). His symptoms remained well-controlled with gradually increased amplitude over the next 3 years (Table 38.3). Interestingly, when we tried to titrate up the pulse width, the patient developed paresthesia of his chest region at 70 μsec.

OUTCOME

This case suggested that GPi DBS may be helpful for dystonic tremor. Specifically, higher frequency stimulation helped not only the dystonic tremor but also the generalized dystonia in this case. Although higher pulse width was associated with paresthesia, we were able to maintain adequate control of his dystonia with a pulse width of 60 μsec. We suspect that this side effect was due to lead location.

DISCUSSION

Tremor is a common presentation of dystonia. For focal dystonia, tremor usually improves with botulinum toxin injections. However, patients with generalized dystonia at times respond poorly to botulinum toxin injections. Medical therapies may be helpful, but many patients don't respond adequately to medications either. Patel and colleagues

TABLE 38.1. GLOBUS PALLIDUS INTERNA DEEP BRAIN STIMULATION PARAMETERS
AFTER INITIAL PROGRAMMING (6/2016)

	Electrode Configuration	Voltage (V)	Pulse Width (μsec)	Frequency (Hz)	Therapeutic Effects
Left GPi	1–	1.0	60	130	Adequate tremor control, improved dystonia
Right GPi	10–	2.0	60	130	

GPi = globus pallidus interna.

recently discussed the choices of DBS targets in patients with essential tremor with dystonic features and suggested that ventral intermediate (Vim) nucleus, GPi, and subthalamic nucleus (STN) are all potential acceptable options.[1] Hedera and colleagues reviewed 10 cases of dystonic tremor and suggested that patients with dystonic tremor and a mild dystonia should be considered for Vim DBS, while the coexistence of severe dystonia and dystonic tremor may justify combined Vim and GPi DBS surgeries.[2] Morishita and colleagues suggested the benefits of Vim DBS for tremor in the setting of dystonia.[3] Our case suggested the possibility of achieving good tremor control with high-frequency GPi DBS. This approach may not be optimal for other patients with coexisting severe tremor and generalized dystonia, and many cases, as in the Morishita series, required Vim DBS. When the tremor is the predominant phenotype, most expert centers now start with Vim DBS.

GPi DBS for dystonia may be used with high pulse widths and low frequencies and also high pulse widths and high frequencies. There are also reported cases of low pulse widths being used for dystonia, so it is important for clinicians empirically to try combinations for maximal benefit. However, our patient had severe dystonic tremor, and during initial programming, his tremor and dystonia symptoms both improved significantly with a pulse width of 60 μsec and a frequency of 130 Hz. Higher frequency settings of GPi DBS may control tremor in many Parkinson disease patients and may also improve dystonia, although notably, low frequency was not tried in our case.

Functional disorder is always a concern in young patients with symptoms suggesting dystonia and psychiatric comorbidities. In addition to dystonia and dystonic tremor, our patient also had nonepileptic spells and cognitive complaints. His initial left arm injury happened when he "blacked out" and fell, though his electroencephalogram (EEG) was unremarkable. He complained of cognitive deficits, including difficulty with concentration, poor executive function, poor memory, and impaired ability to read. He also reported poor job performance. He was evaluated by our behavioral neurology clinic, and his neuropsychology evaluation indicated a complex mixture of somatic focus with overconcern, low positive emotions, low self-esteem, low self-confidence, social withdrawal, and poor ego strength; however, his cognitive function was determined to be intact. His brain magnetic resonance imaging (MRI) study was also reported to be normal. It is important to note here that frequently patients with an organic dystonic disorder may have a coexisting functional disorder. Both the nonepileptic spells and subjective cognitive deficits resolved after his tremor and dystonia symptoms were well-controlled.

TABLE 38.2. GLOBUS PALLIDUS INTERNA DEEP BRAIN STIMULATION PARAMETERS
AFTER SECOND PROGRAMMING (7/2016)

	Electrode Configuration	Voltage (V)	Pulse Width (μsec)	Frequency (Hz)	Therapeutic Effects
Left GPi	1–	1.4	60	130	Improved tremor control, improved dystonia
Right GPi	10–	2.4	60	130	

GPi = globus pallidus interna.

TABLE 38.3. GLOBUS PALLIDUS INTERNA DEEP BRAIN STIMULATION PARAMETERS AFTER LAST PROGRAMMING (4/2019)

	Electrode Configuration	Voltage (V)	Pulse Width (μsec)	Frequency (Hz)	Therapeutic Effects
Left GPi	1–	4.0	60*	130	Adequate control of tremor and dystonia
Right GPi	10–	4.8	60*	130	

*When we tried to increase pulse width beyond 60 μsec, the patient developed paresthesia in the chest region. This side effect may be related to lead location. Otherwise, no side effect has been reported from his deep brain stimulation treatment.

GPi = globus pallidus interna.

PEARLS

- Dystonic tremor may respond to GPi DBS implantation, but in many expert centers, Vim DBS is used if the tremor is the predominant feature. In some cases, GPi DBS will not capture dystonic tremor.
- Although low-frequency GPi DBS is often used for programming in generalized dystonia, higher frequency GPi DBS may also provide tremor control and relief of dystonia. Empirical combinations of pulse width and frequency should be liberally employed to establish the maximal benefit.
- GPi DBS with relatively low pulse widths (60 μsec in our case) could be beneficial in some cases of generalized dystonia, although response is variable across patients.

REFERENCES

1. Patel A, Deeb W, Okun MS. Deep brain stimulation management of essential tremor with dystonic features. Tremor Other Hyperkinet Mov (NY) 2018;8:557.
2. Hedera P, Phibbs FT, Dolhun R, et al. Surgical targets for dystonic tremor: considerations between the globus pallidus and ventral intermediate thalamic nucleus. Parkinsonism Relat Disord 2013;19:684–686.
3. Morishita T, Foote KD, Haq IU, Zeilman P, Jacobson CE, Okun MS. Should we consider Vim thalamic deep brain stimulation for select cases of severe refractory dystonic tremor? Stereotact Funct Neurosurg 2010;88:98–104.

SECTION 5

Miscellaneous

Case 39

Deep Brain Stimulation in Adult Huntington Disease for Treatment of Axial Dystonia

JESSICA A. KARL, KATHLEEN SHANNON, KONSTANTIN SLAVIN,
AND LEO VERHAGEN METMAN

INDICATIONS FOR DEEP BRAIN STIMULATION

Huntington disease (HD) with severe axial dystonia

CLINICAL HISTORY AND RELEVANT EXAM

A 66-year-old man with HD (41 CAG repeats) of 30 years' duration presented with progressive and disabling truncal dystonia. The dystonia interfered with his ability to partake in all daily activities. His wife was his caregiver, and she reported that taking care of him had become progressively more difficult because of the powerful back spasms. The movements were most severe in the sitting position but were also present while supine, standing, and walking. He was unable to sit without falling out of his seat because his back spasms would displace the chair backward. He had to be restrained in his wheelchair. Falling asleep and feeding were challenging because of the constant dystonic movement. Medications, including aripiprazole, tetrabenazine, and haloperidol, were tried without benefit. Bilateral paraspinal botulinum toxin injections minimally reduced the amplitude but not the frequency of movement. The patient was referred to the deep brain stimulation (DBS) clinic to surgically address his primary complaint of truncal dystonia. His Mini-Mental State Exam (MMSE) score was 28/30, and he had no depressive or psychotic symptoms. After multidisciplinary consensus was reached and the patient and caregiver were thoroughly informed about the goals and expectations of the surgery, bilateral DBS of the globus pallidus internus (GPi) was performed. The Burke–Fahn–Marsden Dystonia Rating Scale (BFMDRS) (Movement Scale and Disability Scale), the Global Dystonia Rating Scale (GDRS), and the Parkinson's Disease Quality of Life Scale (PDQ-39) were completed preoperatively and again 24 months after surgery (Tables 39.1 to 39.3).

The preoperative stereotactic magnetic resonance imaging (MRI) study (Figure 39.1) under conscious sedation revealed severe generalized atrophy, with typical atrophy of the caudate nuclei. In addition, the GPi on both sides was severely atrophied to the point that it made confident targeting challenging despite obtaining relatively high-quality 3Tesla stereotactic MRI studies. The procedure was completed in two stages 2 weeks apart. A dual-channel internal pulse generator was implanted in the left subclavicular region (Activa PC, Medtronic Inc., Minneapolis, MN). Body jerks during the study and intraoperatively were of some concern but did not substantially interfere with either the MRI or microelectrode recording (MER). The patient was awake during the procedure. Two MER tracks were made on the left side using a central and a medial track. Both tracks were fairly quiet with few, low-amplitude, pallidal discharges. Monopolar test stimulation in either track revealed low thresholds (4 mA) for (worsening) hypophonia. A reduction in dystonic spasms was observed, and the DBS lead was placed in the medial location. On the right side, one MER track was performed and again was characterized by a few, low-amplitude, pallidal discharges. On this side, the optic track was identified. The right DBS lead was placed in this track, but because of a low stimulation threshold for hypophonia (2 mA), the DBS was repositioned 2 mm anterior. Again, improvement in dystonic spasms was noted, and the threshold for speech-related side effects was slightly higher (3 mA). It

TABLE 39.1A. BURKE–FAHN–MARSDEN DYSTONIA RATING SCALE—MOVEMENT

	Pre-DBS	Two Years Post-DBS	Change (Two Years Post-DBS – Pre-DBS)*
Eyes (max: 8)	0	0	0
Mouth	2	2	0
Neck	6	0	–6
Speech and swallowing (max: 16)	4	4	0
Right arm	12	8	–4
Left arm	8	8	0
Right leg	12	12	0
Left leg	8	8	0
Trunk	16	4	–12
Sum (max: 120)	68	46	–22

*Higher score is worse.

was thought that the degeneration and reduced volume of the target were responsible for the lack of a more obvious GPi MER signal as well as for the low threshold for side effects. It was also considered not practical to perform additional MER tracks because of potential side effects related to the severe atrophy and the mild cognitive impairment. In addition, the consistent MER findings (paucity of neuronal discharges) in all three tracks suggested that additional passes would not likely identify a better physiologic target.

COMPLICATIONS

After surgery, the patient complained of dysphagia and dysarthria. He initially required a gastrostomy tube for feeding and was sent to inpatient rehabilitation.

TROUBLESHOOTING AND MANAGEMENT

Speech and swallowing gradually improved back to baseline over weeks after DBS surgery, and the patient was able to switch back to an oral diet. DBS stimulation was initiated 1 month after lead placement. The patient and his family started to notice significant improvement in the dystonic movement within 2 weeks after stimulation was initiated. The patient's basic DBS programming parameters were optimized 3 months after surgery. Bipolar electrode configuration was chosen

TABLE 39.1B. BURKE–FAHN–MARSDEN DISABILITY RATING SCALE—DISABILITY

	Pre-DBS	Two Years Post-DBS	Change (Two Years Post-DBS – Pre-DBS)*
Speech	3	3	0
Handwriting	2	2	0
Feeding	3	1	–2
Eating/swallowing	1	1	0
Hygiene	1	1	0
Dressing	2	3	+1
Walking	4	3	–1

*Higher score is worse, 0–4 rating scale.

TABLE 39.2. GLOBAL DYSTONIA RATING SCALE (GDRS)

	Pre-DBS	Two Years Post-DBS	Change (Two Years Post-DBS – Pre-DBS)*
Eyes and upper face	0	0	0
Lower face	1	1	0
Jaw and tongue	0	0	0
Larynx	0	0	0
Neck	10	1	−9
Shoulder and proximal arm (L, R)	0, 0	0, 0	0, 0
Distal arm and hand including elbow (L, R)	2, 5	2, 3	0, −2
Pelvis, upper leg (L, R)	4, 6	2, 4	−2, −2
Distal leg, foot	3, 4	3, 4	0, 0
Trunk	10	4	−6

*Higher score is worse, 0–10 rating scale.

TABLE 39.3. PARKINSON'S DISEASE QUALITY OF LIFE SCALE (PDQ-39)

	Pre-DBS	Two Years Post-DBS	Change (Two Years Post-DBS – Pre-DBS)*
PDQ-39 summary index	36.57	21.04	−15.53
Mobility (%)	80.00	16.25	−63.75
Activities of daily living	70.83	66.67	−4.16
Emotional well-being	4.17	4.17	0.00
Stigma	56.3	0.00	−56.3
Social support	0.00	0.00	0.00
Cognitive impairment	31.25	31.25	0.00
Communication	41.67	41.67	0.00
Bodily discomfort	8.33	8.33	0.00

*Higher score is worse.

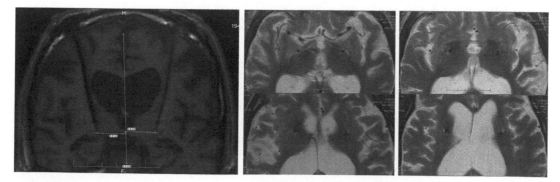

FIGURE 39.1. T1-weighted (*left*) and T2-weighted (*right*) images showing both globus pallidus interna lead tips 19.9 mm from midline close to the optic tract.

bilaterally because of increased dysarthria with monopolar settings. Subtle programming changes have been made at routine follow-up visits to adapt to further disease progression. At 2-year follow-up, the stimulation parameters were: left GPi, 0– 2+, 3.5 V, 60 μsec, 130 Hz; right GPi, 10–8+, 3.1 V, 60 μsec, 130 Hz. The dystonic spasms continue to be controlled at the current time of 24 months after surgery.

OUTCOME

The majority of the BFMDRS, GDRS, and PDQ-39 scales showed sustained improvement 2 years after DBS surgery (see 39.1 to 39.3). The patient has been able to participate in several activities that he was unable to participate in before surgery because of the severity of the dystonic movement. He is now able to sit comfortably without displacing his seat backward. Stimulation has dramatically improved his ability to be seated for meals and other activities. He had a 27-pound weight gain since surgery. His preoperative body mass index (BMI) was 16.1, and his current BMI is 21.7. The patient's cognition has been relatively preserved, with a current MMSE of 26/30.

DISCUSSION

HD is a progressive autosomal-dominant disorder characterized by chorea as well as cognitive and psychiatric symptoms. Dystonia is also common in HD, affecting more than 90% of cases, and more than 50% of HD patients in a recent study experienced truncal dystonia.[1] The prevalence and severity of dystonia increase with disease duration.[1] Tetrabenazine is the only approved medication for Huntington chorea, while amantadine and neuroleptics are used to treat chorea off-label.[2,3] However, no medications have proved efficacious for the dystonia and bradykinesia that become more prominent as the disease progresses. Several reports have outlined the effect of GPi DBS in HD patients with a choreic phenotype,[4–14] but less is known about the effect of DBS in HD patients with a predominately dystonic phenotype. In most HD patients, nonmotor symptoms, such as cognitive impairment, behavioral issues, depression, or anxiety, and motor symptoms related to gait and balance are the major issues, while chorea and dystonia play a relatively less disabling role for the patient. Our patient was cognitively and psychiatrically functioning at a relatively high level, and it was the severe dystonia that was the main cause of his disability and prevented him from performing activities of daily living, sitting in a chair, or even cooperating with his caregiver (his wife). It was not until after detailed discussions with the patient and his wife regarding the goals and expectations of the surgery that we moved forward with the procedure.

This report illustrates that GPi DBS may provide sustained benefit in carefully selected HD

PEARLS

- In HD patients disabled by medication-refractory dystonia, bilateral GPi DBS may be considered so long as there is no neuropsychiatric impairment that would interfere with the patient's comprehension of the potential risks of surgery.
- The patient and caregivers should have realistic expectations of outcomes and be willing to follow through with regular programming.
- The neuromodulation team should achieve consensus to proceed with surgery after ensuring in good faith that the ethical concerns of DBS in an HD patient are outweighed by its potential benefits.
- Atrophy can be an issue in these cases. First, it can make targeting challenging; and second, increasing atrophy over time may decrease the distance between the DBS lead and the internal capsule necessitating programming adjustments.[15]
- Even though it has been reported in HD that chorea responds better than dystonia to DBS,[16] our case illustrates that the effect on dystonia can be quite dramatic, and if dystonia is the main cause of disability, DBS may be considered. Teams should be aware that some cases of dystonia with concurrent juvenile HD have not responded well to traditional DBS approaches.

patients with severe dystonia refractory to other treatment modalities. We are not advocating DBS for HD; however, when specific symptoms known to respond well to DBS, such as dystonia, interfere significantly with a patient's quality of life, and optimal medical management has failed, DBS is a viable option. As was the case in our patient, preserved cognition, lack of significant psychiatric disease, clear goals and expectations, and an involved caregiver are essential for a satisfactory outcome. This case highlights that, while general guidelines certainly have utility, each patient need to be looked at as an individual when it comes to determining the candidacy for DBS.

REFERENCES

1. Van de Zande NA, Massey TH, McLauchlan D, et al. Clinical characterization of dystonia in adult patients with Huntington's disease. *Eur J Neurol.* 2017;24(9):1140–1147.

2. Verhagen Metman L, Morris MJ, Farmer C, et al. Huntington's disease: a randomized, controlled trial using the NMDA-antagonist amantadine. *Neurology.* 2002;59(5):694–699.

3. Reilmann R. Pharmacological treatment of chorea in Huntington's disease—good clinical practice versus evidence-based guideline. *Mov Disord.* 2013;28(8):1030–1033.

4. Moro E, Lang AE, Strafella AP, et al. Bilateral globus pallidus stimulation for Huntington's disease. *Ann Neurol.* 2004;56(2):290–294.

5. Fawcett AP, Moro E, Lang AE, Lozano AM, Hutchison WD. Pallidal deep brain stimulation influences both reflexive and voluntary saccades in Huntington's disease. *Mov Disord.* 2005;20(3):371–377.

6. Hebb MO, Garcia R, Gaudet P, Mendez IM. Bilateral stimulation of the globus pallidus internus to treat choreathetosis in Huntington's disease: technical case report. *Neurosurgery.* 2006;58(2):E383; discussion E383.

7. Fasano A, Mazzone P, Piano C, Quaranta D, Soleti F, Bentivoglio AR. GPi-DBS in Huntington's disease: results on motor function and cognition in a 72-year-old case. *Mov Disord.* 2008;23(9):1289–1292.

8. Biolsi B, Cif L, Fertit HE, Robles SG, Coubes P. Long-term follow-up of Huntington disease treated by bilateral deep brain stimulation of the internal globus pallidus. *J Neurosurg.* 2008;109(1):130–132.

9. Kang GA, Heath S, Rothlind J, Starr PA. Long-term follow-up of pallidal deep brain stimulation in two cases of Huntington's disease. *J Neurol Neurosurg Psychiatry.* 2011;82(3):272–277.

10. Garcia-Ruiz PJ, Ayerbe J, del Val J, Herranz A. Deep brain stimulation in disabling involuntary vocalization associated with Huntington's disease. *Parkinsonism Relat Disord.* 2012;18(6):803–804.

11. Spielberger S, Hotter A, Wolf E, et al. Deep brain stimulation in Huntington's disease: a 4-year follow-up case report. *Mov Disord.* 2012;27(6):806–807; author reply 807–808.

12. Cislaghi G, Capiluppi E, Saleh C, et al. Bilateral globus pallidus stimulation in Westphal variant of Huntington disease. *Neuromodulation.* 2014;17(5):502–505.

13. Gonzalez V, Cif L, Biolsi B, et al. Deep brain stimulation for Huntington's disease: long-term results of a prospective open-label study. *J Neurosurg.* 2014;121(1):114–122.

14. Wojtecki L, Groiss SJ, Hartmann CJ, et al. Deep brain stimulation in Huntington's disease: preliminary evidence on pathophysiology, efficacy and safety. *Brain Sci.* 2016;6(3):10.3390/brainsci6030038.

15. Vedam-Mai V, Martinez-Ramirez D, Hilliard JD, et al. Post-mortem findings in Huntington's deep brain stimulation: a moving target due to atrophy. *Tremor Other Hyperkinet Mov (NY).* 2016;6:372.

16. Velez-Lago FM, Thompson A, Oyama G, et al. Differential and better response to deep brain stimulation of chorea compared to dystonia in Huntington's disease. *Stereotact Funct Neurosurg.* 2013;91(2):129–133.

Case 40

Deep Brain Stimulation for Medication-Refractory Aggressive and Injurious Behavior

OSCAR BERNAL-PACHECO, ADRIANA MARTINEZ PEREZ,
AND MARY FONSECA-RAMOS

INDICATION FOR DEEP BRAIN STIMULATION

Uncontrolled medically refractory aggressive and injurious behavior

CLINICAL HISTORY AND RELEVANT EXAM

An 18-year-old man with past medical history of meningitis, as well as a history of developmental delay, started developing aggressive behavior at 2 years of age. He later developed refractory epilepsy at 3 years of age. As a result, the patient had limited autonomy, requiring assistance for his activities of daily living, including feeding, dressing, and personal hygiene. Physical, occupational, and speech therapy services improved his speech and self-care; however, aggressiveness and epilepsy were difficult to control despite treatment with multiple medications, including typical and atypical antipsychotics and first- and second-line antiepileptics. Issues like impulsive eating and sleep disorders, including wakefulness during the night, also were challenging in his case.

At 4 years of age, when starting day care, his classmates rejected him because of his behavior, which was described as isolated and aggressive. At 6 years of age, he was diagnosed with mental retardation, and since that early age, his mother has been supporting him as his primary caregiver. She was trained to manage his aggression but was physically and verbally attacked by her son on several occasions. Reports indicated that his behavior was directed toward those who interacted with him, for example, his teachers and health care staff. He was known to expose his genitalia in public areas and had also left his house while unclothed, resulting in legal action. Despite nutritional counseling, he continues with impulsive feeding and consumption of excessive amounts of food.

COMPLICATIONS

The patient was evaluated and treated by several psychiatrists, epileptologists, psychologists, and social workers. Multiple medications, including neuroleptics in combination with sedatives and antiepileptics, were ineffective in controlling his behavior. Treatment of generalized epilepsy with antiseizure medications reduced the frequency of seizures to three or four per month; however, his crises were frequently severe and complex. Because of his marked behavioral problems in adolescence, he required a restraint jacket up to 18 hours a day to prevent attacks on other people. There was a failure of high doses of antipsychotics in curbing aggression, which resulted in unlawful public behavior. Because of multiple and recurrent threats to his health and his caregivers, as an exceptional circumstance he was evaluated for deep brain stimulation (DBS) of the posterior hypothalamus (PHyp).

TROUBLESHOOTING AND MANAGEMENT

An institutional ethical committee and review board of the hospital Instituto Roosevelt (Bogotá, Colombia) included an interdisciplinary team of psychiatrists, psychologists, neurologists, and neurosurgeons who reviewed the feasibility of applying DBS of PHyp. We were granted permission to perform the procedure, after gaining the appropriate consent.

The procedure was performed under general anesthesia with stereotactic targeting using a magnetic resonance imaging (MRI) and computed tomography (CT) fusion study. The target

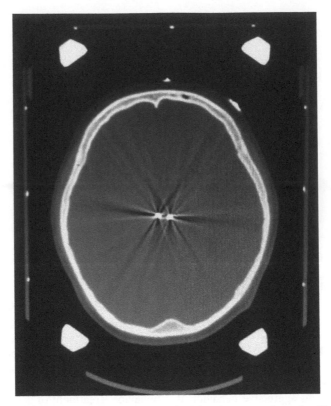

FIGURE 40.1. Computed tomography scan showing the final deep brain stimulation lead location for the posterior hypothalamus.

was chosen based on the report by Sano and colleagues in the 1970s,[1] and although the target was selected for lesioning and not for stimulation, previous reports showed that stimulation in the same target produced a similar outcome, possibly with fewer side effects and lower risk.[2,3] The final DBS lead location for the implant was 2 mm lateral to the border of the third ventricle, 3 mm posterior to the mid-commissural point, and 5 mm inferior to the anterior commissure–posterior commissure line (Figure 40.1). Microelectrode recordings revealed irregular discharges of 4 and 28 Hz, similar to the report of Micieli and colleagues[4] (Figure 40.2). Intraoperative macrostimulation in the surgical target resulted in more than a 10% increase in heart rate, which was congruent with other publications,[3,4] and also we observed mydriasis.[1]

On the first postoperative day, the patient was closely supervised in the intensive care unit. He was observed to be much calmer and quieter, suggesting a microlesion effect because the chronic stimulation had not been activated.

Initial DBS programming was performed 20 days after the procedure. Programming included a continuous increase of the voltage reaching a treshold of 4 V in all contacts, keeping frequency at 130 Hz and pulse width at 60 µsec. Because of the low reliability in the information given by the patient about possible side effects, we decided not to increase the voltage beyond 4 V. Three months after surgery, there was an improvement in his aggressive behavior and attention, with amplitude of 3 V, frequency of 130 Hz, and pulse width of 60 µsec in contacts 2 and 10. The improvement in aggressive behavior was about 70% based on the number of episodes of aggressiveness, impulsivity, and intents of injury reported by his mother. Although he had episodes of anger, he didn´t try to injure others. He also became seizure-free even though epileptologist decided to continue the same medications at the same dosage.

To attempt an improved control for aggressiveness because he still had angry outbursts, the voltage was increased to 3.4 V, keeping frequency at 130 Hz and pulse width of 60 µsec. With this new programming setting, the patient´s mother reported that he became hypoactive and apathetic and had severe loss of appetite with weight loss.

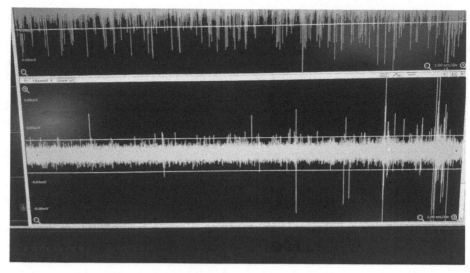

FIGURE 40.2. Microelectrode recordings revealing irregular discharges between 4 and 28 Hz in the posterior hypothalamus.

One month later, he developed an urinary tract infection and subsequent sepsis, requiring hemodynamic and ventilator support in the intensive care unit. The patient recovered completely after receiving antibiotic therapy and nutritional support. The generator was turned off, which restored his desire to eat, and he gained weight; however, he became aggressive and impulsive again, although less than before the surgery.

OUTCOME

Because of vegetative changes and the apathy produced by DBS programming, the concern was inadvertent stimulation of the lateral or ventromedial regions of the hypothalamus. The generator was turned on again, this time with voltage of 3.2 V, keeping frequency and pulse width unchanged, which resulted in resolution of the nonmotor side effects of stimulation.

After 18 months of follow-up, the patient showed excellent self-control, reduced aggressive behavior, absence of seizures, and improved attention. He demonstrated persistent benefit, without tolerance or loss of effect.

DISCUSSION

DBS has been an important option for control of motor symptoms in patients with Parkinson disease, dystonia, tremor, and other movement disorders.[5] Patients with psychiatric illnesses refractory to multiple therapies, such as depression and obsessive-compulsive disorders, have also been treated successfully with this surgical option.[6] For decades, surgical options have attempted, often unsuccessfully, to address complex illnesses (e.g., schizophrenia), but with poor outcomes.[7-9] Focusing on the treatment of symptoms instead of on his primary illness, we had the opportunity to control the symptoms that worsened the quality of life of the patient.[9] In this sense, aggressiveness refers to severe cases of unprovoked aggressive behavior (also described as *erethism*), usually associated with a variable degree of mental impairment and serious brain damage, such as that caused by brain malformations, epilepsy, encephalitis, trauma, perinatal insult, and other causes.[10] Although the most evident manifestation is aggressiveness, other symptoms include hyperkinesia, destruction of objects, and stereotypies with self-injury. These manifestations may be refractory to optimized pharmacologic treatment and to nonpharmacologic management, including electroconvulsive therapy (ECT).[11,12] These patients may require life restrictions, long hospitalization in specialized centers, and multiple medications, increasing the economic, social, and familial burden. More than 60% of these cases are associated with epilepsy, cognitive compromise, and eating, sexual, sleep, and affective disorders. Most of the cases require additional medications, therapies, and other restrictions.[11]

Historically, we have learned that lesions of certain areas of the brain are not enough to treat complex diseases but can be helpful for symptoms such as aggressive and disruptive behavioral manifestations.[1,710] These days, the development of new neuroimaging techniques, neurophysiologic microelectrode recordings, and pathologic studies have collectively facilitated using new pathways and connections in the brain, including the PHyp.[9,10] Thanks to previous reports[2,3,12] and new resources, we partially understand the function of the PHyp in behavior, sleep, attention, and vegetative functions and in thalamic pathways involved in control of seizures. We also are gleaning an idea of how can we help aggressiveness and other symptoms.[13–16] The PHyp is a heterogeneous region of the hypothalamus composed of multiple types of cells with distinct physiologic functions. Anatomically, it lies below the thalamus, located between 1 and 5 mm lateral to the lateral border of the third ventricle and 5 mm inferior to the inter-commissural line, and it borders the rostral end of the red nucleus, the anterior border of the mammillary body, and the floor and lateral walls of the third ventricle. It is located at the crossroads of vegetative, endocrine, and behavioral functions.[9,12] Its neural connections include links to both the direct and indirect pathways, with cortical and subcortical areas, including surrounding hypothalamic nuclei, frontal and temporal lobes, thalamus, and mamillary bodies.

Sano and colleagues reported improvement of the control of aggressive behavior in 10 of 11 patients after lesioning of the posteromedial hypothalamus.[1] In the past decade, Franzini and Torres and their colleagues published series of cases of patients with DBS in the PHyp to control the aggressiveness of patients, all with good outcomes. They also reported control of other symptoms, including seizures[3,13–16] The main side effects of lesioning this area were hypersomnia and tachycardia.[1] The rationale for targeting the PHyp area to control aggressiveness (and epilepsy) has been its neural connections, but we believe that because of the high-level order connections, it may be possible to obtain even more neuropsychiatric benefits, although more observations will be needed. The therapy is also thought to modulate autonomic and behavioral functions and to play a role in epileptogenesis.[13–16] The improvement in attention has been postulated to be a possible indirect result of diminished aggressiveness and injurious behavior. Finally, both high- and low-frequency stimulation have been reported to benefit aggressiveness.[15,16] The main issue with DBS for aggressiveness is that very few cases have been published. For the field to move forward, we will need both more understanding and more data.

PEARLS

- Carefully selected patients with medically refractory severe aggressive and injurious behavior can possibly benefit from PHyp DBS.
- Before considering DBS implantation, an interdisciplinary team will be required to educate the care providers and to create a risk-to-benefit profile. The few available cases and the paucity of randomized controlled trials make this approach highly experimental, and all cases should be reported in the literature. An ethics committee (if available) should participate and provide guidance during the decision-making process, including an appropriately executed consent (signed off by all parties).
- Although epilepsy, attention, and impulsivity can also potentially improve with PHyp implantation, these are usually not primary drivers of the decision to implant. The main goal has been to curb aggressive behavior. More research studies will elucidate the best approaches to the other behaviors and symptoms.
- The postprogramming clinical course can be complicated by stimulation-induced neurovegetative side effects, which should be carefully monitored and addressed. Small changes in voltage and potentially other settings can affect the side-effect profile and outcome.
- Further studies and research will be required to uncover the physiologic and other mechanisms underpinning the action of the PHyp stimulation. These studies could help to establish a longer term safety and efficacy procedure for treating medication-refractory behavioral aggressiveness.

REFERENCES

1. Sano K, Yoshioka M, Ogashiwa M, Ishijima B, Ohye C: Postero-medial hypothalamotomy in the treatment of aggressive behaviors. Confin Neurol 1966;27:164–167.
2. Torres CV, Sola RG, Pastor J, et al. Long-term results of posteromedial hypothalamic deep brain stimulation for patients with resistant aggressiveness. J Neurosurg. 2013;119(2):277–287.
3. Franzini A, Messina G, Cordella R, Marras C, Broggi G. Deep brain stimulation of the postero-medial hypothalamus: indications, long-term results, and neurophysiological considerations. Neurosurg Focus. 2010;29: E13
4. Micieli R, Rios AL, Aguilar RP, Posada LF, Hutchison WD. Single-unit analysis of the human posterior hypothalamus and red nucleus during deep brain stimulation for aggressivity. J Neurosurg. 2017;126(4):1158–1164.
5. Wagle Shukla A, Okun MS. Surgical treatment of Parkinson's disease: patients, targets, devices and approaches. Neurotherapeutics. 2014;11(1):47–59.
6. Williams NR, Okun MS. Deep brain stimulation (DBS) at the interface of neurology and psychiatry. J Clin Invest. 2013;123(11):4546–4556.
7. Faria MA Jr. Violence, mental illness, and the brain: a brief history of psychosurgery. Part 1: from trephination to lobotomy. Surg Neurol Int. 2013;4:49.
8. Faria MA Jr. Violence, mental illness, and the brain: a brief history of psychosurgery: Part 2: from the limbic system and cingulotomy to deep brain stimulation. Surg Neurol Int. 2013;4:75.
9. Barbosa D AN, Oliveira-Souza R, Monte Santo F, et al. The hypothalamus at the crossroads of psychopathology and neurosurgery. Neurosur Focus 2017;43(3):E15.
10. Franzini A, Marras C, Ferroli P, Bugiani O, Broggi G. Stimulation of the posterior hypo-thalamus for medically intractable impulsive and violent behavior. Stereotact Funct Neurosurg. 2005;83:63–66.
11. van Ool JS, Snoeijen-Schouwenaars FM, Tan IY, Jurgen Schelhaas H, Aldenkamp AP, Hendriksen JGM. Challenging behavior in adults with epilepsy and intellectual disability: an analysis of epilepsy characteristics. Epilepsy Behav. 2018;86:72–78.
12. Yampolsky C, Bendersky D. Cirugía de los trastor-nos del comportamiento: el estado del arte. Surg Neurol Int. 2014; 5(Suppl 5):S211–S231.
13. Benedetti-Isaac JC, Torres-Zambrano M, Vargas-Toscano A, et al. Seizure frequency reduction after posteromedial hypothalamus deep brain stimu-lation in drug-resistant epilepsy associated with intractable aggressive behavior. Epilepsia 2015; 56(7):1152–1161.
14. Messina G, Islam L, Cordella R, Gambini O, Franzini A. Deep brain stimulation for aggres-sive behavior and obsessive-compulsive disorder. J Neurosurg Sci 2016:60(2):211–217.
15. Hernando V, Pastor J, Pedrosa M, Peña E, Sola RG. Low-frequency bilateral hypothalamic stimulation for treatment of drug-resistant aggressiveness in a young man with mental retardation. Stereotact Funct Neurosurg. 2008;86:219–223.
16. Franzini A, Marras C, Tringali G, et al. Chronic high frequency stimulation of the posteromedial hypothalamus in facial pain syndromes and behav-iour disorders. Acta Neurochir Suppl 2007;97(Pt 2):399–406.

Case 41

Bilateral Globus Pallidus Deep Brain Stimulation for Dystonia and Dystonic Tremor in Spinocerebellar Ataxia 17

APARNA WAGLE SHUKLA AND PAMELA R. ZEILMAN

INDICATIONS FOR DEEP BRAIN STIMULATION

Tremors, generalized dystonia

CLINICAL HISTORY AND RELEVANT EXAM

A 33-year-old right-handed white male presented with bilateral arm tremors and painful posturing of the neck, arms, and toes. His symptoms first manifested when he was a teenager and became increasingly bothersome by the time he was a senior in high school. He was observed to walk awkwardly; his friends and family commented on his gait to be a "lazy gait." His tremors were more pronounced when the arms were engaged in activities, and both sides were reportedly equally involved. The tremors were observed to improve with either rest or with a glass of wine and were aggravated in the presence of physical and mental stress. The tremors interfered with writing, eating, drinking, and dressing. Painful posturing of the neck and the limbs further affected his activities.

He sought multiple medical opinions for a working diagnosis of childhood-onset dystonia. He underwent treatment trials with several medications, including trihexyphenidyl, levodopa-carbidopa, clonazepam, baclofen, and several rounds of botulinum toxin injections to the neck and feet, with minimal clinical improvement. He was referred to our center for consideration for deep brain stimulation (DBS) surgery. At the time of presentation to our center, he reported symptoms of anxiety, depression, and panic attacks; however, these responded to oral medications prescribed by his psychiatrist. He reportedly had negative genetic testing for DYT-Tor1A dystonia,

a negative workup for Wilson disease, and an unremarkable brain magnetic resonance imaging (MRI) study. The physical examination revealed symmetric moderate to severe postural and kinetic arm tremor with a minimal resting component. There was slight posturing at the wrists. The neck was deviated to the left and tilted to the right, which became more pronounced during walking, in addition to abnormal bending of the trunk to the right, and involuntary toe flexion in the feet (left > right). The remaining parts of the neurologic exam, including cognition, eye movement, and motor system, were unremarkable. We diagnosed him with generalized dystonia with dystonic arm tremor presenting during adolescence, with an unclear etiology, following the movement disorders consensus recommendation that classifies dystonia along a clinical and etiological axis. He underwent an interdisciplinary evaluation at our center by neurology, neurosurgery, neuropsychology, psychiatry, occupational therapy, physical therapy, and speech therapy and was deemed a good candidate for implantation of DBS electrodes into the bilateral globus pallidus internus (GPi). At his 6-month follow-up, there were moderate to significant improvements in tremor and dystonic symptoms.

COMPLICATIONS

Despite these initial improvements in dystonia and tremor, 2 years after surgery, the patient's gait and balance were observed to have worsened further. The patient reportedly veered off in one or the other direction and began to have frequent falls despite using an assistive device for ambulation. He complained of a slurring of speech that was not present before the surgery. He was examined on and off stimulation, and the gait and speech symptoms persisted even when the DBS was turned off. He was diagnosed with new-onset cerebellar ataxia and, together with tremor and generalized dystonia, was considered to have a dystonia syndrome. Although the symptoms were sporadic, the new developments prompted a further workup, including analysis of levels in the serum for alpha-fetoprotein, albumin, amino acids, cholesterol, very long-chain fatty acids, ammonia, transferrin factor, vitamin E, and ceruloplasmin. The urine was checked for elevated levels of organic acids, phytanic acid, frataxin, and lactic acid. A peripheral blood smear looking for an increased number of acanthocytes, serum lymphopoietin electrophoresis, paraneoplastic antibodies, and heavy metal screen was additionally performed. Considering an unremarkable workup, even though family history was negative for symptoms, we proceeded with testing for spinocerebellar ataxia (SCA) panel. He was found to have SCA17 with an unstable CAG trinucleotide repeat expansion mutation coding for polyglutamine tracts in the TATA-binding protein (TBP)—one allele with 22 repeats, and the other allele with 43 repeats.

TROUBLESHOOTING AND MANAGEMENT

The initial DBS settings comprised stimulation with monopolar configuration, 2 to 3.5 V, pulse widths of 90 to 120 (μsec), and frequency of 130 to 180 Hz, and these led to significant improvements in the arm tremor; however, there was only modest improvement of neck and feet dystonia symptoms. Dystonia in the feet was particularly bothersome and significantly contributed to gait difficulties. We, therefore, tried several additional combinations of settings (Table 41.1), including a wide monopolar and bipolar configuration for stimulation contacts, lower stimulation frequencies of 60 Hz, and a higher pulse width (180 μsec). After several programming sessions, we found that a combination of low-frequency and a high pulse width stimulation optimally improved posturing in the neck and feet while maintaining significant tremor suppression in the arms. However, with these settings, the patient reported a weird pulling sensation and heaviness in both legs, which were not felt to be related to the old dystonia symptoms and emerged a few hours after the programming session was completed. These new symptoms were mild but also were reported as annoying and constant. We, therefore,

considered a trial of a cyclic mode of stimulation instead of the conventional continuous stimulation. He was switched over to mode of 1-minute cycles (1 minute on and 1 minute off; cycling duration was empirically selected), with the low-frequency and high pulse width settings remaining the same. These new settings were observed to optimally control the tremor and dystonia symptoms with no simultaneous issues of heaviness and pulling sensations.

OUTCOME

The patient is currently 11 years into follow-up after DBS surgery. He reports significant tremor suppression, a remarkable alleviation of neck dystonia, and a moderate improvement of feet posturing. However, as expected, the gait and balance symptoms related to ataxia (SCA17) have shown continued progression over the years. He now uses a motorized scooter for ambulation.

DISCUSSION

The current case is the first report of SCA17 in the literature that was treated with DBS therapy to address symptoms of dystonia and tremor in this disorder symptomatically. SCA17 is a type of autosomal dominant cerebellar ataxia that results from an abnormal CAG expansion of the TBP gene.[1] SCA17 is rare, with only a few cases reported in the literature.[1] Although the knowledge of the phenotypic spectrum is limited, there are reports to suggest that, in addition to cerebellar ataxia, the clinical phenotype may include dementia, epilepsy, psychosis, and movement disorders, including parkinsonism, dystonia, and chorea.[1] In this case, the SCA17 presented with dystonia, dystonic tremor, and cerebellar ataxia, which manifested almost two decades after the onset of disease.

Although the earlier reports on SCA17 reported 43 as the trinucleotide number cutoff value for clinical symptoms,[2] many later publications have involved patients with lower repeat numbers, as observed in this case.[3] While previous reports discussed focal dystonia symptoms, including writer's cramp and cervical dystonia with CAG repeats of 55, the current case at 41 repeats presented with dystonia that was generalized in distribution.[4]

According to the revised classification of dystonia proposed by the Movement Disorders Society,[5] this patient has a dystonia syndrome. In addition to dystonia, there are neurologic and psychiatric symptoms, including cerebellar

TABLE 41.1. LONGITUDINAL PROGRAMMING SETTINGS FOR BILATERAL GLOBUS PALLIDUS INTERNA DEEP BRAIN STIMULATION

Follow-Up Time	Left				Right			
	Configuration Contacts and Mode	Volts	Frequency (Hz)	Pulse Width (μsec)	Configuration Contacts and Mode	Volt	Frequency (Hz)	Pulse Width (μsec)
1 month	C+ 1– continuous mode	2.5	60	180	C+ 1– continuous mode	2.5	60	180
6 months	3+ 0– continuous mode	3.0	135	180	1+ 0– continuous mode	2.0	135	180
1 year	3+ 1– continuous mode	2.5	135	150	1– 3+ continuous mode	2.5	150	160
3 years	C+ 1– cyclic mode	3.1	60	180	C+ 1– cyclic mode	3.0	60	180
11 years	C+ 1– cyclic mode	3.1	60	180	C+ 1– cyclic mode	3.0	60	180

ataxia, anxiety, and panic attacks. The age of onset is adolescence (13–20 years), dystonia is generalized in distribution, and the disease course is progressive. The patient has a heredodegenerative and an inherited form of dystonia when classified from an etiologic perspective. DBS outcomes for inherited dystonias have been reported previously; however, they mainly involved DYT-TOR 1A, DYT-THAP, and myoclonus-dystonia.[6] While there are few reports of DBS in SCA, these patients underwent ventral intermediate (Vim) nucleus targeting for control of tremor,[7] and no study to date has discussed dystonia, and none has included the targeting of the GPi for control of dystonia.

Another interesting aspect of this case relates to DBS programming. Although the usual trials of electrode configurations, amplitude, pulse width, and frequency titrations effectively alleviated tremor and dystonia, we found that switching from a continuous to cyclic mode of stimulation could accomplish avoidance of delayed-onset side effects of pulling and heaviness. A cyclic mode of stimulation has been reported to extend the battery life,[8] which is not surprising; however, mitigation of capsular side effects likely related to a lower cumulative dose of stimulation has not been reported.

DBS is a powerful therapy, which in this case was observed to maintain symptomatic control of tremor and dystonia and thereby significantly affect the patient's quality of life for nearly 11 years. We acknowledge that we do not understand why cerebellar ataxia manifested shortly after surgery. Whether ataxia was unmasked because of effective control of dystonia and dystonic tremor or the DBS therapy had an adverse influence on the pathophysiology requires further experience. It was more simply disease progression. The current case observations cannot be generalized to all forms of inherited ataxia, and the positive findings require confirmation in more cases with the use of blinded assessments. Nevertheless, a long-term sustained control in SCA17 suggests that DBS therapy is a potential treatment to address the concomitant symptoms of dystonia and dystonic tremor in the setting of SCA17.

PEARLS

- Generalized dystonia and dystonic tremor can possibly respond to DBS therapy even though the underlying etiology is a genetic mutation consistent with SCA17.
- SCA17 can present with a prominent generalized dystonia phenotype even with lower repeat numbers.
- Globus pallidus can be a suitable DBS target for dystonic tremor, but many expert centers will use Vim DBS first if the tremor is the disabling feature.
- Cyclic mode of stimulation increases battery life and simultaneously reduces the possibility of stimulation-induced side effects that may be delayed in onset. The use of cyclic stimulation was a novel aspect of our case.

REFERENCES

1. Toyoshima Y, Takahashi H. Spinocerebellar ataxia type 17 (SCA17). Advances in experimental medicine and biology 2018;1049:219–231.
2. Park H, Jeon BS, Shin JH, Park SH. A patient with 41 CAG repeats in SCA17 presenting with parkinsonism and chorea. Parkinsonism & related disorders 2016;22:106–107.
3. Origone P, Gotta F, Lamp M, et al. Spinocerebellar ataxia 17: full phenotype in a 41 CAG/CAA repeats carrier. Cerebellum & ataxias 2018;5:7.
4. Hagenah JM, Zuhlke C, Hellenbroich Y, Heide W, Klein C. Focal dystonia as a presenting sign of spinocerebellar ataxia 17. Movement disorders: official journal of the Movement Disorder Society 2004;19:217–220.
5. Albanese A, Bhatia K, Bressman SB, et al. Phenomenology and classification of dystonia: a consensus update. Movement disorders: official journal of the Movement Disorder Society 2013;28:863–873.
6. Vidailhet M, Jutras MF, Grabli D, Roze E. Deep brain stimulation for dystonia. Journal of neurology, neurosurgery, and psychiatry 2013;84:1029–1042.
7. Hashimoto T, Muralidharan A, Yoshida K, et al. Neuronal activity and outcomes from thalamic surgery for spinocerebellar ataxia. Annals of clinical and translational neurology 2018;5:52–63.
8. Tai CH, Wu RM, Liu HM, Tsai CW, Tseng SH. Meige syndrome relieved by bilateral pallidal stimulation with cycling mode: case report. Neurosurgery 2011;69:E1333–1337.

Case 42

Deep Brain Stimulation for Disabling "Outflow" Tremors

Troubleshooting Strategies for Tremor Habituation

DANIELLE S. SHPINER, SAGARI BETTE, AND CORNELIU C. LUCA

INDICATION FOR DEEP BRAIN STIMULATION

Medication-refractory outflow tremors secondary to multiple sclerosis (MS)

CLINICAL HISTORY AND RELEVANT EXAM

The patient is a 72-year-old right-handed woman with a history of MS, who presented for evaluation of severe tremors of the upper extremities that were interfering with her ability to feed herself and to write. She also complained of balance problems and falls, requiring the use of a walker to ambulate. Initial examination was remarkable for a yes–yes head tremor, large-amplitude kinetic and postural tremors in the upper extremities, decreased sensation to vibration to the level of the ankles, positive Romberg, ataxia on finger-to-nose and heel-to-shin testing, and wide-based gait. Brain magnetic resonance imaging (MRI) was significant for extensive confluent T2-weighted/fluid-attenuated inversion recovery (FLAIR) hyperintensities throughout bilateral cerebral hemispheres as well as lesions in bilateral cerebellar peduncles consistent with her diagnosis of MS. The patient failed multiple medications for tremor, including propranolol, primidone, gabapentin, topiramate, perampanel, and clonazepam. She underwent unilateral deep brain stimulation (DBS) implantation of the left ventral intermediate (Vim) nucleus of the thalamus. She was instructed to turn the stimulation off at night. Initially, she had an excellent response to the point that she was able to use her right hand to drink water from a cup and was able to write (Figure 42.1). However, this remarkable effect lasted only 1 week before the tremors returned. After multiple adjustments of DBS settings, she regained some tremor relief, but not enough to perform independently her activities of daily living.

COMPLICATIONS

Unilateral Vim DBS produced significant improvement in the patient's tremor—she was able to hold her arm steady and use it to write and to eat. Initial programing resulted in 90% improvement in tremor; however, the benefit was short-lived for tremor suppression. Tolerance to stimulation has been considered a possible explanation for the gradual loss of efficacy of Vim DBS over time. Disease progression and lead location issues are also other possibilities.

TROUBLESHOOTING AND MANAGEMENT

The patient underwent multiple reprograming sessions every 2 weeks and subsequently every 4 weeks for the ensuing 10 months. She had relatively good tremor control at the time of programing by alternating different sites of stimulation. She was able to maintain stable clinical benefits only by alternating different stimulation settings; however, the effectiveness of DBS decreased over time (Table 42.1). In our case, the initial stimulation strategy was to activate multiple contacts simultaneously, followed by alternative stimulation of different sites, which provided similar effectiveness in tremor suppression. As the intensity of stimulation was increased, paresthesias became intolerable, and therefore bipolar programing and, later, interleaving settings were used.

FIGURE 42.1. Writing samples (three trials) of a patient with severe overflow tremor secondary to multiple sclerosis. *Upper panel:* deep brain stimulation (DBS) off; *lower panel:* DBS on 0–, 1– (interleaved), 3+, 5 V, 125 Hz, 90 μsec.

OUTCOME

Multiple programming sessions that alternated activation of different regions along the DBS lead facilitated the more sustained control of tremors. Activation of two contacts with very high frequency and pulse width also alleviated the tremor for brief periods. Alternating the contacts facilitated sustained benefit at 10 months (see Table 42.1).

DISCUSSION

Loss of DBS effectiveness and loss of tremor suppression after an initial adequate control is an important issue in outflow tremors. Tremor prevalence in MS is estimated to be quite high: 46%, with 6% of patients having severe, disabling tremor.[1] Tremors are usually postural, kinetic, or intention tremors, or a combination thereof, with outflow and resting tremors being uncommon.[2,3]

The pathophysiology has not been fully elucidated but is commonly attributed to dysfunction of cerebellar and thalamic pathways[3,4] and likely also involves basal ganglia and cortical connections that may result in an overall hyperactivation of the cerebellothalamocortical pathway.[2] Medical treatment includes a variety of drugs like topiramate, isoniazid, propranolol, primidone, levetiracetam, carbamazepine, and botulinum toxin injections. These observations are based on small studies and case reports.

Surgical treatments for MS-associated tremor include DBS and lesioning. Either unilateral or bilateral Vim nucleus is the most commonly employed; however, the posterior subthalamic area (PSA), zona incerta, subthalamic nucleus (STN), Ventralis oralis anterioris(Voa)/Ventralis oralis posterioris(Vop) Globus pallidius pars

TABLE 42.1. STIMULATION SITES AND PARAMETERS AT DIFFERENT TIME POINTS

Months After Left Vim DBS	Cathode (–)	Anode (+)	Amplitude (V)	PulseWidth (μsec)	Frequency (Hz)	Estimated Tremor Control* (%)
0.5	0, 1	C	2.5	90	180	90
1	0, 1, 2	C	3.0	90	180	80
2	0, 2	C	3.5	90	250	70
3	1	3	4.0	90	250	30
6	0, 1	3	4.0	90	250	50
10†	0	3	5.0	90	125	90
	1	3	5.0	90	125	

*Estimated tremor control is based on assessment by the treating neurologist comparing tremor with stimulation off versus on during the same visit.
†Ten-month program with interleaving between contacts 0 and 1.
C = case; DBS = deep brain stimulation; Vim = ventral intermediate nucleus.

interma (GPi) and prelemniscal radiations are also effective targets.[5,6] Ipsilateral dual lead DBS, usually with the addition of Voa/Vop or PSA targets, has shown benefit and is often considered for rescue therapy in patients with recurrent tremor after single-lead DBS implantation; isolated cases have been reported to demonstrate tremor improvement with initial dual lead therapy. A recent study suggested that dual DBS lead implants in Vim plus Voa/Vop may be useful.[7] In this study, the second lead prevented the worsening encountered 1 week after programming that was seen in our patient.

In patients with essential tremor (ET) and Vim DBS, loss of efficacy of the stimulation over time (disease progression and habituation), even with adjustments to the stimulation parameters, has been described. One study followed 20 ET patients for up to 10 years and demonstrated a decline in tremor reduction with Vim DBS over the long term, compared with more robust tremor reduction in the short term.[8] The study also demonstrated the phenomenon of rebound, or a worsening of tremor after the stimulation was turned off, which reached a plateau at 30 to 60 minutes. The authors noted that assessment of tremor progression as a partial explanation of habituation was confounded by this rebound effect.[8] The effect was more likely disease progression than habituation.

Overnight stimulation shutoff and stimulation holidays have been tried in efforts to combat these effects.[9] In a pilot study of 22 patients with ET and Vim DBS randomized to standard care programming or alternating stimulation pattern programming, the group with alternating stimulation had sustained tremor control compared with the standard care group over a 12-week time period.[9] The overall tremor improvement was 7.3 points (over baseline) on the Essential Tremor Rating Assessment Scale (TETRAS).

Lesioning therapies are again gaining favor, particularly with the advent of MRI-guided focused ultrasound therapy (MRIgFUS). In a review of radiofrequency or gamma knife lesioning of the Vim thalamus for MS tremor, short-duration effectiveness was demonstrated; however, there were persistent side effects in up to 40% of unilateral-lesioning cases.[10]

Mechanism of action

The pathophysiology of re-emergent outflow tremor after DBS is poorly understood. There are some explanations for the loss of efficacy over time: (1) disease progression, (2) severe tremors that may require dual target stimulation, and

(3) compensatory or adaptive mechanisms that induce a rebound tremor in the cerebellar thalamocortical pathway.

Thus far, studies have mostly described disease progression as the major factor for loss of efficacy over time,[11-13] but the literature on suboptimal/loss of benefit early in the disease following DBS adjustments remains scarce.[14,15] Several investigators have reported that "stimulation holidays" temporarily restored the efficacy of Vim DBS and that patients may benefit from intermittent use of the stimulator, usually turning it off during sleep. Another study showed that the systematic optimization of Vim DBS parameters in ET can produce a significant short-term improvement in tremors; however, the effects may be lost over time, suggesting that tolerance to stimulation may perhaps be averted by using alternating stimulation protocols.[9] Reprograming strategies that include use of alternating parameter settings, DBS holidays and adaptive DBS have been proposed and described in a recent review.[16] If these are unsuccessful, repositioning of the leads upgrading the pulse generator or additional lead insertions in the PSA or Vop should be considered.

Lead placement into a suboptimal location could be a possible explanation for tremor relapse (particular for settings that are only effective for hours or days). In our case, the effects were dramatic in the first week after stimulation was turned on. Ideal DBS targeting for disabling outflow tremors has not been well-established and likely depends on the location and severity of the primary lesion or circuit. Given the limited experience and effectiveness of Vim DBS using alternative targets such as the anterior thalamus (Voa/Vop, globus pallidus pars interna (GPi), or (PSA) have also been considered; however, there are limited data. Also, dual lead DBS, with the addition of a second lead in Voa/Vop or PSA targets, may help to alleviate disabling tremors and to avoid rebound.

One possible strategy to avoid early tremor rebound is to provide patients with preset programs with similar effectiveness and to allow them to switch stimulation to a different program, periodically, before tremor relapses. In practice, however, this is difficult to manage because it requires frequent patient adjustments, and therefore compliance can be poor. Advances in technology such as adaptive stimulation, in which the intensity of electricity is dictated by the severity of tremor, can possibly help to offset this limitation. Clinical studies are necessary to evaluate the effectiveness of this strategy.

PEARLS

- Outflow tremor is commonly refractory to treatment with most medications, and the initial effectiveness of DBS may diminish over time.
- Loss of effectiveness or habituation can possibly be reduced by allowing the patient to turn stimulation off at night.
- In cases in which tremor worsening is seen soon after a programming session, an effective strategy is to alternate stimulation sites, similar to a coordinated reset. Additional recommendations may include stimulation-free periods and simultaneous ipsilateral stimulation of different tremor targets using a dual lead approach, as recently published.[7]

REFERENCES

1. Rinker JR, Salter AR, Walker H, Amara A, Meador W, Cutter GR. Prevalence and characteristics of tremor in the NARCOMS multiple sclerosis registry: a cross-sectional survey. BMJ Open 2015;5:e006714.
2. Wilkins A. Cerebellar dysfunction in multiple sclerosis. Front Neurol 2017;8:312.
3. Koch M, Mostert J, Heersema D, De Keyser J. Tremor in multiple sclerosis. J Neurol 2007;254:133–145.
4. Oakes PK, Srivatsal SR, Davis MY, Samii A. Movement disorders in multiple sclerosis. Phys Med Rehabil Clin N Am 2013;24:639–651.
5. Ramirez-Zamora A, Okun MS. Deep brain stimulation for the treatment of uncommon tremor syndromes. Exp Rev Neurotherap 2016;16(8):983–997.
6. Artusi CA, Farooqi A, Romagnolo A, et al. Deep brain stimulation in uncommon tremor disorders: indications, targets and programming. J Neurol 2018;265:2473–2493.
7. Oliveria SF, Rodriguez RL, Bowers D, et al. Safety and efficacy of dual-lead thalamic deep brain stimulation for patients with treatment-refractory multiple sclerosis tremor: a single-centre, randomised, single-blind, pilot trial. Lancet Neurol 2017;16(9):691–700.
8. Paschen S, Forstenpointner J, Becktepe J, et al. Long-term efficacy of deep brain stimulation for essential tremor. Neurology 2019;92:e1378–e1386.
9. Seier M, Hiller A, Quinn J, Murchison C, Brodsky M, Anderson S. Alternating thalamic deep brain stimulation for essential tremor: a trial to reduce habituation. Mov Disord Clin Pract 2018;5(6):620–626.
10. Schreglmann SR, Krauss JK, Chang JW, Bhatia KP, Kagi G. Functional lesional neurosurgery for tremor: a systematic review and meta-analysis. J Neurol Neurosurg Psychiatry 2018;89:717–726.
11. Pahwa R, Lyons KE, Wilkinson SB, et al. Long-term evaluation of deep brain stimulation of the thalamus. J Neurosurg 2006;104:506–512.
12. Rodríguez Cruz PM, Vargas A, Fernández-Carballal C, Garbizu J, De La Casa-Fages B, Grandas F. Long-term thalamic deep brain stimulation for essential tremor: clinical outcome and stimulation parameters. Mov Disord Clin Pract 2016;3(6):567–572.
13. Pilitsis JG, Metman LV, Toleikis JR, Hughes LE, Sani SB, Bakay RA. Factors involved in long-term efficacy of deep brain stimulation of the thalamus for essential tremor. J Neurosurg 2008;109:640–646.
14. Patel N, Ondo W, Jimenez-Shahed J. Habituation and rebound to thalamic deep brain stimulation in long-term management of tremor associated with demyelinating neuropathy, Int J Neurosci 2014;124(12):919–925.
15. Merchant SH, Kuo SH, Qiping Y, et al. Objective predictors of "early tolerance" to ventral intermediate nucleus of thalamus deep brain stimulation in essential tremor patients. Clin Neurophysiol 2018;129(8):1628–1633.
16. Fasano A, Helmich RC. Tremor habituation to deep brain stimulation: Underlying mechanisms and solutions. Mov Disord. 2019 Dec;34(12):1761–1773.

Case 43

Tardive Dystonia and Dyskinesia Responsive to Deep Brain Stimulation

SHANNON Y. CHIU AND IRENE A. MALATY

INDICATIONS FOR DEEP BRAIN STIMULATION

Severe medication-refractory tardive dyskinesia and dystonia

CLINICAL HISTORY AND RELEVANT EXAM

A 26-year-old man presented to our tertiary movement disorders center for management of tardive dyskinesia and tardive dystonia. He had experienced depression and hallucinations after the loss of his father at age 17 years. His depression with psychotic features had been treated over time with haloperidol, risperidone, olanzapine, ziprasidone, aripiprazole, and quetiapine. He first developed tremor in the bilateral upper extremities at about age 24 years, followed by dystonic posturing and hyperkinetic movements of his upper extremities and neck. Specifically, he reported severe retrocollic jerks of the head and trunk with extension and pronation of the arms. Retrocollis included a leftward and backward pulling of the neck. In order to sleep at night, he used a *geste antagoniste* of placing his cellular phone against his left ear to improve the neck and arm movement. His syndrome of progressive dyskinesia and dystonia in the context of chronic neuroleptic exposure was consistent with tardive disorders. He was treated with bromocriptine, tetrabenazine, carbidopa-levodopa, trihexyphenidyl, clonazepam, tizanidine, baclofen, clozapine, and botulinum toxin injections, all without significant benefit. Severe hyperkinetic movements of the neck, arms, and trunk caused an opisthotonic posture that interfered with almost every activity of daily living and thus significantly impairing his quality of life. He was losing weight because the tardive disorders interfered with eating.

He eventually underwent bilateral globus pallidus interna (GPi) deep brain stimulation (DBS) surgery, which led to an overall 50% improvement of tardive movements; he was able to sit in a chair for a longer period of time and walk down the hallway without holding onto nearby objects. However, retropulsion of his upper torso and head as well as bilateral upper extremity dyskinesias worsened over time. Brain computed tomography (CT) revealed suboptimally placed leads (Figure 43.1A and B). It was felt that his severe, intense hyperkinetic movements during his surgery and ongoing frequent aggressive and sudden retropulsive movements of the head likely contributed to a rare ventral lead migration. Notably, the patient's muscle strength and bulk from avid body-building further increased the force of his dyskinetic movements. The patient underwent removal and reimplantation of bilateral GPi DBS under general anesthesia to eliminate intraoperative dyskinetic movements.

Despite the revision, the patient continued to have severe retropulsion of the trunk and neck and an abnormal gait (Figure 43.2A and B). His speech was also mildly impaired; handwriting became more difficult. When eating, he had to prop his elbows and knees against the table to control his movements. A decision was made to offer him bilateral rescue subthalamic nucleus (STN) DBS surgery (Figure 43.3A and B).

COMPLICATIONS

Lead migration (ventral), severe refractory tardive dyskinesia and dystonia, retropulsion, dysarthria, need for dual target lead therapy

(A)

(B)

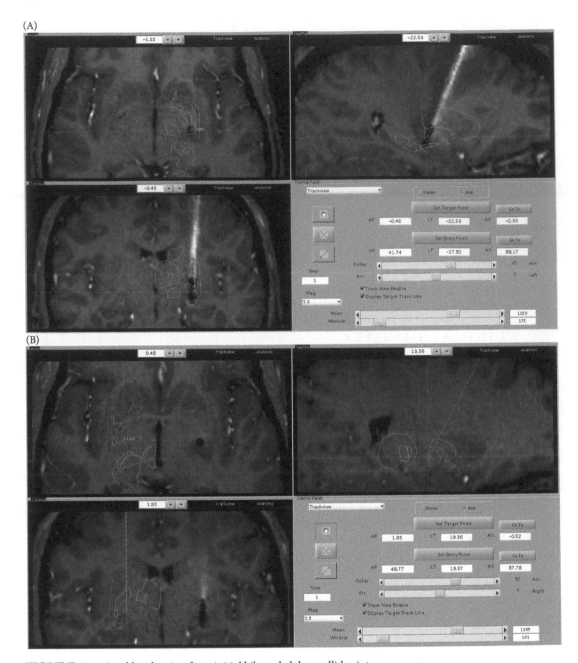

FIGURE 43.1. Lead localization from initial bilateral globus pallidus interna surgery.

TROUBLESHOOTING AND MANAGEMENT

At the time of initial programming, the patient reported improvement of his retropulsion after the DBS procedure, suggestive of a microlesion effect. His 6-month total United Dystonia Rating Scale (UDRS) score was 20, and his Burke–Fahn–Marsden Dystonia Rating Scale (BFMDRS) motor score was 18. With progression of symptoms, his total UDRS score worsened to 27. Unfortunately, he continued to have moderate to severe dystonia 3 months after bilateral GPi revision, with a BFMDRS motor score of 21.5 and UDRS total score of 23, and he also required a high voltage (5 V) on his GPi DBS. He retried botulinum toxin therapy (total 600 units of botulinum toxin type A) without benefit. One year after his bilateral GPi revision, the patient underwent bilateral

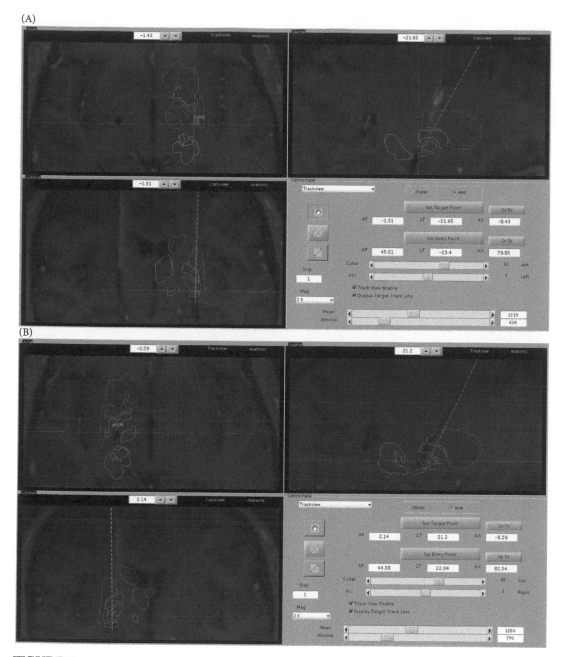

FIGURE 43.2. Lead localization from revision surgery of bilateral globus pallidus interna.

STN DBS surgery. His subsequent 6-month total UDRS improved to 16, and his BFMDRS motor score improved to 6.5, using high voltage (6.4 V bilaterally) with GPi DBS. The STN DBS was set to high frequency (120 Hz) but lower voltage (2 V bilaterally). He was able to perform activities of daily living independently, drive, and walk without retropulsion. He tapered off tetrabenazine. In recent years, he attempted to decrease GPi voltage, but his symptoms worsened immediately; thus, a combination of both GPi and STN targets was necessary to provide maximal benefit. Table 43.1 summarizes his current optimized DBS settings.

OUTCOME

This case illustrates the consideration of concurrent GPi and STN DBS in a patient with severe tardive dyskinesia and dystonia. Our patient's

(A)

(B)

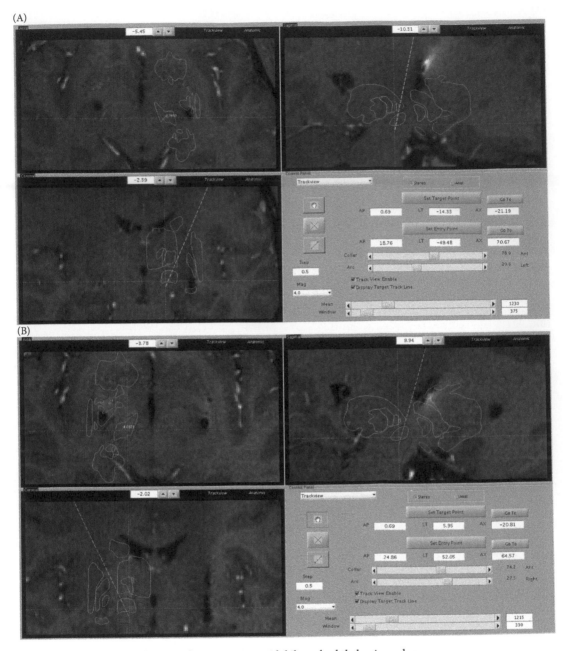

FIGURE 43.3. Lead localization of rescue surgery with bilateral subthalamic nucleus.

avid body-building may have contributed to the increased force of retrocollic and opisthotonic posturing, which caused suboptimal lead location and lead migration (ventral) over time. Ultimately, his disabling dystonic retropulsion and dyskinesia required a combination of both GPi and STN DBS. He continues to follow up in our clinic and has demonstrated sustained benefit for more than 10 years. At his most recent follow-up (12 years after revision of his bilateral GPi leads and 10 years after his bilateral STN surgery), his total UDRS and BFMDRS motor scores were 2 and 1, respectively. He has mild worsening of speech, likely stimulation induced.

DISCUSSION

Tardive disorder is a term that characterizes a group of delayed-onset movement disorders

TABLE 43.1. OPTIMIZED DEEP BRAIN STIMULATION SETTINGS

	Electrode Configuration	Voltage (V)	Pulse Width (µsec)	Frequency (Hz)
Left STN	C+ 1–	2.2	120	180
Right STN	C+ 5–	2.4	120	180
Left GPi	8– 9– 10+	5.9	90	135
Right GPi	0– 1+	5.9	90	135

GPi = globus pallidus interna; STN = subthalamic nucleus.

typically occurring after administration of dopamine receptor blocking agents over a period of at least 3 months, in the absence of other causes.[1] Tardive disorder affects approximately one-third of outpatients with schizophrenia treated with antipsychotics,[2] but it can also affect patients with prior exposure to certain antiemetics or antidepressants, or those treated with neuroleptics for other indications. There are several phenomenologically distinct types of tardive disorder. The classic form is oral-buccal-lingual dyskinesia, often called *tardive dyskinesia. Tardive dystonia* refers to a dystonic syndrome that can affect any part of the body and may include some dyskinesia or other phenomenology.[3] Other phenotypes include tardive akathisia, tics, and tremor.[2] The underlying pathophysiology remains unclear, but proposed mechanisms include (1) hypersensitivity of dopamine D2 and D3 receptors after chronic blockade by dopamine blocking agents, (2) an abnormal balance between direct and indirect pathways in the basal ganglia due to maladaptive synaptic plasticity, and (3) oxidative stress and genetic susceptibility.[4–6]

Chronic tardive disorder can be disabling. Medical management, consisting of anticholinergics, muscle relaxants, dopamine-depleting agents, benzodiazepines, and botulinum toxin injections, is often insufficient or is limited by side effects.[2] In disabling cases refractory to medications, neurostimulation is a potential therapeutic option.

Small case and cohort studies have reported improvement of tardive dystonia and dyskinesia following GPi or STN DBS with reductions in BFMDRS motor and/or the Abnormal Involuntary Movement Scale (AIMS) score.[7–9] A recent review of DBS for tardive syndromes found 117 cases in the current literature derived from four studies on tardive dyskinesia and 30 studies on tardive dystonia.[4] AIMS and BFMDRS motor scores improved across a majority of patients after DBS.[4] The majority of cases targeted bilateral posteroventral GPi; and bilateral STN stimulation was reported in eight cases.[10,11] To date, a French study group (STARDYS) reported class II evidence of the efficacy of GPi DBS in patients with severe refractory mixed tardive dyskinesia and dystonia, based on a double-blind video-based evaluation of 19 patients "on" and "off" stimulation. Improvement was maintained over the long-term follow-up of 6 to 11 years.[9,12] Three class IV studies have similarly reported the efficacy of GPi DBS in patients with tardive dystonia. According to a recently published literature review and proposed treatment algorithm, GPi DBS is currently a level C recommendation for treatment of refractory tardive dyskinesia.[2] More research is needed to evaluate the efficacy of STN DBS and concurrent DBS of dual targets in this patient population.

PEARLS

- Severe refractory mixed tardive dyskinesia and dystonia may respond to GPi or STN DBS and historically have been shown to respond to bilateral pallidotomy. Bilateral pallidotomy is rarely used today because of the risk for corticobulbar worsening.
- When initial benefit wanes, lead location should be confirmed because lead migration is a potential concern. The lead can migrate ventrally, although dorsal lead migration is more common.
- In some severe and refractory cases of tardive disorder, dual lead therapy may be considered.

REFERENCES

1. Fernandez HH, Friedman JH. Classification and treatment of tardive syndromes. *Neurologist.* 2003;9(1):16–27.
2. Bhidayasiri R, Jitkritsadakul O, Friedman JH, Fahn S. Updating the recommendations for treatment of tardive syndromes: a systematic review of new evidence and practical treatment algorithm. *J Neurol Sci.* 2018;389:67–75.
3. Burke RE, Fahn S, Jankovic J, et al. Tardive dystonia: late-onset and persistent dystonia caused by antipsychotic drugs. *Neurology.* 1982;32(12):1335–1346.
4. Macerollo A, Deuschl G. Deep brain stimulation for tardive syndromes: systematic review and meta-analysis. *J Neurol Sci.* 2018;389:55–60.
5. Waln O, Jankovic J. An update on tardive dyskinesia: from phenomenology to treatment. *Tremor Other Hyperkinet Mov (NY).* 2013;3:ii.
6. Westmoreland Corson P, Nopoulos P, Miller DD, Arndt S, Andreasen NC. Change in basal ganglia volume over 2 years in patients with schizophrenia: typical versus atypical neuroleptics. *Am J Psychiatry.* 1999;156(8):1200–1204.
7. Lane RD, Glazer WM, Hansen TE, Berman WH, Kramer SI. Assessment of tardive dyskinesia using the abnormal involuntary movement scale. *J Nerv Ment Dis.* 1985;173(6):353–357.
8. Morigaki R, Mure H, Kaji R, Nagahiro S, Goto S. Therapeutic perspective on tardive syndrome with special reference to deep brain stimulation. *Front Psychiatry.* 2016;7:67.
9. Pouclet-Courtemanche H, Rouaud T, Thobois S, et al. Long-term efficacy and tolerability of bilateral pallidal stimulation to treat tardive dyskinesia. *Neurology.* 2016;86(7):651–659.
10. Meng D-W, Liu H-G, Yang A-C, Zhang K, Zhang J-G. Long-term effects of subthalamic nucleus deep brain stimulation in tardive dystonia. *Chin Med J (Engl).* 2016;129(10):1257–1258.
11. Deng ZD, Li DY, Zhang CC, et al. Long-term follow-up of bilateral subthalamic deep brain stimulation for refractory tardive dystonia. *Park Relat Disord.* 2017;41:58–65.
12. Damier P, Thobois S, Witjas T, et al. Bilateral deep brain stimulation of the globus pallidus to treat tardive dyskinesia. *Arch Gen Psychiatry.* 2007;64(2):170–176.

INDEX

Printed in the USA/Agawam, MA
March 30, 2022

790924.017